How
to Starve Cancer...
and then kill it with ferroptosis

By Jane McLelland

*One Woman's Extraordinary True Story
of Survival, Courage and a Discovery
that could Transform the Lives of Millions*

Dedication

For my long-suffering husband Andrew.
And to Jamie and Sam,
the beautiful bright rays of sunshine in my life.

Jane's life story is remarkable, but what is truly unique is how she intertwines this intimate and heartfelt tale with detailed, specific clinical and scientific pathways along her uplifting journey to cancer freedom.

Embedded in the quintessentially human narrative that Jane describes with such light elegance is a rigorous, evidence based scientific approach. Jane's clinical reasoning is impressive, her experience is compelling, and in the combination of these two elements she has crafted a narrative that, like the anticancer metabolic cocktail she champions, is destined to positively enhance countless lives.

Dr Ndaba Mazibuko, Clinical Research Fellow
King's College London, Care Oncology Clinic Doctor

As a retired scientist who worked in cancer research in both academia and the pharma industry, I can speak with some authority. This book is likely to be a game-changer in the treatment of all types of cancer. The cancer research world is already beginning to move into the direction of cancer cell metabolism instead of focusing entirely on cell proliferation. However, since new drugs take years to go through regulatory processes before becoming available, Jane's approach to existing off-label drugs in combination, should be adopted – especially by a cash-strapped NHS. Please read the book and pass on the word.

George F. Rowland

Brilliant. A truly remarkable book. I just could not put it down. I don't have cancer but worked for a well-known cancer charity. I saw the effects of treatment and how so many are forced to take a route of treatment plans with no choices or discussions about other options or alternatives. I am waiting a couple of weeks then want to read again so I can take it all in! This book is just amazing.

Miriam Horstman

I'm very impressed. In addition to patients, I would also recommend your book for anyone interested in cancer research as your approach to beating cancer is a fantastic start that merits further investigation.

Dr Stephen Bigelsen, stage 4 pancreatic cancer survivor
(in full remission at the time of writing using a supplement
and drug cocktail including chloroquine)

"You have done a magnificent job in your online course… you are providing more relevant information for patients than any other integrative medicine source or platform. You are establishing a way forward that is bringing truly relevant information for people diagnosed with cancer-and their families-and their physicians.

Dr Will Lavalley MD

"Love your course, must have been and is a labour of service to mankind. It is unique, original and ground-breaking, very practical and informative, fuelled by your fiery passion to give those who seek a new possible pathway to work towards health. Thank you."

Dr Etienne Callebout MD

"I just wanted to send congratulations on the course. I've started and it looks terrific. Well produced, professionally presented, as well as being reassuring and easy to follow. Keep up the great work!

Bill Turnbull, former BBC presenter and Classic FM presenter

Anyone who is taking supplements or off label drugs and/or cannabis is blocking metabolic pathways of cancer whether wittingly or unwittingly. The question is...are the correct pathways being blocked using the correct supplement or medication? Jane's book and online video course explain the science behind what she discovered as well as the what, where and when of figuring out which pathways to target. Prior to Jane's published research I think people had some hit or miss luck with certain supplements and medications without knowing they were blocking pathways or why exactly. Jane's book organizes and explains the methodology behind a great deal of what I like to refer to as the metabolic cancer movement. She has saved her own life several times over and is clearly a fighter and an advocate. She is found on YouTube and featured in episodes of Radical Remission, for example. As an RN and an avid clinical researcher I regard her book and course as foundational to anyone affected by cancer regardless of the treatment path that is chosen. I recommend her book and course to everyone.

Suzanne Allison, RN

Acknowledgements

I would not be here today if it weren't for the 'Generals' in this revolution, the many 'Otto Warburgs' who continue to champion the metabolic, epigenetic and infectious theories of cancer. All have been harassed, ridiculed and persecuted for their beliefs as they ride against the entrenched dogma that cancer is merely a result of random genetic mutations, that the disease is just 'bad luck' and that there is little we can do to avoid it.

Writing this book has not been easy, I have tried on several occasions in the past and never got further than a few pages before the emotional pain forced me to put my pen down and abandon it. And writing about the medical treatments without my story makes little sense. So I have had to put my personal feelings aside to tell my story, of how I stumbled across my metabolic cocktail, a discovery that could help so many to starve their cancer, and to stop it in its tracks. And when more trials research my findings, they may eventually be revealed as the cure. Sometimes the answer is hiding in plain sight, we only need to open our eyes and look at the situation through a different perspective to see it.

This would not be a completed manuscript without the help of my supporters; my 'crew' in my Facebook group who have kept sending me messages of encouragement. You know who you are, thank you all for standing beside me, believing in me and pushing me to get this out there. Special thanks go to several of my Facebook crew; Jill Bishop, Jennifer Steil, Jenny de Montfort, Matt Shoard and Gaynor Sheahan, who have given me invaluable feedback on the manuscript. Your enthusiasm kept me going when the task often seemed too big and I was weighed down by research.

And my Facebook group would not exist if it weren't for the Care Oncology Clinic and the sudden flood of information about old drugs, cast aside and forgotten, yet potentially so powerful when used together in the right cocktail.

A huge and grateful thank you to my mentors, Gregory Stoloff and Dr Robin Bannister, founders of the Care Oncology Clinic and all the doctors who work with them, not just for their belief in me, but their tireless work, despite the hostility of many in the oncology profession. And to Dr Pan Pantziarka and everyone working on the ReDo project 're-purposing' old drugs in cancer to bring these cheap neglected medications to the front line in the fight against cancer. Not forgetting the many unsung scientists and researchers out there who provide the evidence for the treatments. This is our ammunition and our weaponry. We are indebted to your work, and I owe you my life.

Huge thanks go to the late Wayne Martin and Dr Betty Rhodes, very much personal heroes of mine; both made me aware of the potential of the old drug dipyridamole. A massive thank you to my guru Dr Etienne Callebout, who prescribed this drug and many useful supplements. You are a true patient champion.

To my oncologist Professor 'T' who prescribed the etodolac and lovastatin cocktail to me. Dr Julian Kenyon who prescribed metformin and administered intravenous vitamin C and ozone infusions to me. And to the late Dr Patrick Kingsley for the Ultraviolet Blood Irradiation and intravenous vitamin C, who also gave me the unquantifiable belief in myself. Dr Wendy Denning, who continues to keep her beady eye on me and supply natural hormones and more intravenous vitamin C as and when I require.

To my friend Travis Christofferson, author of the brilliant *Tripping Over the Truth,* together with whom I hope we can change old, entrenched dogmas with both words and deeds.

Many thanks to Sam Pearce, Laurence Errington and Johnny Burrows for their help with this second edition and to Dr Ahmed Elsakka for his invaluable input and experience with ferroptosis.

To Robin Daly and all at Yes to Life, a fabulous charity and information portal, raising funds to help more people go through the Care Oncology Clinic programme and integrative cancer programmes, and to Chris Woollams for his informative cancer website.

To all who work at the Life Extension Foundation and the Townsend Letter Magazine for Doctors and Patients.

To all the integrative and functional doctors changing the current out-dated medical approach, you bring hope and help to so many by treating the source of the disease rather than merely treating the symptoms. Pioneers. I salute you all.

Mine is a deeply personal and, at times, intimate journey, but to make an impact and effect real change, I realised I would have had to tell my story in its entirety; the ups, the downs, the joy, the agony. But I was not satisfied with just my memoir. After years of research, it was not enough, I knew I had worked out a strategy to starve cancer. So at the end of my memoir, I have revealed my cancer-starving formula and my ferroptosis protocol, despite not being a doctor. The gall of it! So, with a large dollop of courage and a big deep breath, here it is.

Foreword
by Dr George W. Yu,

Clinical Professor of Urological and Pelvic Cancer Surgery,
George Washington University Medical Center,
Aegis Medical and Research Associates
and President of the George W. Yu Foundation for Nutrition & Health

I read Jane's book in one day and took ten pages of notes. It is a wealth of information, yet it reads like a novel, well-organized with many excellent references to put the theme of 'Starving Cancer Cells' as part of a paradigm shift away from traditional cancer protocols.

How to Starve Cancer is a must read for the brave individuals with progressing cancers who want a better choice than just a poor ultimatum, patients trying to navigate uncharted waters with little more than hope. This book will inspire them to take control of their destiny. It is also a must read for medical doctors to understand their patients, diligently searching for answers, seeking help, guidance, thoughtfulness and empathy from us their physicians, just as Jane did with her doctors.

Jane's book centers on 'repurposed drugs' (used for other medical diseases) with impressive cancer research results and clinical outcomes.

In 1971 the father of American oncology, Sidney Farber, explained to United States Congress: 'It is not necessary, in order to make great progress in the cure of cancer, for us to have the full solution of all the problems of basic research. The history of medicine is replete with examples of cures obtained years, decades, and even centuries before the mechanism of action was understood for these cures.' – This is what repurposed and off label drugs are about!

A cancer cell's metabolism is constantly adapting and can first fuel its needs with sugar fermentation, then adapt to use glutamine and eventually even use ketones for its growth and survival. Success depends on a multimodality 'cocktail' approach, used 'sequentially and pulsed' just as with our successful treatments with HIV and AIDS disease. As a surgical oncologist and urological cancer surgeon for thirty-five years I have incorporated many of these drugs along with intermittent calorie restriction and 'metabolic-enhanced' chemotherapy with a gradual and growing success.

Jane is a brave, courageous woman who was plagued with two aggressive cancers with metastatic spread. She used her great passion for research to discover medical treatments on her own, step by step, mistake after mistake, to finally prevail and survive today. Each one of us who develops a cancer will go through much of what she experienced; they should be encouraged by her success to find wisdom when current traditional routes have predicted fatal outcomes.

Dr George W. Yu

'It is not enough to be remembered for one's wealth, knowledge, and achievements. One does not make a difference unless it is the difference in people's lives.' – Joseph Schumpeter, Adolph Drucker The World According to Peter Drucker 1998

'More so, the mark of true achievement and truth is to change the life of the common man who will never know who you are.' – George Yu, M.D.

Contents

Introduction

I was supposed to die. That's what my doctors expected in 1999 when they broke the news that my cervical cancer had spread to my lungs. It was stage IV. There is no stage V. The statistics gave me approximately twelve weeks to live.

Few things are as motivating as the spectre of certain and imminent death. No way was I ready to shuffle off this planet. I was young, only thirty-five years old. I was in love. I desperately wanted to have children. I had professional ambitions. I could not accept that there was no treatment other than the conventional chemotherapy and radiation. I refused to believe I had no future.

Determined to find a cure, I threw myself into research. I was sure that the medical profession was missing something. As a Chartered Physiotherapist, I had a scientific background that enabled me to dig up and assimilate information quickly. Cancer, I realised, behaves just like a parasite. The cancer cells in my body were stealing nutrients, blood and immunity from me and using them as weapons against me. Parasites thrive and reproduce unabated until they either exhaust their food source or kill their host. With cancer, it's usually the latter.

But how could I starve cancer of these nutrients without starving myself? This was the question I set out to answer, using myself as a guinea pig. To my knowledge, no one had done this before. No one had yet come up with a constellation of therapies, using safe old drugs and natural compounds that would attack the abnormal cancer metabolism as well as its genetics, i.e., attack the cells from every direction.

Cancer, I have learned, has several food sources: glucose, glutamine, fatty acids and ketones. It also uses saturated fat to travel around the body.

I knew I would have to starve my cancer cells of all of these if I were to kill them off, especially at an advanced stage of the disease. I would need a large arsenal of weapons. But they would have to do minimal harm to me.

I began a cancer-starving diet, eliminating sugar and other foods that cancer loves to feed on. When that was not enough, I added powerful supplements. Ultimately, it was a combination of common old drugs uncommonly used, the diet and supplements that forced my cancer cells to melt away. When I used all these weapons **together**, they worked synergistically, and their anti-cancer effects were heightened. Boom! My cancer slunk off into remission.

Since 2004 it has not come back.

At long last the concept of 'starving cancer' has become the hot new frontier of cancer research, validating my long-held theories. Several studies have demonstrated the effectiveness of cancer-starving diets. In 2015, I was absolutely thrilled to discover that a clinic in London had begun studying a combination of drugs nearly identical with the cocktail I invented. And their results are impressive. A clinic in Istanbul is also using a combination of methods to starve cancer, again with outstanding results. Pharmaceutical companies are now falling over themselves to develop metabolic drugs to attack cancer.

But solutions exist already, and cost only pennies a day. The medications I took are widely prescribed for other medical conditions. They include metformin, commonly prescribed for diabetes; statins, often used to treat high cholesterol; dipyridamole, given to stroke patients; and an anti-inflammatory drug (aspirin then later etodolac). And in 2007 I took a drug called cimetidine for three months. Cimetidine is available over the counter in many countries for stomach ulcers, but I took it for its immune-enhancing effects. Taking my drug cocktail for just a few months was enough to halt my cancer in its attempts to take over my body.

All these medications are cheap and off-patent, which is why they have largely been ignored by the pharmaceutical industry, despite research supporting their effectiveness against cancer. Pharmaceutical companies are all too often more interested in making money than in curing people. Remember the 1980s, when a diagnosis with HIV was a death sentence? Now, most HIV infections can be controlled with a cocktail of drugs. HIV positive people can lead healthy lives and have near-normal lifespans. This, I believe, could also be the future of cancer.

A fundamental transformation in oncology is long overdue. The number of people to be diagnosed with cancer is predicted to rise 70 per cent by 2030. A new approach is desperately needed if we are to halt this increasingly tragic situation which is set to be a bumper time for the pharmaceutical industry. We are mostly living longer, but not more healthily. This has to change. Taking personal responsibility for our own wellbeing is a necessity.

There are now several trials under way, using old forgotten medications to treat a range of cancers. Sadly, most test only one drug at a time alongside the orthodox treatments, so progress is painfully slow. The elusive cancer stem cells (the initiating cells, which are untouched by chemotherapy and radiotherapy) can be reached and obliterated with many of these medications. This means that in combination with other treatments – given at less toxic doses – they offer the exciting possibility of turning cancer into a long-term chronic disease or permanent remission (i.e., a cure!).

This is the story of how I beat all the odds and forged a unique path, somewhere between complementary and orthodox medicine, not only ridding myself of cancer but regaining vibrant health on the way. On my journey I discovered some simple truths that ultimately led to my approach to beating cancer; starve it, stop it spreading, **then** snuff it out.

I stubbornly clung to life like a Yorkshire terrier refusing to let go of an old shoe, grrrr, and I want to show you how you can dig your teeth in too. If you have been told that nothing more can be done, I am here to let you know that this is almost certainly not true.

Wishing you a healthy, happy and 'revolting' life.

Ten Steps to Starving Cancer

First, the background…

In 1924 Otto Warburg discovered that all cancer cells have an altered metabolism – he was awarded the Nobel Prize in Physiology for this discovery in 1931. The way cancer cells use nutrients for energy has regressed. He noted that the mitochondria (the powerhouses) in the malignant cells stop functioning correctly and the energy is made in the cell cytoplasm instead, reverting to how the cell worked when the atmosphere was anaerobic or lacking in oxygen. Warburg was in fact only partly right. The cancer cell can also upregulate other pathways to maintain its energy needs, including the normal oxidative phosphorylation pathway.

This abnormal metabolism needs huge amounts of glucose and glutamine (an amino acid) and there is also an increase in lipid (fat) metabolism. Unbelievable as it sounds, it took until 2011 for researchers to recognise this and acknowledge the Warburg Effect as a hallmark of cancer. Worse still, the somatic (gene) theory is still accepted by the medical profession as the only driver of cancer. On the other hand, integrative doctors have never forgotten Warburg.

In the 1950s the field of oncology emerged with the use of chemotherapy and radiotherapy that targeted the cell's gene and the cell cycle. This genetic approach was further boosted when it was discovered in the 1960s that the p53 gene was implicated in many cancers. What was not acknowledged was the p53 affected the metabolism, increasing glycolysis (the breakdown of sugar for energy) and glutaminolysis (the breakdown of glutamine for energy) as do many of the main genetic mutations (e.g. BRAF, c-MYC). These metabolic changes trigger further mutagenic changes.

Cancer comprises a genetic component, a metabolic component and abnormal cell signaling. Currently, mainstream oncology focuses treatment on the genetic component; the abnormal cell division and mutated genetic targets, although there have been recently approved drugs to target the immune check points with a small degree of short-term success.

What is less understood is that treating the metabolism in conjunction with these genetic approaches will enhance any other cancer therapy, often reversing 'drug resistance', a common phenomenon where the genes have mutated and become resistant to chemotherapy or immunotherapy.

Research into the cell nucleus, the double helix of DNA (seen as the 'code of life') and decoding the genome through the Human Genome Atlas Project was meant to reveal all the answers. Instead, what was discovered was a random mess. There was no genetic answer to cancer. But the altered metabolism, the increased uptake of glucose and glutamine, was found to be common to all cancers.

Starving cancer is now the 'hot' area of research and drug discovery, even though cheap, off-patent and highly effective solutions exist already. I discovered these on my own between 1999 and 2003, with no assistance from the medical field. They were simply never suggested to me. Instead I had to persuade several medics, complementary and orthodox, to prescribe them.

As the drugs I discovered are off-patent, there is no financial incentive for large pharmaceutical companies to explore them and they continue to be ignored. There is even an attempt to suppress these old drugs because they represent a financial threat to these major corporations and big cancer charities.

With the advent of better detection methods (MRI, PET scans) that showed chemotherapy and radiotherapy shrinking tumours quickly, the mainstream continues to be sold on the somatic theory. It's a rash decision, fed by panic and the hunger for quick results. In the mad dash to get rid of a tumour, the patient is over-treated with high levels of either chemotherapy, radiotherapy or targeted therapies. This approach is doomed to fail – it only makes the patient more resistant to future treatment. Focusing on the DNA does not affect the cancer 'stem cell'. Cancer returns harder and more aggressively than before. The cancer mutates and eventually becomes resistant to these 'targeted' treatments.

Treating the cancer metabolism, on the other hand, alongside targeted approaches, will reach the stem cell and offer the real opportunity for a cure. But these treatments are much slower, taking many months. The patient and the oncologist will both need patience.

*****

By the 1970s two distinct camps had emerged, alternative and conventional. The war between the two has gradually escalated, each camp saying the other is wrong. Now it's at fever pitch, leaving the poor patient in the middle. Who should they listen to and what should they do? All the patient wants is to get better. It is confusing and frightening.

Indeed, neither approach is ideal. Patients are regularly over-treated and poisoned with too much chemotherapy. Furthermore, used on their own, restrictive diets seldom work unless they are very extreme and most patients struggle to follow them.

What I discovered was that the whole is greater than a sum of its parts. In other words, that to combine metabolic and genetic approaches more than doubles the effectiveness of each. They work in synergy, magnifying each other's effects.

So, when you or a loved one are diagnosed with cancer, what should you do? First and foremost, arm yourself with knowledge. Seek the community and the solidarity you need not only to overcome the cancer but to thrive. And remember, no matter what you're told by conventional medicine, there is so much more that can be done.

1. Join my revolution.

My Facebook group **'Jane McLelland Off Label Drugs for Cancer'** (catchy title!) has lots of chat and discussion about various off label drugs. I encourage scientific and peer-reviewed articles and of course stories of personal experience are always inspiring! Search for #positiveprogress on the site to see a long list of others doing well with their protocol, many in full remission from stage IV.

www.facebook.com/groups/off.label.drugsforcancer

I also have my book Facebook group dedicated to 'starving cancer' where I post specific articles on cancer metabolism and speaking events I will be attending where you can come and quiz me in person.

www.facebook.com/howtostarvecancer

Also visit and sign up for blogs and updates on my website which has recommended products and links to doctors who can help put your protocol together.

www.howtostarvecancer.com.

Personal data will never be shared.

If you want to understand the science in a more visual way, particularly if you have 'chemo brain', I now have an online course that will guide you through the key pathways. The first three modules will give you an overview of my approach and the basic principles of how and why it works. Funds from this course will go towards an App and other resources to help future patients.

www.how-to-starve-cancer.teachable.com

2. Attend the Care Oncology Clinic

This ground-breaking clinic has now treated thousands of patients with its off-label drug combination of metformin, atorvastatin, doxycycline, mebendazole and Flarin. All these drugs, their benefits and the ones I used are discussed both in this book and on my web pages.

3. Partner with an Integrative or Functional Medicine Practitioner

You should immediately bring complementary therapy into your treatment. The right practitioner can check your micro-nutrient status, work on gut issues (leaky gut, dysbiosis), recommend supplements and intravenous vitamin C or other treatments if necessary.

4. Partner with a nutritionist

You should find a nutritionist experienced with intermittent fasting, ketogenic, low glycaemic, macrobiotic or reduced-protein diets (e.g., the Paleo Diet). He or she should tailor your nutrient intake to your personal requirements, ensuring that the diet is neither unnecessarily complex nor too extreme as the combination of everything you will be doing will help reduce the need for severe dietary measures. Fasting for long periods may make cancer more aggressive as it is adaptive. Although there are only a few specialised oncology nutritionists now, your own knowledge of what fuel your cancer prefers (the glutamine: glucose: lipid ratio) will guide food choices and help you starve your cancer. I hope to create trained H2SC (how to starve cancer) coaches in the future to help with guidance on this. For instance, virtually all cancers respond to a reduced glucose intake, glutamine-fuelled cancers require a lower protein intake and fat-driven cancers (e.g., prostate, melanoma) may need to avoid high fat ketogenic diets. Reducing saturated fat is also important for every type of cancer.

5. Educate your oncologist.

Go to *www.howtostarvecancer.com* or my Facebook group, download the relevant articles and show them to your oncologist. It is vital to keep your oncologist on side. Emphasise that you want to combine genetic approaches with metabolic approaches. You need a collaborator, not a dictator! Sadly, most oncologists currently do not agree with a combination approach, for myriad reasons. Find one that does (see my website *www.howtostarvecancer.com* for an up-to-date list – oncologists who initially resist may eventually be won over).

6. Exercise

Recent research by the diabetic community shows that appropriate exercise can dramatically enhance cancer therapy. The secret may not be about how much exercise you do, but rather **when** you take it. A brisk walk fifteen to twenty minutes after eating pulls out glucose from the blood and redirects it to the muscles. This effectively starves the cancer-cell micro-environment.

7. Monitor your blood glucose and blood markers.

You need to track your blood glucose to find out how well you metabolise carbohydrates, just as diabetic patients are told to do. Insulin resistance can strongly influence the chances of success. Invest in a continuous blood glucose monitoring system for at least 2 weeks.

Have your cancer antigen markers taken regularly and make sure you track them. I plan to create an App for this and for providing potentially useful drug and supplement suggestions.

8. Sleep and de-stress.

The right amount of sleep at the right time, together with lowering stress, will improve immunity while also reducing cortisol and insulin resistance. Yoga, meditation, exercise, even beta-blockers such as propranolol (which is a very effective cancer-growth blocker) can all help improve your chances of beating cancer.

9. Keep hydrated.

Good hydration levels are important to lower the glucose concentration of the blood. Raised salt levels change the osmotic potential of your blood, encouraging the growth of pathogens. This creates inflammation around the cancer cell (the 'terrain'), and inflammation drives cancer growth.

10. Don't give up.

Continue with a good low-glycaemic diet, the supplements and the off-label drugs, incorporating extra virgin olive oil,[1] (See my website for the best brand, quality is important). Avoid alcohol until the cancer is under control and markers are stable and normal; then one unit per week of either wine or a spirit (not beer) may be permitted with vigilance. Be

---

1   Olive oil contains oleic acid, a monounsaturated fatty acid (MUFA). This stops progression in some cancers (e.g., HER2) but can be used by highly metastatic cancer to stimulate progression by a process called fatty acid oxidation which we will discuss in Part 2. Red sage or Danshen will block the fatty acid oxidation while retaining the other benefits of olive oil. Article Source: High Metastatic gastric and Breast Cancer Cells Consume Oleic Acid in an AMPK Dependent Manner
Li S, Zhou T, Li C, Dai Z, Che D, *et al.* (2014) High Metastatic gastric and Breast Cancer Cells Consume Oleic Acid in an AMPK Dependent Manner. PLOS ONE 9(5): e97330. https://doi.org/10.1371/journal.pone.0097330

strict about avoiding smoke and carcinogens, especially those that affect your hormonal balance. It is imperative that you monitor your blood glucose and track your triglyceride levels. Specific supplements, exercise and drugs will keep insulin and glucose levels low. It is possible to live with cancer, even when advanced, though you may need to develop a long-term approach (like living with diabetes).

The major barrier to achieving the above ten steps is that your cancer diagnosis must come from an oncologist and most are currently not supportive of the combined metabolic and genetic approach. I have witnessed some oncologists sabotaging results when the patient is showing healthy improvement, by increasing the dose of chemotherapy, effectively killing the patient. Some refuse traditional treatment altogether if the patient includes off label drugs in their treatment programme. Or the oncologist suggests a trial where the inclusion criteria means the patient must stop all metabolic drugs. I have witnessed many patients with rampant disease stabilise while on the Care Oncology Clinic drugs, then be forced off them for a trial and deteriorate rapidly. Combination treatments work. When more data is released from the Care Oncology Clinic, they will show success at an unprecedented level. The early data on glioblastoma already shows a doubling of survival time.

Until the metabolic approach is accepted as standard of care, arm yourself with knowledge and seek the help you need. Yes, it's a tough road, but like me, you can make it too.

It is my aim to inspire you with my story and my discoveries and to convince you that there truly is more hope than you may think.

Take action. Do not be passive. Doing nothing is not an option.
Starve your cancer. Stop it spreading. Snuff it out.
Hello brand-new you.

'It is in the nature of revolution, the overturning of an existing order, that at its inception a very small number of people are involved.

The process, in fact, begins with one person and an idea, an idea that persuades a second, then a third and a fourth, and gathers force until the idea is successfully contradicted, absorbed into conventional wisdom, or actually turns the world upside down.

A revolution requires not only ammunition, but also weapons and men willing to use them and willing to be slain in the battle.

In an intellectual revolution, there must be ideas and advocates willing to challenge an entire profession, the establishment itself, willing to spend their reputations and careers in spreading the idea through deeds as well as words.'

Jude Wanniski, The Way the World Works, Touchstone Books 1978

Join my revolution. Spread the word.

My online course, research articles, podcasts, interviews, blogs from survivors will be on my website.
www.howtostarvecancer.com

Lively discussions, peer-reviewed medical articles to download, inspirational patients (my Facebook family)
www.facebook.com/groups/off.label.drugsforcancer

Research on starving Cancer and ferroptosis on
www.facebook.com/how-to-starve-cancer

The patient-led metabolic revolution is in full swing!

Although more doctors are embracing the cancer-starving approach, there are still too few doctors per patient, and a cumbersome resistance to change from within the medical community which is slowing progress in this area. Thank heavens for the Care Oncology Clinic and some fabulous open-minded doctors out there. I love seeing the positive progress reports from patients; remissions appear on my Facebook group almost every day. Even more gratifying are the emails I receive from practitioners all over the world, from Korea to Canada.

One doctor in Nashville, thrilled with his results, wrote to me and likened my revolution as the 'third invasion' by the British of the USA. The first needs no explanation, the second was the Beatles and the third he describes as little old me, taking on the power and might of the world of oncology. That makes me feel like I should resemble Joan of Arc, armour-clad and shouty, which is an image I am not sure I should embrace!

So, while I am back at HQ working out the strategy for my continued invasion, you are the foot soldiers for this revolution. It takes a bit of pluck on your part to enter the hallowed turf of the consultant's room and then ask for some low toxicity drugs to complement your treatments. It is well worth sounding out your doctor's view on, for example, metformin, before you go all in for help with the entire Metro Map, particularly as the reaction can be somewhat unpredictable. On one occasion a patient had the book grabbed from her hands by her doctor who then stood up and made as if to wipe his bottom with it while uttering the words, 'That's what I think!'

The annual straw poll in my Facebook group reveals that 30-40% of oncologists tolerate the inclusion of off label drugs, 10% are fully supportive, the rest remain outright hostile. This may in part be because there is the moral and ethical dilemma of new drug trials – if you want to enter a trial, the conditions are that you halt any other drugs or supplements, no matter how low toxicity. The Pharmaceutical companies stand to make millions (the oncologist also receives substantial funding) while using the patient as a guinea pig, barely a thought given to the ethics of denying a stage 4 patient treatment choice. Keeping your oncologist on your side is important but this book redresses the balance and places the power of healing firmly back in **your** hands.

'Carry on with whatever you're doing because it's working,' is routinely heard by my tribe when they show an unusually good response to conventional treatment, with no curiosity from their doctor as to why this might be so.

In this second edition of *How To Starve Cancer* I provide a few more key metabolic pathways cancer uses to feed itself; I have added fat, glutamine and lactate transporters on my new Metro Map. Also included is the proteasome (a 'shredder' to break down proteins) and the cysteine-glutamate antiporter that draws cystine, an amino acid, into the cancer cell to make cysteine and glutathione. The cysteine is an important defence system cancer uses to combat free radicals caused by chemotherapy, radiotherapy and intravenous vitamin C . Blocking the xCT pathway is critical for creating ferroptosis, a newly discovered form of programmed cell death using iron, which cancer loves. This is an exciting area and ferroptosis is especially useful in many of the really chemo-resistant cancers such as glioblastoma, pancreatic, triple negative breast cancer, ovarian, mesothelioma, sarcomas to name a few. Ferroptosis is not really known, even by other leaders of this metabolic revolution and it requires a different approach as it is a 'Kill Phase' to be done separately to a 'Starve Phase'. I have spent months researching ferroptosis to provide you with the unique diet, supplements and drugs for this exciting new solution.

So now you have my book, please READ IT! Don't skip Part One as many do, thinking all you need is the information in Part Two. Then wonder why you are lost and you haven't grasped the basics. If you are in a hurry (most patients have far more time than they realise) then there is always my online course on *www.how-to-starve-cancer.teachable.com* to explain why cancer behaves as it does and how to starve and kill it. The course will help simplify what, why and when. I am also creating an App to help patients work out their combinations, but that is taking up masses of my time and App developers don't come cheap!

Cancer is overwhelming, that is the nature of the beast, and if you have no medical knowledge then please find a doctor as soon as possible to help you as you cannot do this protocol alone. There is a growing list on my website. Do not expect the wealth of information in here to magically seep through your fingers by osmosis into your brain without reading. It is your user manual. Use Post It notes, highlighter pens, whatever it takes to help you assimilate the information. Getting better requires some measure of effort on your part and a basic level of understanding of how cancer works – but don't panic if it mostly goes over your head first time you read it. You don't need to understand how each pathway works in detail, all you need to understand are the important fuel lines, as blocking these will slow growth and buy you time to explore additional treatments. I may mention strange unfamiliar supplements, drugs and medical terms that you have never heard of, but have patience, after a while it will gradually all start to make sense.

Since my first edition, many of you have shared your survival stories – a truly wonderful gift for others with a similar cancer who feel all hope has gone. I have some inspiring video testimonials in my Teachable online course that are free to view, posted by patients who have overcome tricky cancers like pancreatic cancer and triple negative breast cancer, so please do check them out.

To every patient who is marching alongside me, helping this metabolic approach become accepted by the mainstream, I cannot thank you enough.

Part One

The Discovery of
My Metabolic Protocol

Chapter One:

Maracas

'Come on, wake up!' I heard the words faintly as I tried to open my eyes. I had had another fractious night, taunted by nightmares. Just as I had finally fallen into a deep sleep, someone was nudging me awake.

'It's 6 o'clock. You need to get up. We have to get down to the coast by 8.' My husband Andrew gave me another affectionate prod.

'Okay, I'm moving,' I lied. Then I remembered why I had to get up. I was going racing! I grinned in the dark. Excited but still groggy, I pulled the covers off and headed to the bathroom.

The last time I had sailed with the team – in a reckless attempt to lead a 'normal' life – I hadn't yet finished my six months of chemotherapy. I had not been fit enough. During the first race I had very nearly thrown up all over the spinnaker and my arms had felt like lead while I packed it into a sail bag down below. I hoped I would feel better this time. I desperately needed to feel better.

Nine months earlier, in the summer of 1999, I had been diagnosed with stage IV cancer. Nearly five years after the primary cancer was diagnosed in my cervix, it had spread to my lungs. My illness and the relentless rounds of chemotherapy had led to my spending the winter hibernating, struggling to get through each day. Now I was emerging with the spring, making a conscious effort to fight the exhaustion that drained my strength. I had decided that a bit of exercise might fight the fatigue away.

Grabbing my Ziplock bags of supplements from the kitchen, which were all botanical extracts apart from a low-dose aspirin, I headed for the door, stuffing them deep into a pocket out of sight. Andrew was waiting at the wheel and I slid gratefully into the passenger seat. It takes an hour and a half to drive to Lymington. Perhaps I could catch a few more zeds on the way.

Trying to swallow supplements while on chemotherapy had been difficult. I had ignored my oncologist's advice not to take anything at all and had done my own research. Some supplements, like EGCG from green tea and curcumin, found in turmeric, enhanced chemotherapy. Now that I had finished those dreadful infusions, the number of supplements I was taking had skyrocketed. I wanted all the help I could get. And they might just make the difference.

When we arrived, the crew were gathered on the dock. My friend Louay was carrying an armful of t-shirts. Everyone in the twelve-strong team was handed one with his or her crew nickname on the back.

My husband opened his, emblazoned with his nickname, 'SPOTTER'. With his boat-nerd ability, he can instantly tell from a distance the make, model and engine size of any boat, as well as who built her, when, and how well (yawn). I giggled and wondered nervously what Louay had in store for me.

'Jane, this one's for you,' he said with a grin. As I turned the shirt over, I saw it: 'MARACAS'. I laughed. 'Damn it! I thought you hadn't noticed all the pills!'

Louay looked at me incredulously. 'You have to be joking. We've all seen those little Ziplock packets you take everywhere. And that green muck you drink? If you were trying to hide it, you failed miserably.'

Bother. I hadn't been quite as discreet as I thought. These pills and the green drink – what I liked to call my 'primordial soup' – were my lifeline. I had wanted to keep my illness a secret, a private nightmare. It was unfair to drag anyone else into it. I was terrified about my future, which, if I listened to the medics, would be extremely short. But how ridiculous to think I could hide anything from twelve crewmates on a 48-foot boat! There were no secrets, no matter how hard I tried.

Mixing up the daily drink – spirulina, chlorella, and all manner of pulverised shrubbery – and organising daily sachets of supplements took some time. But it was a small price to pay for getting out of the house and living a bit. It was surviving. Please God, I silently prayed, don't let this be my life forever. It was so hard to stay upbeat and positive with all the uncertainty.

I hated drawing attention to my problems. I couldn't bear the thought of my teammates treating me as an invalid, as someone to be pitied. I wanted to continue to be Jane, their rugged and quirky sailing buddy. I wanted them to joke with me as they always did, not to ask anxiously how I was feeling. I understand that some people are proud of their chemotherapy baldness and lymphoedema stockings – their surgery scars are badges of honour. Not me. I just couldn't see it that way. My mild right-leg lymphoedema, caused by extensive surgery to remove my lymph nodes, remained hidden under long skirts and trousers.

Fortunately, unless I pointed it out, most people didn't even notice. And when my hair fell out with all the chemo, I did not wear a scarf or hat. Too obvious. I wanted to look as normal as possible. Even though they were unbearably itchy, I wore wigs partly because I wanted to deny even to myself that anything was wrong and partly because even I was shocked when I caught sight of my hair-free noggin in the bathroom mirror. It made me catch my breath. Even after several months, the horror at my reflection hadn't got any easier.

As soon as my hair had started to drop out (in great big handfuls), I had rushed out and bought some decent wigs in Selfridges. I bought three at once, in three different styles. When I wanted to feel glamorous, I could wear the long wavy wig. Sporty? The bob. Everyday? The mid-length straight hair. 'Which wife would you like today?' I would ask Andrew as I got dressed in the morning. It certainly confused the builders who were extending our attic at the time when I came downstairs with short hair one day and long hair the next.

I used the shortest wig for sailing because it was easier to wedge on under my cap. Sailing was my passion. It was helping me to keep my sanity when I was perilously close to despair. Being so surrounded by a team of close buddies, laughing at each other's stories and competing in intense racing was a help, even if only for the briefest time. The activity and friendship took my mind off the pain, disfigurement, and the loss of who I once was. And death. I was desperate to believe that this was not my last season racing on the boat.

While I was thoroughly exhausted by my treatments, I was keen to pretend that nothing out of the ordinary was happening. It was business as usual. I forced myself to carry on sailing, even though on race mornings I wanted nothing more than to dive back under the bedclothes. Once out with the team, I insisted on throwing myself into the action on board, despite some crewmates' concerns that I wasn't up to it. With the benefit of hindsight, I realise that this might have been selfish, slowing the team down. I was taking much longer to get myself back up on the rail and to keep the boat level than the others.

Upwind, I would be down below, packing the enormous spinnaker, usually on my own. It can be awkward packing a sail the size of a tennis court into a few feet of space, especially when the boat is constantly changing direction, keeling over at a 45-degree angle. It was exhausting even if you weren't poorly – particularly if it had got wet. When we reached the top mark and turned the boat to run downwind, I was the 'trimmer', constantly checking the set of the spinnaker, ensuring that we were sailing as fast as possible.

I loved the feeling of exertion, the wind on my face, the ozone, and the sting of the spray as the boat cut through the water in a gentle sway. It soothed my worries, this game of chess on the water, working out the shifting wind directions and the tides. Tactics and strategy were more Andrew's field, but all of us on board needed to be aware of where we were and what we needed to do to get ahead and stay there – and to prepare for sudden manoeuvres.

Sailing has been in my blood for generations. My father owned a succession of boats in Guernsey, where I grew up. Sailing on a little 26-foot yacht with my elder sister Suzie was one of my earliest memories. We mostly cruised around the other Channel Islands, especially Herm and Sark, but some summers we nipped over to Saint-Malo in Brittany, on the north-western coastline of France. It was a heavenly childhood, one I associated with sparkling seas and stunning island beaches.

Even amidst the frantic activity during a race, there would be moments of quiet and calm, with just the soothing sound of the waves as a backdrop. I would often become lost in thought, trying to recapture that long-lost stress-free feeling of pure bliss from my youth. It was gratitude tinged with sadness that my love of sailing, the sea and of life itself might soon come to an untimely end.

In my teens I had been desperate to take a more active part in yacht racing. Sailing with my father was immensely frustrating because he was very old-fashioned and never let me touch any winches or ropes (I was a girl, after all). Eventually I gave up, worked during the holidays, saved up and bought myself a windsurfer instead. I loved the challenge of learning this new skill and I became a total surfing bum, never off the beach in the summer. But the competitive spirit inside me still wanted to race boats.

The opportunity came in the form of a lovely sailing boat called *Assuage* (affectionately known as *Sausage* by our opposition). *Assuage* was a 42-foot Swan, a boat known for its solid yet streamlined design, the perfect marriage of safe cruising and speed. She had come over to Guernsey to compete in the Swan European Sailing Championships in the early 1990s and she needed one more crew member. I leapt at the opportunity. Once I was on board, they weren't getting rid of me!

Sailing on *Assuage* was brilliant fun. For years, my weekends and holidays were taken up racing around the south coast of England. I was also lucky enough to sail in Antigua, Majorca and Sardinia and to compete in many offshore races to France – even in the notorious Fastnet Race. My uncle had drowned during that race in the great storm of 1979, so I had always been reluctant to enter. By the time I talked myself into it, our team had racked up an impressive list of trophies. It was still a hobby, but it was also a complete contrast to my day job as a Chartered Physiotherapist with the seriously ill.

I had initially worked in neurology. Much of my time was spent rehabilitating people who had suffered head injuries and strokes. I helped them relearn how to use their bodies, to move their hands and legs. It had been physically demanding. Later, I specialised in orthopaedics and sports injuries. Many high-level athletes became dependent on my expertise.

Despite sailing with Andrew for many years on *Assuage*, it had taken us ages to get together. He hadn't liked my former boyfriend and I hadn't liked his former girlfriend, so we had rarely socialised. We'd made some poor choices, but eventually we both ditched our partners. A year later we found ourselves snogging outside the Cherbourg Yacht Club after a boozy day, celebrating a win after a rough offshore race.

You might expect sailing to be a supremely healthy hobby, but this is far from the whole truth. Sure, we got exercise and fresh air. But we were also consuming copious quantities of chocolate bars and quick carbs during the races, then downing serious amounts of rum and Coke in the evenings. The good was very much outweighed by the bad. Our crew mantra was, 'Eating is cheating'. Leaving the bar to eat a proper meal was frowned upon. It makes me wince to even think about that now. Clearly there were more than a few significant errors in my lifestyle choices. Looking back to my days as a physiotherapy student, when I believe the cancer may have begun, I can see that my diet was terrible. A good meal involved a pile of mashed potato, melted cheese and bacon. Green vegetables? What green vegetables? Idiot.

Now that I had terminal cancer, the fear of death that haunted my every breath could be shaken off briefly in the heat of the action. But then, with regular and hideous force, the reality of my diagnosis came back and smacked me full in the face. It was as if the Grim Reaper were standing right behind me all the time, an ever-present spectre, breathing down my neck, waiting for the right moment to strike.

When the team started to plan sailing events for the next season, my first thought was, will I still be here then? It made me immensely sad to think about the future, a future in which the world would go on as before, but without me.

I now took my diet seriously. Gone were the so-called 'energy snacks' and the sugar-fuelled drinks. The crew got used to my bringing odd snacks on board and never questioned my low-carb choices. Sailing was more to me than just a frivolous bit of fun. I could forgo all those sugary foods easily. All I craved was just a little return to my old life, and if that meant a complete change of diet and knocking back a handful of supplements, that would be a small price to pay.

So, there I was, on that bright April day in 2000, less than a year after my diagnosis of a secondary – and terminal – cancer. Despite recently finishing chemotherapy, I still had a PICC line in my arm that led all the way up a vein into my chest. I had kept it in place for intravenous vitamin C infusions. It was fully bandaged to avoid being damaged, but even so, this was not the best attire for a race! Wearing my Maracas tee-shirt under layers of waterproofs, I left the dock with my crewmates and headed out to the start line. The sun was shining, and the wind was a steady 15 to 18 knots. Breezy. Perfect.

On the first beat, we found ourselves pounding upwind in a close tacking duel with another boat. A quick tack led to a scramble from one side of the boat to the other. During a tacking manoeuvre the crew must get across the boat, in windy conditions, as quickly as possible. This meant ducking my head under the guardrails before rushing across the deck to sit out over the rail on other side.

Squashed together, it was hard to get out from my position. In my hurry, I misjudged the distance and felt the guardrail scrape off my sailing cap. As if in slow motion, my hands reached out to grab it – but it was already swept away by the wind, over the side of the boat, still attached to my wig. 'Nooooo…,' I cried, watching in dismay as they floated off together down the Solent. 'Bugger,' I said, watching my lovely locks disappearing like a drowning rat under the waves.

Andrew was looking at me with an expression that implied asking whether we should go back. Well, only for a millisecond. We all wanted to win and turning back would have been disastrous. It was never an option. 'Leave it!' I yelled.

Everyone else was staring at me, stunned. It was the first time that anyone had seen me bald. The cold wind whipped past my ears. Suddenly I felt vulnerable, exposed. I put my hands to my scalp, trying to cover up its nakedness. I was mortified. A crewmate saw my look of horror, took off his own cap, and gave it to me without a second thought.

'Well, get back on the rail! We have a race to win!' he shouted with a grin. How I loved him – and the whole team. They didn't care about my baldness or my illness. They were still going to treat me as me. Indeed, we did have a race to win. This wasn't a jolly on the river with gin and tonics! Moments later we were all back on the other rail, roaring with laughter.

I have been called many things, but 'Maracas' was the nickname that stuck during my many years of racing with *Assuage*. I rattled with pills as I took them several times a day. It meant lots of complicated planning (and I am first to admit being organised is not my strongest suit!), but I managed.

Looking back now at that long list of supplements, I can see that it contained several mistakes: doublings up, unnecessary items, and at times even cancer-promoting ones. I had started to fight back, but I had a great deal more to learn. Rough winds and rocky waves were nothing compared with the turbulent journey that lay ahead of me.

Chapter Two:

A Spot of Bother

I was first struck with cancer in 1994. That makes it sound like a sudden event, but it wasn't. No cancer happens overnight. For years I had been seeing a consultant for abnormal cervical changes.

Cervical cancer is totally preventable and treatable if caught early and given proper attention. I had trusted the gynaecologist to do his job and I had naturally assumed that he was treating me correctly. I had been given a colposcopy a few years earlier in 1989 when a few mildly abnormal cells had been found. After several return visits to the hospital and years of repeatedly being told that there were no more abnormalities to be seen, I thought my worries were over and I assumed the problem had been eradicated for good.

But I was wrong. A repeat smear performed at my local doctor's surgery had shown the problem had returned as 'severe dyskariosis', a sign that further treatment was warranted.

However, the gynaecologist at the hospital had told me that my biopsy, within the same four weeks, had shown no such abnormalities. Surprised by this contradiction, I wondered who I should trust, the GP's results or the hospital's? My instinct was to trust the hospital and the specialist; surely a biopsy was more reliable than a smear?

My GP told me that there were a few cases where abnormal tissue reverts to normal. 'You might be one of the lucky ones,' he said. Perhaps I was.

He asked if I wanted to be referred to another hospital. But this South London hospital was a main teaching hospital. A relative had trained as a doctor there. Surely it was one of the best? I stayed put, little guessing the fate to which I was consigning myself.

Like anyone diagnosed with a potentially serious illness, I was desperate to believe that my body was capable of healing itself, so I convinced myself that I had indeed reversed the abnormal changes on my own without surgical intervention.

I shudder when I think back to those visits to that South London hospital. It was during my last visit that I became suspicious of the specialist's behaviour and his overly casual, indifferent demeanour. Every time I saw him, he prescribed a progestin tablet for the symptoms of 'spotting', but I had no idea that this is a synthetic form of progesterone which raised my risk of breast cancer and may have made the cervical cancer worse too.[2] Not only that, but it also raised my risk of blood clots and cardiovascular disease, so progestin may have poured fuel on the fire. The specialist dished them out like candy.

Put simply, he wasn't doing his job correctly, a fact that would be confirmed four years later in 1998, when there was a national recall of over a thousand of his patients. All the women recalled already had moderate or severe abnormalities detected by a standard smear test. They were each sent a letter stating that there were 'grave concerns' about the screening. Women given the 'all clear' were going on to develop cancer. I knew nothing of this at the time but became increasingly concerned when repeated visits over a year revealed worsening symptoms.

---

2   Fournier A, Berrino F, Clavel-Chapelon F. Unequal risks for breast cancer associated with different hormone replacement therapies: results from the E3N cohort study. *Breast Cancer Research and Treatment*. 2008;107(1):103-111. Progestin raised risk significantly whereas progesterone did not.

On my last visit I was begging him for a hysteroscopy, an examination of the uterus that might tell me why I was continuing to have spotting. He replied without even looking at me:

'I'm booked up. You'll have to wait until after Christmas for that.'

Wow. Really? It was only September. I somehow doubted he couldn't fit me in between September and January. This didn't sound right.

'But I'm losing weight. Believe me, it's most welcome, but it's going from places I have never lost it before. I am extremely worried. I simply must get this sorted out. It hasn't got any better.'

Because I had just started seeing Andrew, I had initially convinced myself that it was the first flush of love causing me to shed the pounds. But the pattern of weight loss was different. I **never** lost weight from my inner thighs. The supermodel 'thigh-gap' eluded me no matter how many inner-thigh exercises I performed. And yet this normally stubborn fat was disappearing before my eyes.

Without looking up, he went on, 'You really are worrying over nothing. I'm sure we can sort this out with more progestin.'

'But it isn't helping!' I protested.

Was the NHS in such a bad state that I had to wait until next year? What if I did have cancer? I had already had treatment for early cancerous cell changes and now I had other classic symptoms, not only the unusual spotting that was getting worse, but the weight loss. Surely this was urgent?

He gave me a thin smile devoid of any hint of compassion. 'Extra bleeding between periods is very common. But I will make another outpatient appointment for you in two months' time.'

Two months' time? For just another chat? This was totally unacceptable.

Years later, following the recall of his patients and an ensuing enquiry, I was to learn that this doctor typically biopsied only 64 per cent of his patients with cervical changes, against a national minimum guideline of 90 per cent. These women had come to his clinic with abnormalities, all needing further investigations to rule out cancer. A review of his colposcopies also found those to be inadequate. Of the 64 per cent he did biopsy, far too little tissue was excised to make a valid diagnosis. No wonder my problem had returned. The enquiry was to find that as many as nineteen women with advanced cancer were misdiagnosed or incorrectly treated. The rate of cancer in his patients was 34 per cent above the average.

I knew nothing of this at the time, but a nasty thought occurred to me. I wondered if there were doctors who allowed cancer to progress on purpose. I blotted it out. Surely not. Weren't all doctors interested in getting patients well? Didn't they take the Hippocratic Oath? But what if a doctor had made a serious mistake when treating a patient, and instead of owning up to it and risk being sued and losing their licence, they stuck their head in the sand by persisting with inadequate treatment? Dead patients don't sue. Might there be doctors out there who weren't giving their patients the medical attention they needed, knowing they had a life-limiting disease? I dismissed the thought. I was being ridiculous.

But his apparent indifference to my pleas was enough for me to decide to go private. I'd had enough. I knew there was a problem and he was not taking it seriously enough. My health was at stake.

I flew back to Guernsey with these grim thoughts and worries nagging away at me, but I convinced myself he was probably right. I was by nature a worrier and I was panicking over nothing. The tests at the hospital so far had been clear, hadn't they? But why had he not done any more biopsies? What if he had biopsied the wrong area? Incompetence would be easy for any gynaecologist to cover up. Who would ever know? It was his word against the patient's. The courts always took the side of the expert.

I busied myself back at work in my clinic and made an appointment with a private gynaecologist locally. This problem needed to be sorted even though the gynaecologist at the hospital had suggested it wasn't anything to worry about. Apart from anything else, I had a new boyfriend, with whom the spotting was a bit of a passion killer to say the least. It was embarrassing and inconvenient.

When the specialist in London learned that I had arranged a private referral in Guernsey, he totally changed his tune. In his referral letter, he insisted that treatment was urgent and that a hysteroscopy should be performed immediately. It was as if it had been written by a different person. He had never said anything like that to me. He hadn't even given me a biopsy for nearly a year.

Why this sudden change? Although it was all highly suspicious, I had little choice but to put my faith in the system. What else could I do?

The hysteroscopy took place on a Thursday afternoon and I remember waking up to find lots of medics peering over me, looking concerned. I told myself that was probably normal after anaesthetic.

The following day, Andrew flew over to visit me. I had the weekend to forget all about it. I was sure by Monday the results of the operation would reveal little more than minor changes that might at the most need another colposcopy. I had no reason to believe otherwise.

It was a beautiful crisp autumn evening as I waited in the Arrivals hall for Andrew, an irrepressible grin on my face. I was sure he was the one for me. I was so looking forward to spending the weekend with him, walking on the cliffs, sailing on my Dad's boat, going out and visiting friends. The flights and phone bills between Guernsey and London were costing us both a small fortune, but we didn't care. It was money well spent.

One of my former boyfriends had initially been charismatic and charming. I had thought he was a keeper. But then he began going out every evening and what started out as verbal threats gradually became physical. He was always very remorseful the next day and he would promise to make it up. But things got worse.

I hate confrontation but I was not willing to let myself be abused. I argued back, which only exacerbated the situation. One evening, he told me never to leave, grabbed me around the throat, and what happened next I will describe as a 'window incident'. Fortunately, I was unharmed, but shocked to the core. Never leave? I was **done**. I packed my bags the next day and ran back to the safety of my island home. I didn't think my ex would dare come and threaten me surrounded by my family.

Andrew, his polar opposite, was exactly what I needed. He was calm and dependable, kind and thoughtful, not too bad-looking and a top sailor to boot. It was an irresistible combination. He had already talked about the longer term and was making it clear he was keen. No arguments, no violence – things were looking up.

After settling back in Guernsey, I had found myself a great job in a private physiotherapy practice. It was a busy clinic, and I was earning good money. And Guernsey was beautiful. A ten-minute drive after work would take me to the marina, where I could leap into a boat and go out sailing for the evening.

But I still wasn't sure where my relationship with Andrew would lead me. I didn't know whether I would have to give up my Guernsey paradise to live in London, and I didn't know whether I wanted to. Nor did I know where he would want to start a family. If we had kids, would I have to bring them up in England or would he be prepared to live in Guernsey? I turned it over in my mind as I paced around Arrivals. My hopes and dreams, the two of us, building a future together.

And then there he was, running to give me a big warm hug. 'Hi, darling,' he said as I took his hand and led him to the car. It was a short journey back to the rented house I shared with another girl. On the way he tentatively asked about my operation the day before.

'I really don't want to talk about it. Can we just forget about it and go out for supper? There's nothing I can do about the result so let's not give it a moment's thought.'

But that was not to be. We pulled into the drive and as I looked up at the house, I saw my flatmate Carol-Ann hurtling down the steps to meet me. Before I had even stepped out of the car she blurted out, 'Jane, your GP has been looking for you! He was here half an hour ago.'

What? At 7 o'clock in the evening on a Friday? I looked at Andrew with horror. We both knew that this was not a good sign.

'I have to phone him,' I said, my voice trembling. I ran upstairs, shut my bedroom door and dialled. My doctor was insistent he had to come and see me. 'No, please just tell me now,' I begged. 'I know it's bad news, otherwise you wouldn't have driven over. I can't wait, I need to hear it.'

So reluctantly he told me. He had talked to the gynaecologist who had just operated on me. I would need a hysterectomy. It was cancer.

He said that they had already arranged an operation the following Tuesday at Hammersmith Hospital. The surgeon had called in a favour with one of his friends in London to get it done quickly. I wondered if they thought it must be quite aggressive to have progressed so fast without anyone noticing. Or had it been ignored? I was too overwhelmed by the diagnosis to ask.

My head was spinning. I tried to compute his words, but it felt as if I were overhearing a conversation with someone else. This couldn't be happening.

I put the phone down, stared at it for a minute and then I began to sob uncontrollably. My world had imploded. I was thirty. I had cancer. I hadn't had children and now it seemed I never would.

I must have stayed in my bedroom for over an hour. When I finally came downstairs, I managed to stammer the one word: 'cancer'. They had already worked that one out. My smeared make-up and puffy red eyes told the story. Andrew hugged me and suggested we get some fresh air.

Wrapped in warm clothes, we drove to a coastal path and sat in the moonlight on a bench overlooking the cliffs and the sea. I was in shock. So was Andrew. This shiny, happy new relationship was suddenly not so shiny. We had been together for only two months. Would our fledgling relationship survive this unexpected challenge? I was deeply distressed by the diagnosis and what it meant to both of us.

I was young. I would survive. I felt certain of it. Cervical cancer if caught early was perfectly curable, I had been told. Well, I could only hope it was still at that stage.

But I would never carry my own children. Perhaps someone could carry them for me? I had heard of surrogacy arrangements. I would still have my ovaries. The subject of death only briefly occurred to me. I had so many other worries. How badly would the operation affect my sex life? Would I still be able to have my own biological children using my eggs? I didn't even want to discuss these things with Andrew. I was too terrified that he would now turn his back on the relationship. Already it felt like an invisible curtain had come down between us. This diagnosis was going to change everything.

Andrew was saying very little. I was unable to guess his thoughts, too consumed with my own. He had not seen this coming. He had no experience of dealing with such a situation and felt completely out of his depth. If we had been sailing and the mast had come down or the rudder had fallen off, he would have been the first to know what to do. But dealing with a distraught thirty-year-old about to lose her womb to cancer?

While I was obsessing about my infertility, he was worrying about how serious it might be. It was comforting that he didn't want to lose me. But I wondered if a self-protective instinct was kicking in, keeping him from growing closer to me. If he were shutting me out, my situation would be far worse. A depressing sense of isolation began to descend on me.

Only hours into my diagnosis, I was realising that cancer's effects extend far beyond physical illness. I tried reassuring him that I didn't feel as if I were dying, but I could see that he was not convinced. A diagnosis of cancer means different things to different people. Some take it far better than others, but this diagnosis had implications for both of us. It would ruin our sexual relationship, certainly in the short term, and I had no idea about the long term.

The gynaecologist at the South London hospital had told me only a few weeks earlier that there was nothing to worry about. He had always reassured me that cervical cancer grew very slowly. I had been proactive, having a colposcopy and going for check-ups. So surely I must have caught it early enough? I ignored the niggling doubt in the back of my mind that it might have been growing for years and that perhaps he had failed to do his job properly all this time.

As we sat there looking out to sea, I convinced myself everything would somehow work out, that I would eventually land on my feet, even if my plans had to be altered. I could save my ovaries, maybe have them frozen. Then perhaps find a surrogate to carry my child. I had to get through an enormous operation the following week, but I was young. I would cope with this.

Death was not my immediate concern. It was having children that mattered to me. A happy home filled with kids' laughter was what I had always dreamt of. Somehow, no matter how difficult, I had to find a way to make that dream come true.

The rest of the weekend passed in a different mood. We cancelled plans to meet friends, but still went sailing. Andrew and I made practical arrangements, but the passion in our relationship had vanished. In its place was fear and worry. My feelings ranged from disbelief and anger to intense sadness and beyond. It all seemed so unfair. Just when I thought I had found my 'happily ever after'.

I knew I had to break the news to my parents. They'd be devastated, especially as they'd been concerned about the way I had been treated at that South London hospital. I couldn't face telling them in person, so in the end I chose to do it over the phone. I could tell that Mum was very distressed, but she immediately offered to travel to London with me on the Monday, to help me prepare for the operation on Tuesday. Our relationship had at times been difficult, as mother-daughter relationships can be, but I welcomed her support. I didn't want to refuse her company even though I knew it would be extremely hard for her.

Mum had been diagnosed with early-stage breast cancer a couple of years earlier, but she had kept her treatment to herself, telling us all it was just a 'spot of bother'. We weren't very good at sharing our feelings, but I knew she would be deeply traumatised by my diagnosis and my loss of fertility. She was really hoping to become a granny and was disappointed that I had kept on calling off engagements (two, to be precise). I never told her about the 'window' incident.

I had very basic knowledge about cancer, just what I'd been taught as a physiotherapy student, but it seemed obvious that the early decisions were crucial. Some doctors and surgeons were better than others, too. I had already learned this, at great cost. I worried that my choice could determine whether or not I survived.

I was being pushed into surgery without any time to think or to check my surgeon's background. If diagnosed with an aggressive and rapidly-growing cancer, it is important to be able to make educated decisions fast, but I was given no opportunity for spending time on research. Was it so aggressive that I could not even wait a week? All the urgency made me wonder just how bad it might be. All I had was a basic computer but no Internet access in 1994. It was impossible to explore ways of saving my ovaries or to prepare for the extensive surgery.

When I arrived at the hospital on the following Monday, the surgeon seemed nice enough. I had a long list of questions for him, not least the subject of saving my ovaries. I was desperate that they should be spared. I wanted to know what would happen if the cancer was worse than everyone thought.

He told me that if the cancer had progressed to any lymph nodes, I would need chemotherapy and radiotherapy. He did not offer suggestions about saving my ovaries, but I knew that those treatments, especially radiotherapy to the pelvis, would put them at risk of shutting down. I asked if he could perhaps freeze one of the ovaries if, when he opened me up, he thought I might need further treatments. He looked at me and nodded sagely. Was that a yes? I assumed it was. He quickly moved on to the operation and the risks.

The next day I woke up groggily after the seven-hour operation. As soon as I saw the surgeon, I needed to find out exactly what he had done. 'Did you freeze my ovaries?' was my first question. I was desperate for reassurance. It was a shock to learn that no, he had not. Perhaps he thought the cancer wasn't too bad. But when the histology results came back, they showed that the cancer had spread to a great many of my lymph nodes.

As he told me this, I was shaking with a mixture of fear, fury and disappointment. There was no question that chemotherapy and radiotherapy would follow, and these would switch off my ovary function forever. Why hadn't he frozen one of them as I'd requested? How could he have just brushed this request aside?

As I lay there, I realised that all was not completely lost. I had a window of a few weeks before the chemotherapy started. I would see if I could still find a fertility specialist, anyone to help me save my chance to become a mother. Time was of the essence and it was ebbing away fast.

The operation had been huge, and two weeks went by before I could even get myself discharged. While still an in-patient, my surgeon recommended that I see a well-known fertility specialist on the ground floor of the Hammersmith Hospital.

My hopes were instantly dashed. He didn't think anyone would be able to find my ovaries and, in any case, he felt surrogacy was too cruel and emotionally challenging for the surrogate mother. I had taken my sister Suzie along, and despite her noble offer of her own womb, the fertility specialist told me quite bluntly that nothing could be done. It was the harshness of his tone that was so shocking. I was so distraught I could hardly walk out of his clinic. I staggered back up to the ward, held up by Andrew and Suzie, wracked with grief. My children were gone forever, and I was powerless to get them back.

Infertility tortured me. Everywhere I looked on the street or on TV, I saw babies, children and happy families. Every advert seemed to be about nappies or infant milk formula. Unless I shut myself away from civilisation, I was constantly confronted with my loss. There was no escape. The pain of infertility hurt like a knife plunged into my chest. Every day when Andrew went to work, I lay on the bed and sobbed with despair and grief for the children I was never going to have. My hopes and dreams for the future lay in tatters. I felt empty. Shattered. I felt I had died already.

Anger built up inside me. I felt violated by the first gynaecologist, further admonished by the specialist at Hammersmith, robbed of my femininity, my womanhood, as well as the family I had always wanted. I wanted to sue, but this would be impossible if I wanted to get well. That task alone would take everything I had. Allowing emotions to surface, the anger and my deep sadness would not be helpful. I knew stress would potentially make things worse.

'Chemotherapy is only for a couple of months, to sensitise your cancer cells to radiotherapy,' my oncologist had said.

'So if it sensitises the radiotherapy treatment, why is there a gap of a month between the two treatments? Why don't you give the treatments closer together?' I asked, confused. It made no sense to me.

'Well, you might be right, but for now we don't have the evidence. There have been no trials on using them together.' Surely it would be better to combine them? It seemed illogical.

Even though it was a short course of chemotherapy, I lost most of my hair and was violently sick. I couldn't be sure it had shut down my ovaries, but I knew without any doubt that the intense radiotherapy that followed would.

When the first rays of radiotherapy had passed through me, effectively wiping out any chance that my ovaries would work again, I had wept on the radiotherapy table. The radiotherapists milled about, unsure what to say to help, offering tissues. 'Are you OK?' they had asked. Of course I bloody wasn't. I wanted to rage, to shout and scream. 'Do you know what you've done? Murderers! You have killed my future children!' They were only doing their job, of course. It was not their fault. Instead, I lay there in silence, tears rolling down my cheeks.

My hormones plummeted to zero. I hadn't been warned about that. I plunged from being a hot-headed, hormonal thirty-year-old into instant menopause. Few will understand what that's like. It's bad enough for many women when their levels of oestrogen dwindle naturally with age, but for a flirty spirited young female to be stripped of her hormones overnight was nothing short of traumatic. Without any warning the flashes would set my body on fire at the most embarrassing moments. Every night I was so drenched with sweat that I'd have to rip off the covers and dash to the shower.

Ovaries produce not only female hormones, but a small amount of testosterone as well. Because I was such a sporty character, I think I had more than my share. Without my normal mix, my mood was low, my sex drive was understandably zero and my skin was pallid and dry. In the longer term, my hair might become thin and I ran the risk of osteoporosis and heart disease. Gloomily, I assumed that as no-one had offered me hormone therapy, it meant that I should avoid it. Perhaps the hormones were implicated in driving the cancer. My mother's breast cancer had been oestrogen-driven.

At least I no longer had periods, but this was no compensation for all I'd lost. My mood was now permanently low. I no longer had any zest for life. No mojo. Nothing. Hormones play a huge part in defining who you are as a person. Without them there was little left of 'me'.

When I looked in the mirror, I no longer recognised myself. I vaguely resembled the old Jane, but the person staring back looked different. And I felt different. I was nearly bald and had gained a stone and a half thanks to steroids, several courses of antibiotics, and comfort eating. Where was the upbeat, carefree sailing and surfing chick? Had she gone forever?

My relationship with Andrew was thrown into turmoil. We found ourselves in a completely unexpected situation neither of us had prepared for. I knew he was finding it hard to allow himself to get close to me. While I understood, it was incredibly painful to accept. He would say things I found unsympathetic and hurtful, like 'Will you always be resentful and angry?' Well, yes, if you put it like that, I will be. I was upset that he seemed unable to understand or empathise, or to give me the time I needed to overcome the devastating diagnosis. Looking back, I realise that I must have been suffering from a form of post-traumatic stress disorder.

I didn't feel that my low mood was in any way unjustified. I had every right to be upset, furious, eaten up with grief. It had a disastrous effect on us as a couple. We couldn't talk about the future; we couldn't make plans. We had no idea what lay ahead. Conversations were stilted and superficial. After a few months our relationship began to cool and slowly break down. We were having real difficulties. For Andrew the concept of fatherhood was not paramount. It wasn't woven into his being, as motherhood was for me.

Thanks to the surgery, sex was not what it had been. Necessarily there were a few months of abstinence and when action eventually resumed it was agony. It was incredibly depressing, but I tried to put on a brave face. I didn't want him to know just how painful it really was. Thankfully he was a kind and considerate lover, but I had no idea whether it would ever be 'normal', pain-free and pleasurable again. The doctors assured me that things would improve slowly, but this aspect of our relationship made me incredibly insecure. Why would anyone want to stay with me?

In the past, I had never had any trouble getting and keeping boyfriends. I'd been engaged twice. I had never been desperate to be loved and needed. Relationships had been on my terms. But now, all that, it seemed, had changed. I was no longer a 'catch'. Instead, I was on the scrap heap, spurned by the opposite sex. I felt despair at how much cancer imposed itself on every facet of my life. It was overwhelming having to deal not just with the illness but with the emotional and financial complications that came with it. I lied about how I was feeling to keep friends and relatives happy; I listened and allowed others to have a say in my treatments. I constantly worried about keeping it all together in front of everyone, putting on that mask, pretending I was fine when all I wanted to do was just to cry. And turn back the clock.

My relationship with Andrew became so difficult that, with huge reluctance and a heavy heart, I decided we needed some time apart. I was aware that I was becoming too needy and suffocating with talk of children and a future. He could not see how much I was striving for hope and he wasn't ready for these discussions.

Despite my instinct to stay, I knew I had to find my feet, to find a way to be strong and show I could manage on my own. I was too reliant on him. He had to conclude that he still wanted me in his own time. It hurt me deeply, but once again I found myself leaving a relationship, running away, booking myself on a flight back to Guernsey, back to my island sanctuary. I told him I was going home to my parents and back to work.

But I didn't want my parents to see the depths of my grief and despair either. I rented a cottage on my own, resisting their help even though the treatments had made me weak and tired.

Being alone did nothing but make my mood sink further. I felt so isolated, so misunderstood. Magnifying my misery, my knee, damaged from a ski accident, now became so painful that I could hardly walk. And the other leg was showing signs of early lymphoedema, because of all the lymph nodes removed during surgery, a chronic condition that causes swelling in bodily tissues. I was an inflammatory mess, a hormonal mess, my body little more than a scarred piece of wreckage.

My whole world had fallen apart. I knew I would never be completely fixed again. I felt lost, in a body I no longer recognised, thinking thoughts that had never been there before. I was consumed with grief, not just for the devastating loss of my future babies but also the loss of myself. I just wanted to die.

At my lowest point, I found myself on the phone to the Samaritans. Once I put the phone down, I felt ashamed. How had it come to this? Was I truly suicidal? I could never subject my family and friends to that kind of pain.

No. I gave myself a stern talking to. Self-pity was no way to get better. Where was Jane the Fighter? The woman I had been before cancer? Was I really going to let this kill me? Would that incompetent specialist win? I needed to find something in my life that gave me joy. I needed meaning and fulfilment.

I tried briefly to go back to work as a physiotherapist, a job I used to love. But patients complaining about the most trivial problems just irritated me. My compassion had vanished. I had stupidly thought the job might help distract me, but how could I be sympathetic about a sprained ankle when I was dealing with cancer? It was hopeless.

I quit and instead focused on selling *BATHrobics*, a fun bath-time exercise book I'd created before becoming ill, which so far had been selling well through bookshops and the Innovations Catalogue.

The book turned into a flip chart that stuck over the side of the bath with a rubber sucker. This novel and practical design proved very popular. I turned my energies to promoting it and driving up sales. Ironically, I had just started writing a new exercise ritual for pregnant mothers when I'd become ill. I made the decision to finish it and publish it before the end of the year, torture though it was. I was determined to find a way to be a mum and vowed that one day I would give *BATHrobics for Pregnancy* to a surrogate carrying my baby. I would make it happen. It was the only way I could handle the pain.

There was still little joy in my life. Fortunately, my passion for sailing and the sea came to the rescue. I went out sailing in the evenings in Guernsey and travelled back to the UK at weekends to race with *Assuage*. Gradually I felt my inner strength returning. I was getting fitter. At long last a doctor prescribed some hormones to replace those I had lost. I began feeling more like the old me.

Andrew started to see that I was still the same person underneath the misery and that the grief-stricken creature before him was, deep down, still the woman he loved. After sailing one day, he took me out for supper.

'It's going to take a while to get you back up, with all engines firing,' he said. 'But I'm here, right by your side, to help you through all this. I believe in you and I love you. I really want you to come back to London and live with me.'

I cried with relief. Thank God! I wanted to forget about the cancer so badly, to move on with my life, to patch up my broken body and fix what I had lost. But losing my fertility was beyond my ability to fix and the subject of children was still hanging between us.

I continued to cry every single day, on my own, when no-one was looking. When I went for check-ups, it was hard to hide my feelings and my grief. The medics were understandably concerned for my mental health. They offered me Prozac, but I refused. No antidepressant was going to hand me back my fertility or cure my lymphoedema. So instead, they sent me to counselling. I was doubtful that this would help but willing to give it a try.

The therapist listened to my problems, occasionally offering the odd platitude, but her main job during these sessions was to supply endless tissues as my grief came out in torrents. She was genuinely nice, but she offered no practical solutions. Andrew, who accompanied me a couple of times, was a large part of the solution. Ultimately, therapy just compounded my issues, particularly as Andrew was immoveable about children. I knew he was worried about the prospect of ending up a single parent. Even so, I knew he was by my side, solid as a rock.

Surrogacy required us to be married and he seemed averse to this subject too. His lack of commitment was killing me. Deep down, was he a romantic who just needed to do things in his own time? My situation demanded the comfort of knowing. I wrestled with my inner voice, which was telling me at times to walk away. My former self would have had no problem with this, but infertility and cancer made decisions far more complicated. I wanted to see this through, to keep going and get back to where we were at the beginning, if that was possible.

What I hadn't realised was that the doctors had been far more honest with him than with me. They'd been upbeat and positive to my face, giving me the impression I would survive, while telling Andrew and my family a different story. This, it turns out, is not uncommon for cancer patients. They are often the last to know of the seriousness of their situation.

A turning point came one evening when Andrew and I were at home. We had just watched a movie, I was tired and was just about to get off the sofa and head to bed when he turned to me and held me back.

'I've been thinking a lot about kids. I'm sorry I found it so hard to discuss before, but I've decided I'm ready,' he said.

'What! Really? You really want children? You're not just saying that to cheer me up?'

'Believe me, I've thought about it non-stop! I have always wanted children. I know you've not been given the all-clear yet and I'm still worried about you. I've had to think about the worst-case scenario. But I think I could handle being a dad on my own if it happened again.'

I threw my arms around him and vowed I was not going to die. No way. This was what I had been hoping for. We were planning a future! The relief was immense. We stayed up late discussing the options. Andrew thought that adoption would be the best route, although I strongly favoured surrogacy. In his eyes, we would be coming at the problem together, that somehow having his genes and not mine in our child would be selfish if we pursued the surrogacy route.

What he didn't realise was that choosing him **included** choosing his genes, that what made Andrew **Andrew** was part of the equation. If I were to select a biological mother then wasn't I, in effect, selecting both sets of the baby's genes? The child would still be my creation.

Still, I knew the process of surrogacy would not be easy. Would anyone take on a woman who'd been through cancer?

I didn't want to rule out any options, limited as they were, so I wrote letters and waited. I contacted the adoption agencies and despite Andrew's concerns, I wrote to COTS (Childlessness Overcome Through Surrogacy), the surrogacy organisation founded by Kim Cotton in 1988. I expected to have a battle with the agencies, guessing that they would probably refuse me on health grounds.

I wasn't wrong. A refusal from an adoption agency soon arrived, stating that I needed to be clear of cancer for at least five years before I could even be considered. This was exactly the response I'd been expecting.

In five years I would turn thirty-five, too old for the agencies' strict criteria to be considered anyway. Yet again time was not on my side. It seemed too young to me – lots of women were becoming mums at forty – but there it was. In fact, Andrew had a much better chance of adopting as a single male than we had as a married couple.

While apologetic, the letter went on to argue that the child might suffer further emotional loss on top of what he or she had already gone through if I were to die. I understood this view and realised there was little point in contesting this decision. Even so, I couldn't help looking through the pictures of the children again, their little faces staring up into the camera, so desperate to be loved. My heart bled. I could have offered them a stable, safe and loving home. I would never get anywhere with their rigid rules and blinkered attitudes. Angry, I threw the letter in the bin.

With adoption out of the equation, I persuaded Andrew to focus his energies on surrogacy. He still worried that it was an inequitable arrangement, but with no other available options he was on board. Surrogacy, I hoped, would eventually provide the missing pieces in my life.

And so began the task of finding a suitable surrogate and perhaps an egg donor too. COTS was a young agency and getting ourselves onto their books took ages.

The public largely viewed these arrangements as not only bizarre but risky. Biased and sensationalist press articles didn't help. One story I read was about a surrogate who had kept the baby. This was something that worried us too. How far could you trust anyone in these circumstances? The article suggested that the problem stemmed from ignoring the pregnant surrogate, leading her to think the baby wasn't wanted enough. It didn't seem to have anything to do with an emotional bond between the mother and the baby.

Since that report, more background checks on surrogates had been put in place, so finding women prepared to take on such an extraordinary act of selflessness, having them properly assessed to verify their good intentions, all took time. I would spoil my surrogate rotten if I ever found one.

I knew I should be waiting until the magical five-year 'all-clear' mark before we started this process but there was no harm in exploring how to go about it in the meantime. I had already quietly gathered information without telling Andrew. I desperately needed this scrap of hope.

COTS finally sent through a list of possible surrogates with their profiles: where they lived, their age, weight, education, work, hobbies, etc. One Thursday evening I was busy leafing through some of the profiles and reading the COTS newsletter, when my phone rang.

It was my dad. He never called; it was always Mum. I knew something serious must have happened.

In a broken voice, he told me that my mother's breast cancer had spread and was now in her liver. I nearly dropped the phone. I knew that once the disease reached the liver, lungs or brain this meant only one thing. She was stage IV, terminal, and only sixty. She was far too young to die.

Chapter Three:

Tell me the Truth!

I instantly felt a strong sense of solidarity with my mother. I knew how alone and isolating it felt to be diagnosed. Even worse, she was now facing a death sentence. I could only imagine how terrible this was. I immediately began a frantic search for anything that might help her, knowing full well that time was not on her side and conventional medicine on its own would be futile.

The Internet in 1996 was sparsely populated, but there were a few stories of people surviving cancer by adopting a radical change in diet. The more I looked, the more I began to wonder why some of these treatments and altered diets weren't suggested or explored by more cancer patients.

As I delved into the world of alternative treatments, I began to uncover facts about cancer that no-one had ever told me. For example, I learned that glucose feeds most cancers and that IGF-1 (an insulin-like growth factor hormone found in high levels in dairy and meat) was implicated in driving its growth.

Wow. Why hadn't I known this before? Cancer cells have many glucose receptors on their surface to 'feed' them glucose and give them the enormous amounts of energy they need to replicate. Reading further, I learned that they're always hungry. Their insatiable appetite for nutrients helps them carry out their relentless proliferation, giving them both the building blocks and the energy to keep on doubling in size. It seemed all the focus for conventional treatments was on the genetic mutations and division in the cell nucleus. What about targeting the altered metabolism too? Why was this not addressed?

I learned that cancer doesn't survive in oxygenated environments. It prefers anaerobic conditions and a process called glycolysis (a breakdown of glucose in the cytosol, not in the mitochondria) to 'ferment' and grow, a bit like the way yeasts ferment. This 'fermenting' process is a grossly inefficient way of making energy, almost as if the cell had reverted to primitive times when the world had no oxygen. I learned how cancer sends messages and signals to build new blood vessels to feed itself (a process called angiogenesis) and that it needs other factors to feed its exponential growth. And I discovered the importance of maintaining a functioning immune system, ironically something that's ruined by too much chemotherapy. None of this had ever been discussed with me.

As a fully trained physiotherapist, I felt I should have known all of this or learnt it when I was diagnosed. I felt I'd been very remiss, but it seemed that even the medics themselves didn't understand these facts or at least disputed their importance. When I questioned them, they told me that diets had never been shown to help. I asked if there had ever been any trials. There hadn't. Trialing diets was notoriously difficult. But that was no proof they didn't work, right? And what about targeting the immune system? No use. The immune system was so overwhelmed by cancer that it failed to treat it as an invading force. Believing the cancer to be just another part of the body, the immune system no longer attacked it, so there was little point targeting it. This seemed a defeatist argument to me. But perhaps the tumour needed to be 'switched off' somehow to allow the immune system to be switched back on. I wondered how that could be achieved, and whether slowing or turning off the altered metabolism of cancer could help to give my mother a fighting chance.

Oncology was not a specialty I'd been familiar with as a physiotherapist. As a result, I had placed all my faith in my colleagues in the medical profession to get me well. At the time I hadn't even questioned the treatments I was given. I spent little time researching how effective they really were or whether there were complementary therapies that might help. I had naturally assumed I was getting the best treatment possible. I believed the doctors' reassurances that I'd be cured.

Over the following weeks, as I watched my mother die, the burden of my grief only intensified. It was a depressing realisation that the oncology profession was not tackling cancer on enough levels. My emotional state must have been massively detrimental to my immune system, and I felt guilty that my own cancer diagnosis must have, in turn, deeply affected my mum. Nothing I said could persuade her to cut out or reduce sugar and high glycaemic, refined carbohydrates in her diet. And taking supplements was not something she was prepared to do.

In any case, I think it was probably too late to rescue her. Like many of her generation, she worshipped her doctor. She blindly did everything he told her, like eating cake and biscuits to 'feed her up' and 'give her energy'. I was the only one telling her to try something different. But I was merely a physiotherapist, while other members of my family are doctors. They weren't overtly against what I was saying but I felt they thought my efforts were misguided and of little value.

It was frustrating and painful to see my mother wasting away, but by this time there had been too much damage to her body from both the cancer and from the chemotherapy. Slowly, she grew weaker and weaker until she was bedridden and one evening in early October, she finally died peacefully at home with me, my dad, and my brother holding her in her last moments.

Even though it was a peaceful event, it was devastating to witness. I will never forget it. I had felt so helpless and powerless. Again, I hit rock bottom. Modern medicine had let me down, and now it had let my mother down too. Death suddenly felt very real indeed, no longer something that happened to other people. I was still in my early thirties and suddenly I wasn't feeling as invincible as I had when I first got cancer.

I knew I had to do more research and prepare myself if cancer came back. Thanks to the confusing and misleading grading and staging of cervical cancer, only now did I begin to realise that my 'stage Ib' cancer was in fact stage III, as it had been in many of my lymph nodes. I was only one step away from a terminal diagnosis of stage IV.

In the months after my mother passed away, not only was I grieving her loss deeply, but I was haunted by visions of myself on that deathbed. Instead of seeing her, I imagined myself lying there, staring into the distance, drawing my last breaths.

This was a loud wake-up call. I needed no further encouragement. The shock and trauma of this experience made me look at my life through fresh eyes. I had too much to live for. I didn't know it at the time, but her death was going to save my life. Her passing became the platform for a turnaround in my own health. I began to modify my diet, exercise more, research more, and pay more attention to the fact that my body had suffered cancer. I had focused all my energy on infertility but now I no longer tried to brush the disease under the carpet as if it had never existed. I knew my health demanded my full attention, that cancer was a lesson to which I had so far refused to listen.

I had to reduce my sugar levels at the very least, so I cut out many simple carbohydrates like bread and sugar (although at this stage I didn't take it far enough) and I removed dairy and most meat, which both contain the IGF-1 hormones that drive cancer growth. I rarely ate red meat anyway, but now I cut out foods I personally found inflammatory, such as potatoes, tomatoes, rhubarb, grapefruit, and strawberries. I felt these were too acidic and they seemed to stimulate an inflammatory reaction in my body. I could tell. I'd just been through a knee operation for a ski accident and my joint would make it abundantly clear the next day if I'd made a dietary error. Inflammation seemed to be a driving force for cancer and if what I ate sparked inflammation in my knee, might it spark further cancer?

Monitoring my diet this carefully meant paying close attention to how food affected me, whether I felt tired afterwards, whether I was bloated or had joint pain. I eliminated foods and made lists of everything I'd been eating to try to work out which foods didn't agree with me. It was very much trial and error, and it took some time to sort out which foods were a problem. Today, tests exist to detect IgG antibodies, so the offending foods are easily identified. This is far simpler than my initial hit-or-miss approach, which was time consuming and inaccurate. Wheat and dairy, it appeared, were the worst offenders. I swapped normal tea for green tea and began juicing. I cut right back on alcohol and started popping more supplements. If the cancer came back, I sure as hell was going to be prepared. I was already hoofing glucosamine supplements for my knee, but I increased my intake of vitamin C and other vitamins.

It turned out that the glucosamine sulphate was a good thing. It's a great prebiotic, excellent for maintaining a healthy gut, a fact that is still largely unknown and I was to discover it is also a matrix metalloproteinase inhibitor (more on this later, but in short, it helps halt cancer progression). But I realise with the benefit of hindsight that I may have fuelled my disease by taking certain antioxidants like the tocopherol form of Vit E. I had assumed by taking these I was preventing a 'metastasis', where the cancer sends out a mass of little satellite cells and strikes in a new zone of the body. What I had yet to learn was that supplements for cancer **prevention** were totally different to those you need when you already have cancer. The assumption I had beaten it would turn out to be entirely wrong.

By the end of 1998 I started to get a nagging cough. I'm not the kind of patient who runs to the doctor at the merest tickle, but I was worried. I knew enough about my cancer now to know the lungs were the most likely place for it to spread. So naturally I found this new complaint extremely stressful. I was on high alert.

The doctor told me I had a chest infection, that was all, but one round of antibiotics failed to clear it. I tried another course, which again failed, so I decided to adopt the tactic of waiting for it to clear by itself. It didn't. Every time I went back to the doctor, I was prescribed another round of antibiotics and another bug would be revealed, as if I were peeling back the layers on an onion, with one infection hiding another.[3]

Two months later, I was still coughing badly. No longer content to accept it was just another infection, I went back to the doctor and asked for an urgent X-ray. My GP duly obliged and that afternoon I walked up the road to the Chelsea and Westminster Hospital's radiology department, my X-ray request clutched in my hand, with trepidation about what it would reveal.

I told the radiographer I'd been treated for cancer already and that I feared it might have spread. I asked if she could please take a lateral X-ray too, as the GP had put only one view on the request form. A 'lateral view' is side-to-side. Another angle helps rule out anything suspicious. About thirty minutes later, she came out smiling, saying it had been looked at and there was nothing to worry about, it all looked perfectly clear, a lateral view was not needed.

Phew! I really should try to stop worrying, I told myself. I was behaving like a typical cancer patient, getting anxious over every niggle and ache. But I had been let down by tests before.

---

3   In 2020 I was finally diagnosed with cystic fibrosis, which explains a lot!

Another two months on and the cough was still coming and going. My nagging doubt continued to grow. I'd started legal proceedings against the first gynaecologist and the South London Hospital and my trust in the medical profession was at an all-time low. Why had my lungs suddenly started giving me all this trouble, and why couldn't it be fixed with antibiotics? I was constantly dismissed as a 'worrier' by the surgery.

Then one Sunday afternoon in August, after a coughing fit, I tasted blood in my mouth. Whoa! Had it really been blood? I said nothing to Andrew but quietly took myself upstairs to cough into the basin in the bathroom. Right in front of me, as clear as day, was a big streak of blood. Oh God. Could this mean anything else? I sat on the edge of the bed trying not to panic. Think, Jane! Had I eaten something that'd scratched my throat? I coughed again and there it was, even more blood. Shit. Shit. Shit.

I called Andrew upstairs. He stared at the blood but somehow remained calm. Perhaps he didn't quite understand. Even after I explained the seriousness of what he was looking at, still an expressionless face. He would be great at poker. Often I found his outward lack of emotion irritating but in a time of crisis like this his logical, calm and practical approach was incredibly useful.

We sat there trying to figure out the best course of action. Where should we go? I could no longer trust the Chelsea and Westminster Hospital. I had a suspicion my X-ray there had not been read correctly. We decided to head back to the Hammersmith Hospital, where I'd had all my previous treatments in 1994-5.

It was a longer drive and I would have done anything to avoid ever entering that hospital again. The memories and the trauma of it all had left me with a deep-seated fear and loathing of the place. Reluctantly, we headed back to the grim, dilapidated building, the Hammer House of Horror.

In Accident and Emergency that Sunday evening, the staff were trying to deal with hordes of demanding and angry patients. An elderly man who'd clearly had a lot to drink had accidentally cut his finger off. He was charging about shouting and accusing everyone of being useless, his finger in a bag of ice. Perhaps they were being useless. Hard to tell. Someone surely should get him into surgery straight away.

The blood kept coming to my mouth every time I coughed. How long would we have to wait? After about an hour we were seen by a young and nervous junior doctor who led us into a cubicle. He asked the usual medical history questions, then tried every vein he could find in my arms and hands to get a blood sample. He was about to move down to try my feet when I suggested someone else should maybe have a go. Andrew has never been good with blood and needles, and he had to leave the cubicle as he was feeling faint. 'Man up!' I teased through the curtain. I was feeling like a pincushion.

After that, I was sent for an X-ray. I was still telling myself it must have been something rough I'd eaten at lunch. But the blood was still there, it hadn't stopped. It had got worse. As my business advisor used to tell me, 'There is nothing worth worrying about unless you're going to die. And if you're going to die there's no point worrying.' It was a mantra that somehow didn't fit the context of illness, where the real possibility of pain and suffering lay ahead, but I decided he was right, I'd stay calm and positive until we knew exactly what we were dealing with, if anything. Stay in the present, Jane. Deep, slow, calm breaths.

I made sure the radiographer took both a posterior-anterior (back-front) as well as a lateral view. Then Andrew and I sat down and waited. And waited. A junior doctor came out to see us. He looked seriously concerned. 'I just have to get someone else to check this,' he said. Fine, I wanted it checked properly. Even if he came back saying it was clear I was going to get a copy and at least another opinion. I wanted to be 100 per cent sure there was nothing there. I had lost faith in relying on one voice on anything to do with cancer.

We started leafing through magazines and tried not to think about it too much. Still, we occasionally addressed the question, 'What if?' I braced myself for any bad news and decided whatever the outcome I was now knowledgeable enough about stage IV cancer that I was at least going to be able to have a go at beating it. Knowing where to start digging for information was something I had already tackled. I had a head start.

We waited and waited. A couple of hours passed. 'Okay, this is normal for a busy outpatient department,' I said to myself. It was just typical NHS, too many patients, too few staff. It was now about nine o'clock in the evening and Andrew was getting peckish. I was too worried to eat and I didn't want him to wander off and leave me on my own in case we were called. We sat there trying to stay upbeat. But the staff on the desk were acting strangely. It looked as if they were quietly talking about us. I told myself I was imagining it and tried to ignore them.

Why were they taking so long? Where were they? I already knew the answer, but I continued to deny it to myself.

Finally, a doctor made his way over and asked us into a side room. I held Andrew's hand and squeezed it. We looked at each other and silently acknowledged that this was not a good sign. If the X-ray had been all clear we would have been sent on our way ages ago, not been made to wait and then pulled in here. I took a deep breath and summoned up every ounce of bravery I could muster.

Once inside I perched on the edge of the bed, trying my best to act normally. He shut the door and came straight out with it.

'Unfortunately, it appears there is a shadow in your right lung.'

I already knew. He stuck the X-ray up on the viewer and showed us the slightly irregular round lump in my right lung. Yes, there it was, cancer. It had come back, and I knew without him saying so that I was now stage IV, so-called terminal or incurable. Try to stay calm, Jane. Looking down, I saw my hands were shaking uncontrollably.

'How many tumours can you see?' I asked, my voice quite composed despite the turbulent emotions inside me. 'Well, we can't be sure it's a tumour. We need the results of the blood test to be sure, and a biopsy of course,' he said.

'Look, I'm a physiotherapist and I know it's almost certain to be a tumour. I've had cervical cancer, the most likely place for a secondary is in the lungs and now I'm coughing up blood with a shadow right there. Please be honest with me! The chance of it being anything else is extremely remote. How many tumours can you see?'

The doctor looked at me silently for a few seconds and realised there was little point trying to fudge the information as they normally do, or to break the news gently in half-truths, not being completely honest with the seriousness of the situation.

'Well, yes, it is most likely a tumour, but the good news, if there is any, is that it looks like there's just the one, although it is bigger than a golf ball. The bad news is, I'm afraid you're going to have to stay in hospital. We're worried you might need emergency surgery if a major vessel bursts, so we've arranged a bed on one of the wards.'

Whoa. Okay, that hit me like a punch on the nose. They thought I might be close to popping my clogs at any moment? Shit. Andrew looked at me and I murmured, 'I'm going to be alright, don't worry. I'm sure they're just being over cautious.' Although I really had no idea if they were. It may seem strange that here I was, having just been diagnosed with terminal cancer, and taking it far better than I had five years earlier. Losing my womb, my womanhood and the family I'd always craved more than anything else in the world had been far worse.

I would usually describe myself as an emotional train crash. I cry at the most pathetic adverts on the TV. But a strange calm came over me in that dingy hospital room. I felt a surge of strength, a new purpose and meaning flow through me. The survival instinct was flooding through my veins. I was being reborn.

I knew what I had to do. And it didn't involve crying, taking a passive role or relying solely on the medical profession. I had been let down too often. I'd had such faith in the NHS and the medical system as a physiotherapist and been so sure I'd be looked after and put back together. It was a painful and bruising lesson to discover just how ineffective it could be at times.

In the end, it had come as a depressing realisation that cancer treatments were not nearly as effective as they make out in the mainstream press. The 'game changers' rarely were. The system was inherently flawed, set up to benefit the pharmaceutical industry rather than the patient. Patients were routinely let down by a lack of proactive treatment. Prevention did not seem to exist. Rather, it was a matter of waiting for the cancer to come back, for the axe to fall, before they got off their backsides to treat you with their latest array of toxic chemicals.

The doctor asked what my last squamous cell marker had been. 'My what?' He said I could have had blood markers that might have shown up any progression, but I had never been offered one. Ever. Why? It was so simple and non-invasive. Why had no one ever suggested them? Where was the proactive approach in all this so-called care?

When the doctor left us alone to work out what we wanted to do, I put my arms around Andrew and we just hugged in silence for several minutes. I had no clothes or toothbrush with me for an overnight stay.

'Come on, you'd better run home and get my things,' I said.

'I don't want to leave you,' he said. 'I can't go back home tonight while you're all alone after what he's told you. It's not right. I want to stay with you.'

'Look, I really don't feel that bad. I'm sure they are just being ridiculously cautious about the whole bursting blood vessel thing,' I said, trying to sound reassuring. 'We can get through this. Let's take it one day at a time.'

I was quite surprised I was even able to speak without sounding panicked. An inner strength had emerged that I had no idea existed. I'd never felt stronger. I felt I was rising from the ashes. I could do this. I was sure of it. I was being faced with the greatest challenge of my life, and I would face it full-on, with bravery. Time to 'man up,' as I had told Andrew to earlier.

With this terminal diagnosis, suddenly everything came into focus. Despite all the grief that had overcome me before, I realised I could not waste another ounce of energy on that destructive emotion. I had to channel everything into survival. Dying was not an option. It might seem an obvious thing to say, but I've met many patients who accept their fate with little resistance. Almost with a shrug of acceptance. 'Well, I've had a good life,' they say, conceding that it's over without even considering a fight. That somehow bad luck had dealt its card and there was little they could do.

No, I had too much living left to do. I was still only thirty-five and I resolved to investigate everything I possibly could. There was said to be no cure, but I was sure the answer had to be out there, perhaps buried in old papers or an overlooked study. I would somehow find it.

I refused to see myself as a wounded soldier limping to my untimely demise. I was a fighter, back on the front line. Although I was carrying many deep scars physically, mentally and emotionally, they were not enough to stop me from picking myself up and walking back into the fray.

Was I ready? Bring it on.

Chapter Four:

Collaborators not Dictators

It took a lot of persuading to get Andrew to leave me at the hospital that night. To be honest, I nearly refused to stay. The warmth and comfort of my own bed, the normality of being at home, the reassurance of waking up next to him were the only things I wanted at that moment. But the situation was apparently life threatening. So reluctantly Andrew drove home, gathered up some clothes for me, and sped back to the hospital to meet me on the ward.

It was after visiting hours, but the staff showed some compassion and allowed him to stay for an hour. I had a side room to myself, which was a relief. The last thing I wanted was the hurly-burly of a ward. I needed space to think. I was still coughing up the blood, a nasty reminder of what was going on inside. Otherwise, physically I didn't feel that bad.

Mentally, I was terrified, of course. What if they were right and I burst a major vessel in the middle of the night and needed emergency life-saving surgery? Andrew was equally terrified, but we chose to think about other things, practical stuff, organising ourselves to deal with this enormous change in our circumstances.

Our wedding had been planned for three months' time. The church, the reception, everything was booked, invitations had been sent out. I realised with dismay that there was a good chance I was going to be given chemotherapy yet again. Not only would I feel sick, but I would also be bald, which – let's face it – is not the best look for a bride. It wouldn't be the wedding I had always dreamed of, looking gorgeous, healthy and radiant. Bugger this cancer. It had ruined my chance of a family and now it was ruining my wedding too.

We'd have to postpone. We would wait until we knew just how far the cancer had spread before breaking any news to anyone except for my sister Suzie, a doctor. I would talk to her. She had been amazing at helping me through the first time, although I knew I'd relied on her too much and hadn't done enough research for myself. She knew little about complementary treatments and I knew that orthodox medicine alone would not be enough to save me this time.

At eleven o'clock that night, the staff nurse came in and said she really was sorry, but she couldn't allow Andrew to stay any longer. We had a long hug. It was so hard to let go. 'I promise I'll be fine. I have a phone. I'll text you first thing tomorrow.' He struggled to leave, lingering at the door. After the doctors had put the fear of my imminent death in his head, he wasn't sure if this was the last time he would see me.

'Go on, go home! I'm absolutely fine!' He slowly turned into the corridor, blowing me a final kiss. I was left alone with my thoughts.

Back at home, Andrew got straight onto the Internet and looked up the statistics and my chances of survival. In 1999 no one could source information at the click of a button on a mobile. For me, stuck on the ward that night, it was probably a good thing, but for Andrew it was a different story. I don't think he got any sleep that night.

Sitting there alone in my hospital room, five miles away from home with no depressing statistics to ponder, I was already starting to feel more upbeat. I decided I wanted to see the X-ray taken months earlier at the Chelsea and Westminster Hospital. I needed to know if the cancer had been present then, as I was deeply suspicious that it had been missed.

From that we could work out what the tumour 'doubling time' was, how fast it was growing. I had learnt quite a bit about cancer looking after my mother but nowhere near enough. Why had I not known about the blood tests?

Amazingly, I slept well. By the time the doctors crowded into my room first thing in the morning, I was smiling and cheerful. Honestly, there must have been ten of them, all full of morbid fascination to see this thirty-five-year-old with stage IV cancer. I felt like a prize exhibit.

I think they were more than a little surprised by my upbeat attitude. Perhaps they thought I hadn't quite grasped the gravity of the situation. Well, I was still alive, wasn't I? I hadn't bled to death during the night. That was a good start.

They looked carefully at the X-ray and decided the major blood vessels were a sufficient distance from the tumour for them not to pose an immediate threat to my life. So, I could go home provided I came back later that day for more tests. Hooray! I wasted no time checking myself out of the Hammer House of Horror. I phoned Andrew who immediately drove over to collect me.

The relief of being back home was overwhelming. After cuddling my two gorgeous cats I allowed myself to cry for the first time. Big sobs came from deep down as I buried my head in Andrew's arms. But as I cried, I knew I had to get to work. I didn't have time to feel sorry for myself. I needed to be in control. I too wanted to know what the statistics said. Andrew told me not to look but I needed to know. What I saw shook me to the core.

Everything the doctors did to me from this moment on could affect my chances of survival, and too many mistakes had been made already. This time I was going to play a big part in my treatment choices, whether the doctors liked it or not!

I had been too traumatised and depressed by my diagnosis the first time around to be able to do anything other than agree to suggestions and meekly and submissively take the first path offered. I had been too passive and too desperate to get rid of the cancer.

This time it was going to be different. It was my body they were treating. I was going to run the show and the doctors were going to play important parts but not the lead role. That part was mine, thank you.

Many doctors are a little affronted by a patient armed with a long list of questions, particularly about alternative treatments. And if you dare mention diet then expect a quick and scornful dismissal (don't even think about bringing up the subject of nutritional ketosis – it sounds too similar to ketoacidosis – your doctor will immediately tell you to avoid it!). Oncologists are, for the most part, in a league of their own, certain that they know what's best for you with a 'My Way or the Highway' approach. Despite this mostly dogmatic attitude, instilled by years of training, I knew there were some super ones who were prepared to listen to the patient and respect their wishes.

Good oncologists even acknowledge that patients can be their greatest teachers. But I have come across too many who are arrogant, who seem to enjoy belittling those in their care. This does nothing for the confidence of the ordinary patient, who is made to feel ignorant and stupid in the presence of their superior medical knowledge. All it does is feed the oncologist's ego.

Attitudes are slowly changing, but even today I know a doctor whose coffee mug reads, 'You are confusing your quick google research with my six-year medical degree', which he'll leave strategically on his desk before meeting the incurable hypochondriac. Social media and the Internet have meant many patients now become experts in their own disease.

There is no doubt that there are doctors who are highly skilled and knowledgeable, who understand their patients' diseases. They appreciate the ways in which drugs can interact with each other, and they are aware of the course of the cancer, the statistics and the conventional options. They are there to help guide you through the medical minefield with its confusing terminology and hidden pitfalls. I have great respect for their knowledge. Despite this, it seemed to me that my oncologist was missing the bigger picture.

I was going to have to become my own expert. I would need to learn all the medical terms if I was to understand the research, be treated as an equal, and have the doctors listen to me, rather than treat me as a patient with a lump that had to be shrunk. And I would have to learn fast. Time, the doctors reminded me, was not my friend. But I already had a great deal of medical knowledge – that was a bonus. And I had already learned much about cancer from researching for my mother. Terms such as 'angiogenesis' and 'apoptosis' were already familiar.

I was never going to turn my back on conventional treatment completely, but there had to be other options to the surgery and chemotherapy. It seemed medical progress had made little headway for decades. To survive, I needed to take the treatment further than anyone had done before, to add things to my treatment not only to address the genetic mutations but the metabolic problems that went with it, an area that seemed to be ignored by the mainstream, despite Otto Warburg's research dating back to the 1920's.

To beat it, I had to know my enemy. I had to discover its every little nuance, exploit its weak points, its Achilles' heels, and hit them all together. I would tackle it from every angle I could, whether with conventional drugs, supplements or alternative therapies. There had to be more to it than just surgery and chemo.

As a physiotherapist, I had been trained in science and evidence-based medicine. I knew that elsewhere, combinations of drugs were being tested, such as for HIV infections. Several different drugs with different actions were being used together, a combination sometimes called a drug cocktail. Cancer was a complexity of abnormal pathways and cell signalling, so where were the combinations to match it? They didn't exist.

When I spoke to my sister the following night, she tried to keep upbeat despite being clearly upset. 'Oh no. You have another spot of bother,' she said, using Mum's phrase for her cancer. A spot of bother. Was she being dismissive? No, she was trying to minimise the emotional impact. 'Yes, let's just think of it like that, an irritating little problem, a disobedient child that needs a time out. Not some invincible foe.'

I started to formulate my plan. I drew out a map of how I was going to attack it. In the centre, I made a little jagged circle, the 'Spot of Bother', and then drew arrows hitting it from every direction. From the North whizzed the surgery arrow. From the South, chemo attacked. But those two arrows were not enough. I knew it had also to be hit by arrows from the East, West, and everywhere in between. I even visualised it in 3D.

One thing I knew for sure was that my diet would need even more drastic changes. Cancer wanted glucose. Lots of it. If I could reduce this, at the very least it would weaken its defences. Surely this made logical sense? I ignored the medics telling me that diet would make no difference. How could it not?

During the first three days after I'd started coughing up blood, I had been given CT scans and ultrasounds and was prodded and poked by various staff of the hospital. By the Wednesday of that week I had been 'staged'. The search for other tumours was over. To my immense relief, there were none, but I was still diagnosed with stage IV. The realisation that I had only one 'spot of bother' made the diagnosis that bit easier to accept. I had been convinced that if the cancer had been lurking inside me all this time, it must have spread elsewhere.

Had I been lucky or had my change in diet since my mother died already helped slow it down? The disease at this stage was normally rampant and aggressive. I knew that whatever I'd been doing must have had an effect. This was strangely reassuring amidst all the gloom. I was certain my low sugar intake and the supplements I'd taken must be helping. Diet makes no difference? Rubbish. I'd already proved to myself that it did.

The oncologist also wanted to take a biopsy from my tumour. No way was I going to let them do that! What the hell for? Just to prove it was a tumour? That was investigation for the sake of it. It was highly unlikely to be anything else and it wouldn't make the slightest bit of difference to my medical plan. They were still going to remove it surgically.

As far as I was concerned, they could wait and perform the histology after it was cut out properly. I did not want to risk breaking the capsule surrounding the cancer, thus increasing the likelihood of it spreading elsewhere. Surely this was common sense? To my mind, biopsies were a sure-fire way to mess with the body's attempt to contain damage.

Tumours have a kind of fibrous capsule. A tumour the size of a tip of a pencil can contain billions of cancer cells and surgeons do their utmost not to spill those when operating, especially during lung surgery. I was aware by now that post-surgical metastatic spread was a widespread phenomenon, something surgeons never mention to the patient, or even seem to acknowledge. I didn't want any more tumour cells whizzing around my body looking for another cosy place to live.

This difference of opinion led to a heated 'discussion' with the doctor for a good thirty minutes. I told him in no uncertain terms that they'd leave it alone. In the end we reached a compromise. I allowed him to take nearby sputum sample by bronchoscopy but told him that on absolutely no account was he to break into the tumour. He got the message. I was starting to feel as if I might have some control, that perhaps I would be allowed a voice in this medical merry-go-round, but my goodness it was not going to be easy.

I was not seeing eye-to-eye with the oncologist I had been allocated at the Hammersmith Hospital. I can't even remember his name, as he lasted only two visits. He had been brusque, dismissive and scornful of my point of view. Stuck in his rigid, blinkered approach, he wasn't able to answer many of my questions and seemed resentful that I was asking them at all. It wasn't long before he got the flick off my team.

I wanted to find the professor who had treated me first time round. She had moved out of London to Guildford, an hour away, but I knew she would be worth the trip. I would rather make the longer journey for someone who knew me and was more likely to tolerate my difficult and awkward behaviour. She listened and she respected me. I needed a collaborator, not a dictator.

It had been a revelation that between the primary and secondary diagnosis, on any of my routine six-monthly visits over the past five years, a simple blood test could have been taken to detect changes. I felt despair that the system had failed me on so many levels. Now the test came back showing high levels of the squamous cell carcinoma antigen – around 190. A normal reading was under 150. The higher the number the more active it was. So a reading of 190, while bad, was not terrible. I felt sure my diet and healthier lifestyle was keeping the reading lower than it could have been. Perhaps it really was starving the cancer of what it needed to grow.

I contacted the Chelsea and Westminster Hospital and got hold of the X-ray they'd taken of my lungs. When I showed it to my oncologist, she could clearly see the tumour. I felt I could not let this go without comment, so I wrote to the hospital manager. Surprisingly, I received a contrite letter of apology, but at least they had admitted guilt.

Getting hold of the X-ray was not to say, 'I told you so', although the temptation was huge. I wanted to show the medics just how much bigger it had grown over time. Sure enough, there was a tumour in the same place, a little smaller, but there. Once I knew where it was, it was easy to spot. It should have been obvious to any decent radiologist. And it had not grown rapidly since the last X-ray, not at the rate I feared, which also meant I was doing something right.

Given that I had lived with it for several months, I was not in an enormous panic. Perhaps I could control my tumour with an even more radical diet and supplements. I took big positives out of this. I decided I was not going to be rushed into any treatment or surgery. I needed to do further research and take my time before I let the medical profession loose on my body again. I made the decision to wait a few weeks before I had surgery, to take stock and prepare myself for the battle ahead.

My other siblings were understandably shocked when we broke the bad news. I have two younger brothers as well as an older sister. Going through Mum's illness had brought us all quite close together. My new diagnosis coming so soon after we buried our mother was a blow to them all. Would they have to suffer that anguish and heartbreak once again?

Although we were united in the fight against cancer, having doctors in my family made my route to health more complicated because we held different views. They had been sceptical about what I'd suggested to Mum, so I decided I wouldn't discuss my 'complementary' plans with them, in case they put me off or influenced me in some way. I wanted to be entirely responsible for my decisions if I decided to take a different path. I was open and receptive to their ideas and suggestions, but I would try to steer my own course. They decided wisely to let me do my own thing without offering any judgement.

Suzie, I later learned, had quietly informed the family that she thought I was unlikely to survive a year. I am so glad I didn't know this. Being told would have been worse. Fortunately, no-one ever said it outright to me, even though I'd read as much online. Twelve weeks had been the average. Predictions like that can become self-fulfilling, particularly from someone in the medical profession. That damn white coat is just too powerful.

I have often wondered whether patients should be told by medics how long on average a person with their stage and level of disease has to live. On the one hand, it is deeply depressing. Also, every patient is different. Many go into a protective cocoon from which they never emerge. On the other hand, it's important to know just how deep in the quagmire you're standing, so you can take the appropriate level of action.

Armed with some knowledge already, I was tough enough to know my statistics. No-one would fight this as hard as I would. I was going to defy that death sentence. I could see that as cancer progressed it became harder and harder to treat, becoming more and more resistant to conventional therapies. By stage IV, the oncology profession regards the disease as unstoppable. Oncologists remain convinced that the fight is futile, that treatments will ultimately fail, that we're merely 'delaying the inevitable'.

I needed to try something drastic. Throwing a bucket of water onto a raging fire is not enough to put it out. It was an urgent situation that required an immediate response. Stage IV in most cases means you have a year or less to live, if you stick to orthodox definitions. Stage III means you generally have at least a year to live, with the possibility of overcoming the cancer completely – if you're lucky. The bigger the cancer is, the more aggressive it is and the further it has spread means the response must be proportionally greater. And, I surmised, that meant that cancer needed to be attacked from more angles. Was this not common sense? I could not understand why oncologists persisted in their mono-therapeutic approach, attacking merely the genetic angle and not the metabolic.

It was clear that I had lots of work to do. Monotherapy meant treating every single cancer patient like a guinea pig in one great big experiment. We all buy into trials because we're sold the belief that it's 'for the greater good'. But a disease as complex as this demands an equally complex solution: combinations of metabolic **and** genetic approaches. The metabolic approach was not even acknowledged, it was as if it had no importance at all. And what of patient choice? A stage IV patient is defined as 'terminal' or in the 'final stage'. Were we not allowed any say in our treatment decisions? In the manner of our deaths? Were we just pawns in a system that serves the pharmaceutical industry?

I was not going to let fear guide my decisions.

Chapter Five:

A Cancer Sherlock Holmes

And so began my quest for answers.

I didn't limit my search to alternative treatments, as many patients do. I couldn't turn my back on conventional treatment altogether. In fact, many useful areas of conventional oncology seemed to be completely ignored. I became a 'PubMed' explorer, scouring endless published medical articles. A cancer 'Sherlock Holmes', piecing together clues and trying to make sense of the confusing and complex picture.

Research had focused primarily on the activity of genes in cancer. But what about the rest of the tumour, like the growth factors it used to fuel itself? These growth factors, like IGF-1 and Vascular Endothelial Growth Factor (VEGF), were clearly linked to inflammation and metabolic changes which sugar, meat and dairy intake would only make worse. It seemed to me that oncology researchers' focus on genetic changes blinded them to the overall picture and led them to ignore the general health of their patients. Cancer was a systemic disease; markers were detectable in the blood, so it affected the whole body. It was not just a 'lump' to be excised.

Patients often talked of being 'healthy' before getting cancer, but this was almost never true when you dug a little deeper. There were always prior infections or gut issues or both. In the medical literature, I came across references to cyclo-oxygenase or COX inhibitors being useful for cancer.

I had no idea what the heck these were when I first started looking, but I sure as hell would made it my business to find out.

COX (cyclo-oxygenase) was an enzyme linked to inflammation. COX seemed to be involved in the process of helping to stimulate new blood vessel growth around the cancer, stimulating Vascular Endothelial Growth Factor (VEGF). These new blood vessels brought nutrients to the cancer to allow it to keep increasing in size, to fuel its growing biomass. With my troublesome and often swollen knee, I wondered if I had low-grade inflammation throughout my body. Perhaps that's why it was so slow to get better. I had little doubt I had an inflammatory component to my disease and my gut instinct told me I needed to damp this down.

I wasn't sure if a simple anti-inflammatory would stop this enzyme. Indeed, aspirin was a COX 2 inhibitor and a Vascular Endothelial Growth Factor inhibitor. It seemed like a good idea to me – all I had to do was walk to the pharmacy and get it over the counter. I couldn't understand why it wasn't mentioned or implemented already by my doctors.

'How much does my tumour express COX 2?' I asked my thoracic surgeon who was soon to operate on my lung.

'My goodness,' he said in a somewhat condescending tone, 'you **have** been doing your homework.'

'Yes, I have. I want to know if you think I could take it,' I said, slightly affronted by the implication that it was beyond mere laypeople (he'd forgotten I was a physiotherapist) to investigate these things, let alone attempt to understand them, and then muster the sheer audacity to use their special secret language.

'There's not enough evidence to suggest it's useful,' he said.

'Surely surgery causes inflammation? Wouldn't an anti-inflammatory before and after surgery be useful in that case?' I pressed on, not in the slightest bit fazed by his dismissiveness. I had read that tumour markers invariably shot up after surgery. Was this rise caused by inflammation? Or spillage of cancer cells into the blood? Or a dampening of the immune system? Or quite possibly all of these?

'Well, I would be very worried about stomach bleeds,' he added. 'I don't advise it. It's up to you if you want to take that risk, but if you do take it, I don't want you taking it too close to your surgery as it makes you bleed more.'

Fair enough. I wondered if another non-steroidal anti-inflammatory like ibuprofen might be better in the run up to the surgery as it wasn't a blood thinner like aspirin. He thought this would also be risky. It seemed illogical. Or was he really saying that anything I tried would be futile anyway?

I wondered what the real risk of taking aspirin was. Other non-steroidal anti-inflammatories carried a higher risk of stomach ulcers. As far as I was aware, aspirin seemed to be liberally prescribed for stroke and heart attack prevention. If it was good enough for them, it was good enough for me. I resolved to look up the stats when I got home.

I made the decision to take aspirin at a low dose despite his negativity, but his words wormed their way into my psyche in a way that would prove catastrophic years later. Indeed, if only I had known the risk with aspirin was a mere 2% which, compared to my **100%** risk of dying otherwise, would have made it an easy decision. Any improvement in my survival odds was surely a risk worth taking! Besides, keeping the cancer cells circulating would be better than letting them stick to my blood vessel walls and set up camp somewhere new.

I continued to probe.

'Okay... this surgery. I know that right now it's only one tumour, but I'm really worried it might come back sometime in the future and I might have more tumours next time. Have you operated on more than one tumour before?'

'Oh yes. Many,' he said with a reassuring smile.

'How many have you taken out at one time?' I had a macabre curiosity.

'Oh... about twenty!' He said this with obvious pride. Crikey. Twenty! Was there any lung tissue left after that? I wanted to know just how skilful he was.

'Did the patient survive?' I immediately regretted asking this question. I knew the answer before he shook his head.

Again, the reality of my situation hit me like a train. I was going to die.

If I was going to die, I might as well enjoy myself feeling well while I could. Coughing up blood was a constant source of alarm, but otherwise I really didn't feel ill as such. Tired, but not ill. I knew it was the upcoming barbaric treatments that would mess me up and make me feel terrible, not the tumour itself.

I continued my questioning, putting on my brave I-can-defeat-this face, trying not to stammer with fear or look shaken by this revelation.

'Andrew and I have just married. Would it be okay if I delayed the operation for a few weeks while we have a honeymoon?'

'I'm sure that'd be a good idea. Go ahead and I'll book you in for the end of September.'

Wow. Five weeks away. An age, particularly when I only had a mean survival of twelve weeks. Either he didn't give me much hope and thus wanted to grant me one last holiday, or perhaps he genuinely felt I could afford some time to relax. I decided, probably incorrectly, it was the latter. My brain refused to accept he thought my chances were zero. It was all too depressing. In any case, I felt it was important to prepare for the onslaught of surgery. Five weeks would be time well spent. I was definitely in no rush.

As I left the hospital, I'd already decided the conservative approach was not for me. He hadn't given me a straight yes or no about the aspirin and, like all risk-averse doctors, had erred on the cautious side, but sod it. I had stage IV 'terminal' cancer. My developing theory was that anything that might weaken the tumour had to be a good thing.

Attack from every angle. That was my mantra. This was war. No question I was going to take aspirin! The doctors found it easy enough to recommend high dose chemotherapy. Why was it so hard to recommend humble aspirin if my gut was okay? Was he just blindly accepting what he assumed was my predetermined fate, that any intervention, no matter how small, was ultimately a waste of time? Perhaps he worried about the heavy hand of the General Medical Council coming down on him because of the lack of a randomised clinical trial? The gold standard which ensures no doctor steps out of line. God forbid doctors should try anything innovative like low dose aspirin to help a dying patient!

It was true that we'd just got married. Four days after discovering the tumour in my lung, I had realised there was no point waiting until my hair grew back to hold our wedding. I had no idea how I might respond to chemo, if indeed I decided to have it. Also, if I was brutally honest with myself, I didn't know how much time I had left on the planet. I had to be realistic as well as positive. Despite my best efforts, I might not be around in six months. My feeling was we may as well go ahead and tie the ol' knot.

Having confirmed that Andrew did still want to marry me despite this new diagnosis, I followed up with 'how about this Saturday?' I wanted to be married but I didn't want the distraction of planning it. My dreams of a fairy-tale wedding were already shattered and I kind of needed it out of the way. I had a bigger task ahead that demanded my full attention.

I was delighted to hear Andrew respond, 'Great idea! Let's do it!' So I took it upon myself to organise the event last-minute, having only just finished cancelling the arrangements back in Guernsey. I think Andrew was mightily relieved, to be honest. He hates big parties (I love them) and was not relishing the idea of a huge event dominated by my massive family. A quick registry office affair was much more up his street, even though it wasn't mine.

'I'll book it then,' I said, glad to have something positive to do in the midst of so much depressing news.

I phoned the Chelsea Registry Office, but because it was such a popular venue, and this was August, it was completely booked up. The Fulham Registry Office was also fully booked that weekend. But after I put the phone down, I ran over there in person and had a little chat with the registrar face-to-face. After I callously played the 'terminally ill card', he slotted me in between two other brides who can't have been too chuffed about the wedding assembly line they found themselves on that day.

Andrew's only two tasks in the whole event were to (1) turn up and (2) bring a ring. The second half of this extensive list he somehow managed to completely forget.

'You do have the ring, don't you?' I asked on the morning, innocently assuming he'd gone shopping as we discussed the day before while I was having the bronchoscopy. The look on his face was akin to realising a tarantula was running up his leg and if he moved the wrong way, he might be dead.

'Um… ah… oh.'

Without another word, he turned on his heels and dashed out the door. He told me later he frightened the life out of the cleaner in the jeweller's (who had yet to open) by bashing on the door so loudly while she was hoovering, she thought it was an attempted robbery. Fortunately, he had my engagement ring for size, so, quick as a flash, the jeweller sorted it out. Andrew came back looking very sheepish, but I was not cross. We laughed! He was understandably a little distracted by recent events.

Our wedding day was beautiful. The sun shone, we drank champagne in the garden and were joined by twenty-three of our close family and friends, some of whom had flown over from Guernsey. We had cocktails outside in our garden, a case of pink champagne arrived, courtesy of my fabulous aunt Jane in Guernsey, then we all walked over the common to the Registry Office.

After the ceremony, we headed off to lunch in a French restaurant in Pimlico. There were tears of joy, problems forgotten, more drinking (at least by everyone but me) and much merriment.

This photo was taken that day in 1999. I have the lung tumour, but I really don't think I look unhealthy. I certainly didn't feel it. I bought the dress hurriedly on the Thursday afternoon (my real wedding dress was only half made) and the flowers were chosen the evening before. It's amazing how much you can arrange in a couple of days. All this less than a week after my diagnosis of terminal cancer.

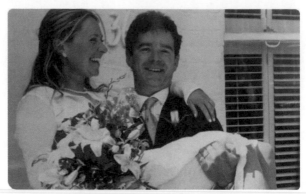

Married!

Do I look weak and defeated? No. In that picture is a strong determined Jane. (And a particularly strong new husband).

The evening finally ended in a fabulous art deco suite in Claridge's, bigger than most London flats. This had been a complete surprise, arranged by our lovely friends – we thought we were going back home. I felt happy and blessed to have such support and love. What followed was quite some party. We had to nudge people out of the door at 2am.

I woke up the following morning a married woman. It felt good.

But with the wedding over, it was back to the serious business of research. As every cancer patient soon realises in this situation, it is an exponential curve of discovery. I was convinced the clues to survival were out there if only I could find them. I could not believe that after all these years of medical and scientific advance, there weren't drugs or treatments that could destroy my cancer.

It was 1999. We flew people to the moon, landed rovers on Mars, connected the world via the Internet, built the International Space Station, and we had the spectre of genetically modified food. How and why did we not have a cure for cancer?

Chapter Six:

No Stone Unturned

'Good God!' Andrew cried in horror as he picked up a receipt from the Health Food shop. I'd left it casually – carelessly – on the kitchen surface. 'I knew you'd be a high maintenance wife,' he added with a grin.

"I know. Sorry,' I said sheepishly as he looked through the bill.

'Well, as long as you really need them all and you're not just creating expensive toilet trips,' he said, watching me expertly swallow five supplements at a time.

He was right, of course. How could I be sure they'd do anything? It was impossible to know if they contained mostly filler or if they really had the correct amount of active ingredient it displayed on the label. How much lead, cadmium, arsenic and other nasties did they contain? It was so hard to tell. I bought quality brands I felt we could afford and kept my fingers crossed. Even if I only absorbed a little, it might be enough to tip my body back into health and make the difference between death and survival.

Every time I read about some exciting new supplement to target cancer, it went into my cocktail, another addition to my Spot of Bother Chart. What I had failed to learn at this point was that there's a clear distinction between supplements that **prevent** cancer and supplements that **treat** it. There is a tipping point in cancer development, where some antioxidants useful for prevention (vitamin E in tocopherol form and N-Acetyl

Cysteine aka NAC, a precursor of glutathione, a master antioxidant) then switch allegiance and support the enemy, helping to promote and fuel its resistance to apoptosis (death), effectively making it immortal. I was to learn this later. In these early days, I simply took the lot.

Over the next few months, between hospital visits, my head was stuck into every reference book I could find, discovering, learning, trying to decipher fact from fiction. Hearsay and anecdotes were not enough to convince me to try something. I drove my oncologist and integrative doctors mad with questions, almost to the point of mental combustion. I rifled through endless scientific papers. There had to be real hard scientific evidence. Although there was often no real 'science' behind the stories, anecdotes of survival against the odds were also a kind of therapy for me. I bought as many of these as I could, looking for any kind of recurring pattern that linked them. I was desperate to find clues that it was even possible.

Every unusual disappearance of the disease was described as a 'spontaneous remission' by the medics, a deprecating term when you realised the herculean effort involved to achieve it. Each appeared to be linked with a radical change in diet. Cutting out sugar was a common theme. While these worked for some cancer patients, few anti-cancer diets I investigated seemed to go far enough in lowering glucose. The term *ketogenic diet*, a more extreme low glycaemic diet, had not even been coined in those days. Bizarrely, some diets still included honey and pizza, bread and other starchy foods, foods I would class as high glycaemic, as they released a lot of glucose. As a result, they still raised insulin levels. Surely these would be disastrous for cancer patients.

This was the diet espoused by Professor Jane Plant in her bestselling book, *Your Life in Their Hands*. Her focus had been on lowering IGF-1 by cutting down on meat and dairy. Professor Plant's diet suggested a swap from sugar to honey, which seemed illogical to me. How would that starve the cancer of glucose? Sugar is sugar in all its guises, honey included.

My Spot of Bother Chart thus far only had treatments I'd heard about while researching for my mother. It was 1999 and information was still hard to come by. Now Facebook is awash with 'cures' and Functional Medicine doctors ready to share the latest trend. In fact, it has now become too confusing to track.

Back then, with a bit of digging online I found the Gerson diet, macrobiotics, proteolytic enzymes, bitter almonds, and intravenous vitamin C. I hadn't been radical enough with my diet, but I was not convinced that Gerson took the whole low sugar approach far enough either. Potatoes were allowed for a start – they were definitely on my banned list! Not only would they potentially elevate insulin and glucose levels, but they were also part of the nightshade family of plants and could cause gut reactions. While potatoes are alkaline foods and neutralise acidic foods, they can also cause inflammation, something I knew to be a major factor in my cancer. Today, you can buy kits to test yourself for inflammatory reactions to food with just a few drops of blood. Interestingly the Gerson approach seemed to work best for melanoma patients. What was so different about this cancer? Was it metabolically different to other cancers, less driven by glucose? It turns out that most, but not all, are more driven by fat and Oxphos, less glycolysis (why they respond better to immunotherapy) – so a traditional ketogenic diet may be a potential disaster for melanoma patients – unless combined with inhibitors of other pathways too.[4]

4   Aloia A, Müllhaupt D, Chabbert CD, Eberhart T, Flückiger-Mangual S, Vukolic A, Eichhoff O, Irmisch A, Alexander LT, Scibona E, Frederick DT, Miao B, Tian T, Cheng C, Kwong LN, Wei Z, Sullivan RJ, Boland GM, Herlyn M, Flaherty KT, Zamboni N, Dummer R, Zhang G, Levesque MP, Krek W, Kovacs WJ. A Fatty Acid Oxidation-dependent Metabolic Shift Regulates the Adaptation of BRAF-mutated Melanoma to MAPK Inhibitors. Clin Cancer Res. 2019 Nov 15;25(22):6852-6867. doi: 10.1158/1078-0432.CCR-19-0253. Epub 2019 Aug 2. PMID: 31375515; PMCID: PMC6906212.

Cancer diet books in 1999 focused mainly on either macrobiotics or Gerson. I thought both had their merits and pitfalls, but the low-glycaemic approach of macrobiotics with its emphasis on whole high fibre complex carbohydrates seemed to make more sense to me. The seaweed element, disgusting as it sounded, was probably useful; I'd wondered if I might have an underactive thyroid and I wanted to boost my iodine levels naturally. Seaweed was said to do just that.

I instinctively felt my focus should be on starving the cancer, but there was very little information about keeping blood glucose low. I could find no information on this specific to cancer.

A diabetic friend of mine had discussed low-glycaemic diets with me when I treated him with physiotherapy. I had saved him from major back surgery. At the time I had been researching for my mum and as a thank you, he gave me a book by a Frenchman called Michel Montignac. Michel Montignac was the first to actively promote a low-glycaemic diet to the public years. It was called *Eat Yourself Slim*. Perhaps my friend was really just telling me I was a fatty!

Montignac's diet method became immensely popular in Europe in the 1990s. It was designed for weight loss, to avoid cardiovascular disease and diabetes, but not for cancer. He had been a seriously chubby young man and had ended up working for the pharmaceutical industry. He realised that it was the high glycaemic foods that caused weight gain and health problems. He was the first to expose the hoax of calorie counting. The quality and choice of what you ate was far more important than counting the energy input versus the energy output. Je Mange donc Je Maigris (I eat but lose weight) was his most popular book. It certainly seemed like a good idea to adopt the low glycaemic principles.

I discovered that eating fat on its own was apparently not a problem for insulin and glucose levels.[5] It wasn't the demon it was made out to be for cardiovascular health. I memorised the glycaemic value of different foods, the amount of insulin released by the pancreas to deal with the sudden spike of glucose released after a meal. And I learned about how food preparation and the method of cooking could make big differences to the glycaemic index.

Reducing blood sugar was my primary focus but I worried about the type of fat I ate. High-fat diets had been linked to cancer too. As if to prove the point, I discovered Michel Montignac had died at the young age of 63 of prostate cancer. His heart and insulin levels had been perfect. I was to learn that prostate cancer is driven by fat and branched chain amino acids (such as leucine found in meat and dairy) until it becomes hormone resistant when it then becomes more glucose driven (unless driven by a PIK3CA mutation and PTEN loss, mutations that make it more glycolytic).

Low-glycaemic diets made perfect sense to reduce blood glucose. I still lacked any further specific information on how precisely to starve my cancer of the nutrients it craved. But lowering glucose and saturated fat seemed to be critical. I was concerned that high fat diets might be too taxing on my liver and gallbladder.

Je Mange donc Je Maigris was a forerunner to the more famous Atkins diet and the recent *Eat Fat Get Thin* by Dr Mark Hyman, who has gone further into healthier fats – from eggs, nuts, and avocados to olive oil and coconut oil. Both books are focused on losing weight; they weren't written for cancer. Beware the saturated fat content of eggs and coconut oil. Eggs are linked to colon, ovarian and prostate cancer because of the

---

5   I now know that is not entirely true. The influence of ceramides, waxy substances, can strongly affect insulin resistance. Sokolowska E, Blachnio-Zabielska A. The Role of Ceramides in Insulin Resistance. *Front Endocrinol (Lausanne)*. 2019;10:577. Published 2019 Aug 21. doi:10.3389/fendo.2019.00577

high cholesterol levels and many recommend no more than two a week if you have any type of cancer. Cancer nutrition needs specialist attention beyond weight loss and heart disease. The principles of the low GI diet, though, were the real message. The book taught me which foods raised glucose and insulin (high-glycaemic foods); how to best combine foods; how to best prepare foods; and that slow cooking was preferable to both speedy cooking and overcooking.

Simple carbohydrates – refined grains, sugars, some fruits – trigger spikes in glucose and insulin levels. The liver then converts excess carbs and fat to more fat. This was my problem. Slower-release carbohydrates, in contrast, do not lead to an insulin or glucose spike. Fat without sugar just gets shuttled out of the body (through the reverse cholesterol transport system, I would later learn).

But I still wasn't sure about fat. Too many of the omega-6 oils (sunflower, canola) routinely used for cooking encourage angiogenesis – the growth of new blood vessels around a tumour to provide it with nutrients. These went on my banned list.

Perhaps the rising levels of cancer incidence in our society comes down to a lack of sufficient omega-3 fats in our diets to balance the dominance of omega 6. Found in fish, these damp down inflammation and help put the brakes on cancer. Did some saturated fats help drive cancer, then? Coconut oil was saturated. Could it be trusted? It became the 'oil du jour' in those days, and an integral part of a ketogenic diet. Coconut oil may in part be good – the Medium Chain Triglycerides (MCT) part – which makes up 13-15% of coconut oil, but the rest might be less beneficial. I decided to stick to quality extra virgin olive oil (EVOO) and small amounts of butter to cook with. Grass fed butter contains an important ingredient called CLA (conjugated linoleic acid) which has been linked to lower rates of cancer. I also took CLA as a supplement (sea buckthorn oil may be a better choice).

Researching cancer treatments was as clear as mud, particularly if there were no proper trials conducted or if the data had been manipulated.[6] I was learning that gut health was crucially important for the immune system, but I was more than dubious of those coffee enemas encouraged by the Gerson Protocol. I worried that while they allegedly 'cleansed' the colon, which was probably a good thing, that if the enemas were done to excess (and the Gerson diet seemed to suggest conducting them three times a day!) then you might also be losing valuable nutrients or electrolytes, like magnesium as a result.

According to the Gerson diet, the enemas could encourage more glutathione to be released by the liver, which I soon learned might actually help cancer progress. This may be a problem if you have liver metastases whereas they may keep the liver functioning well if you don't. This is mere speculation and there is no research. Like most patients I've met, I made the common mistake of thinking that glutathione would be beneficial for cancer. I tried coffee enemas but switched to straightforward colonics after my chemotherapy, using boiled and cooled water only.

Proteolytic enzymes are a large part of Gerson therapy and would do me no harm, as far as I could tell. They would at least help me to absorb food better. The suggestion was to take these between meals, as this supposedly dissolved the outer fibrin shield of tumour-associated macrophages that protected the cancer from destruction. I was not sure if this was the reason they worked. Cancer had been often linked to parasites. Perhaps they helped get rid of parasites in the gut by dissolving their protein membranes. Not that I knew I had any at this stage. Bitter almonds or laetrile seemed interesting as they might reduce something called catalase that is part of the defence system of cancer. Could they help to selectively kill my cancer?[7] Every time I found something that looked useful there was something conflicting in another book or website.

---

6   See **Doctored Results** by Ralph Moss.

7   I later discovered that I had **Blastocystis hominis**, a common gut parasite

I bought many books, subscribed to integrative cancer and health journals, and spent weeks in the library, sipping green tea, popping my ever-expanding quantities of supplements and knocking back (as quickly as possible) my revolting 'primordial soup'. I scoured medical journals, PubMed, and Medline. I read many self-help books and huge tomes on alternative cancer therapies, desperately looking for clues. Dr Ralph Moss and Burton Goldberg were fascinating and informative on complementary treatments. How many of these might help me? Iscador, a mistletoe treatment, seemed interesting for boosting the immune system, a therapy regularly used in Germany. Coleys toxins? Essiac tea? I left no stone unturned. But what had the best evidence? Intravenous vitamin C at high doses seemed to have good evidence for increasing oxygen (hydrogen peroxide) around a tumour in contrast to its better-known antioxidant effects. That would help kill it.

I wondered what might happen if I combined chemotherapy with intravenous vitamin C. Would it boost its effects and help maintain my immune system? I was tempted to have a go at alternating the two, but in the end fear of the unknown got the better of me. I decided to leave the IV vitamin C until I had finished chemo and perhaps the supplements would be enough to maintain my immune system.

After visiting Dr Etienne Callebout, a very knowledgeable integrative doctor, my Spot of Bother Chart was filling up nicely. I collated all the information and went with my gut, as well as with my research, on what I felt would work best for me.

Dr Callebout wanted to do a full examination, send off a stool sample for a thorough analysis of my gut bacteria and take a blood specimen to evaluate my vitamin, amino acid and fatty acid status. But as soon as he learnt I was to have chemotherapy he decided there was little point until I'd finished. These blood and stool tests went on my 'to do' list. I would wait for a month post-chemo to allow my poor body to settle.

Dr Callebout also guessed I was low on folate, as I had been given methotrexate chemotherapy when I was first diagnosed. Folate is necessary for the de novo ('from new') formation of a nucleoside, a building block of DNA, specifically thymine. Methotrexate in effect 'starved' the cancer of this vital B vitamin needed to create a new daughter cell DNA.

Interesting. Was it safe to add folate into my regime again? Dr Callebout said if I was not taking methotrexate or 5FU then I should supplement with B vitamins – these were essential for detoxifying my body of excess 'bad' oestrogen (oestradiol), which I knew to stimulate cancer growth. He also recommended I take the B vitamin niacin, even though it gave me an odd flush for a few minutes. This happens to most people who take it. It is totally normal and does not suggest toxicity.[8] I now believe niacin should be part of most cancer protocols – it helps starve cancer by reducing fat. Niacin can increase HLD while lowering cholesterol LDL and triglycerides.

I was now taking many supplements I hoped would target and block different cancer pathways and growth factors, angles ignored by conventional medicine. I was soon on a first-name basis with the owners of my local health food store – I'm quite sure I single-handedly kept them in business. All further receipts went promptly into the bin, out of Andrew's sight.

At first, I found it hard to believe that potentially useful treatments were forced into obscurity. Yet the more I researched, the clearer it became that many studies were biased, that data was often hidden, and that methodology was frequently twisted to confuse the results. As my knowledge grew, so did my realisation that cancer was first and foremost a business. Anything that didn't have a patent was belittled by the industry, particularly by some of the big cancer charities.

---

8   No-Flush Niacin brands are now available.

Survival with alternative approaches seemed to be littered with failures, but then so were conventional ones. I guessed this may have been partly because patients often started to look for complementary therapies too late. Generally, the longer cancer is present, the harder it becomes to treat. So I kept an open mind.

I noted that people tended to throw their faith behind just one modality. Nowadays people are not only terrified by chemotherapy, with more patients refusing it than ever before, but there seems to be an obsession with cannabis oil, regardless of the strength of the THC or CBD content. I see many patients using cannabis, DCA, or the ketogenic diet to the exclusion of anything else. It seemed obvious to me that combining approaches was far more effective.

But combining treatments requires a huge dollop of courage. What will the interaction be? Is it safe? Targeting different cancer pathways at the same time were surely the way forward, but a patient needs the guidance of a qualified doctor experienced in nutritional and medical interventions. The growth in numbers of Functional Medicine Practitioners is a relief to all cancer patients. However, most people cannot afford this kind of help, and with a shortage of integrative oncologists, many go it alone on a wish and a prayer.

The first rule in war is to Know Thy Enemy. This rule underpinned everything I did. I had to put fear of the unknown aside. This was 'no time for feak and weebleness' as my sister used to say when I was feeling drained. She was right. A lot of it was in my head. Stay strong, stay positive, and never give up looking for answers. I was convinced they were out there, even if neither the conventional nor the complementary side had the complete answer. What else had I missed, that neither side were using?

A hallmark of cancer is that a patient's white blood cells fail to recognise their own cancer as the enemy. Cancer seems to switch them off. They needed to be woken up again. Might it be possible to reactivate the immune system in some way? If each treatment I discovered weakened and 'switched off' a different part of cancer's armour, adding them all together might eventually allow my immune system a chance to gain the upper hand. Could it then deliver the final punch?

Still unsure about chemotherapy, I came across a new option called insulin potentiated chemotherapy. The insulin made the cancer cells more permeable to chemo, so you didn't need as much. It was reportedly getting a lot of success. Still, I didn't like the thought of all that extra insulin. It might make the cell more permeable to glucose too. I decided to put it on the backburner if everything else failed.

Andrew and I sat down and had a chat about how we should handle the problem of having so many options and no clear roadmap.

'The only way is to approach it scientifically,' I said. 'We need to know how all these different options actually affect my cancer. I'm getting blood markers taken now. Maybe they'll show what's working and what isn't.'

Andrew set up an Excel spreadsheet and we began plotting my blood antigen marker levels on a chart. Although there was likely to be a bit of variation, I might be able to spot a trend when I began a new line of treatment. I wanted to approach it with my decisions based on evidence, not guesswork, even though I knew I could be making mistakes. I was aware it could all go horribly wrong and time could run out before I'd discovered anything.

Hunting for reliable advice on the Internet is as confusing as trying to sail in thick fog with no radar. And potentially as dangerous. I came up against conflicting and alarming advice, especially about the use of supplements, vitamins, and juicing. Trying to extrapolate the truth can be difficult.

For this reason, Dr Google can be your foe. Half an hour on Cancer Research UK (the aim of which is get more patients into trials – it's 'Big Pharma' thinly disguised as a search on Wikipedia will show you. Its founder, Jimmy Wales, has long been a staunch critic of alternative and complementary therapies) will have you running a mile from anything unconventional. Pharmaceutical companies do not want you to try anything other than their unholy trinity of chemotherapy, radiotherapy, and surgery or the latest targeted drugs and immunotherapies. I had to dig deeper. Much, much deeper.

Big Pharma would rather you didn't know about a natural substance until they've worked out a way of copying the beneficial effects with a lucrative patented drug. At the time of writing, if you look up 'disproven cancer treatments' on Wikipedia you can see two major cancer charities in action. Quick, before they change it! One of these charities has tried for years to patent a synthetic formulation of resveratrol while denying that this supplement is of any help despite easy-to-find research that proves just how useful it is.

The same is true with hydroxycitrate, a supplement that mimics fasting and improves the effectiveness of chemotherapy. The same charity is happy to tell you that a diet or short-term fasting is dangerous, despite burgeoning evidence to the contrary. What about stage IV terminal cancer? Isn't that more dangerous? The advice is not to try any diet or supplement until there's an effective, patented drug available.

Debate and contention were just as evident in 1999 as today. Back then, research did not fall into my lap at the touch of a button. There was no Facebook, no support groups, no Internet chat rooms, no list of resources from helpful charities like Yestolife.org.uk. All I had were journals, books, and medical sites like PubMed and Medline.

Only a couple of weeks after my diagnosis and intense research, I was brimming with new knowledge and ready to take a much-needed break. We flew off for a few days' belated honeymoon in Majorca, soaking up some essential vitamin D, taking the rest of my supplements with me in their ziplocked sachets. I was quite sure I was going to be stopped at security and forced to explain why I was carrying this suspicious looking stash.

Andrew had booked us into the honeymoon suite of a four-star hotel. Our room opened out onto a private pool. We were greeted by rose petals strewn over the bed in the shape of a heart. It was a relaxed, soothing atmosphere. The husband had done well! Tick.

It was just what I needed. For five days, I meditated and swam every day, went on long scenic walks and ate a healthy low carbohydrate Mediterranean diet doused with lots of extra virgin olive oil. It was heaven.

This was a pre-surgery strategy I can highly recommend to anyone who can afford it. Having surmised I was not about to drop dead from the tumour, that it wasn't pushing on vital arteries or any other life-threatening structures, I took my time to make sure I was in a fit state for the operation, mentally and physically. I knew what treatment traumas lay ahead.

Delaying my surgery was a decision I will never regret. The knee-jerk reaction of almost every cancer patient is to want to remove a tumour as soon as humanly possible. The thought that they're harbouring a parasitic alien creature in their bodies means they can't book themselves in for surgery fast enough. Panic influences far too many early decisions and patients often feel bullied into early operations. Having evaluated the dangers of my situation, I decided I needed time to allow the aspirin, my radical diet and the supplements to get to work. I was not going to be rushed.

Surgery replicates the inflammatory process of mass 'apoptosis' and subsequent fibrinogen (scar tissue) production and this suppresses important T cells and Natural Killer cells, exactly the ones your body needs to knock out the cancer. It triggers an inflammatory reaction in the body, one reason I felt non-steroidal anti-inflammatory drugs like aspirin were so important. Tackling the problem of post-surgical metastatic spread is an area still ignored by mainstream medics despite its huge potential for massive improvement in survival outcomes at little cost or toxicity.

Science has revealed that my decision to take aspirin perioperatively was correct. Anti-inflammatory drugs used for two or three weeks **before** surgery and then for up to a year after, have been shown to massively improve survival statistics. Around 90 per cent of cancers are not immediately deadly, but cause death by metastasising. Cancer patients regularly live with large tumours, so it was stopping further metastases that was important. Low dose aspirin (75mg) prevents metastasis by about 20 per cent[9], and greater gains can be made in some inflammatory cancers with short term stronger NSAIDs up to 70%. Instant improvements in survival prospects through these simple interventions continue to be overlooked by surgeons who pride themselves on the idea that good surgery is the main reason that cancer patients survive. They could vastly

---

9   Peter C. Elwood *et al.* **Aspirin in the Treatment of Cancer: Reductions in Metastatic Spread and in Mortality: A Systematic Review and Meta-Analyses of Published Studies.** *PLOS ONE*, 2016; 11 (4): e0152402 DOI: 10.1371/journal. pone.0152402

Benish M, Bartal I, Goldfarb Y, Levi B, Avraham R, Raz A, Ben-Eliyahu S. Perioperative use of beta-blockers and COX-2 inhibitors may improve immune competence and reduce the risk of tumor metastasis. Ann Surg Oncol. 2008 Jul;15(7):2042-52. doi: 10.1245/s10434-008-9890-5. Epub 2008 Apr 9. PMID: 18398660; PMCID: PMC3872002.

improve statistics if they would only add an anti-inflammatory before and after their excellent surgical skills.[10]

I knew my natural defences needed to be at their highest during surgery. Why give my already stressed body all that extra work?

After the negativity of my surgeon, I still had my worries about gastric bleeding, so I asked my GP for his thoughts. He was a little more encouraging.

'Lots of people take low dose aspirin to prevent heart attacks and strokes so it should be okay,' he said after a little thought.

'Would taking an antacid help protect my stomach?' I asked.

'I'm not sure about that. We don't like to suggest taking more than one drug at a time and I don't know what effect it would have on your cancer, so best not,' he added.

If only I had discovered cimetidine (or Tagamet) at this time. This was in widespread clinical use for gastric ulcers, and was the first antacid on the market. It used to be freely available over the counter in the UK and has since been shown to have enormous potential, attacking cancer through multiple pathways. Long term use of antacids has been linked to gastric cancer though, but a short-term hit could have been a great help especially pre and post op.

When I discovered cimetidine in 2007, many years later, I took it for three months for its immune-boosting effects and I still occasionally take

---

10   Retsky M, Demicheli R, Hrushesky WJ, Forget P, De Kock M, Gukas I, Rogers RA, Baum M, Sukhatme V, Vaidya JS. Reduction of breast cancer relapses with perioperative non-steroidal anti-inflammatory drugs: new findings and a review. Curr Med Chem. 2013;20(33):4163-76. doi: 10.2174/09298673113209990250. PMID: 23992307; PMCID: PMC3831877.

it. Cimetidine, I realise now, would have also helped protect my stomach from the aspirin and may have provided a bigger anti-cancer punch if I'd taken them together. The downside is that this anti-histamine inhibits a detoxifying liver enzyme (cytochrome P450), meaning it increases the dosage of any other drug you may be taking. But this could be used in a beneficial way too, increasing either the plasma level of a drug or delaying clearance to maintain the anti-cancer effects in the body.

One of its potential uses may be post-operatively. If you are a patient recovering from surgery, there is a critical period of seven days when you experience a surge of T suppressor cells. These subdue levels of your white cells called tumour infiltrating lymphocytes (TILs), which are the good guys that fight your tumour cells. Suppression of these allies is one reason cancer may flourish after surgery in the inflamed environment, the effects becoming visible about 10 months after surgery.

Cimetidine helps reverse the suppression of the T suppressor cells, which in turn helps keep the levels of tumour infiltrating lymphocytes up. If I had discovered this vital piece of evidence before my lung operation, I have little doubt I would have taken cimetidine immediately after surgery for those critical seven days.[11]

Cimetidine is also sometimes effective against Epstein Barr Virus, even when the virus is latent, and this is implicated (along with the HPV virus and MMTV) for activating many breast cancers. When the patent lapsed, cimetidine went out of fashion in the UK and unless you have friends in either Canada, the US or Germany where it's still available over the counter, it can be hard to obtain.

---

11   Long term use of cimetidine (over years) has been linked with cases of gynaecomastia (enlargement of the breast) and hyperprolactinemia, as it lowers testosterone altering the hormonal balance, so perhaps it has a hormonal component that some cancers should steer clear of. But short-term use for a few months, in my opinion, outweigh those potential negatives.

Ranitidine (Zantac, an H2 inhibitor) and cetirizine (H1 inhibitor) are both readily accessible antihistamines that can be bought over the counter. These may be useful for both their antiviral and anti-cancer effects, boosting tumour infiltrating lymphocytes, and helping to protect the gut from gastric bleeds, possibly working best together. (As always, check with your health practitioner) but neither are as potentially as useful as cimetidine.

Perhaps I should have been more confident about my aspirin use, which I took cyclically, a few weeks on, a few weeks off, having been put off by my surgeon. A study[12] by Professor Peter Elwood at Cardiff University's School of Medicine, looking at the overall risk of stomach bleeds using aspirin had shown there was no increased risk of death from stomach bleeding in people who take regular low-dose (75mg) aspirin, and that the spontaneous bleeds from non-users were far more dangerous.

Elwood hoped his study would make doctors more comfortable prescribing aspirin. Other research papers agree. Low doses of aspirin, given alongside chemoradiation, boost the effects of this therapy and increase the five-year progression-free survival (86.6% vs 67.1%) with a lower risk of metastasis.[13] Generally caution is needed giving aspirin alongside chemotherapy as this could increase the risk of bleeding but there are benefits to adding it to radiation therapy. My rationale was, and still is, that all these little additions were not just cumulative but if they worked on different pathways, they would synergise and multiply each other's effects. If I approached from all these different directions, I wondered if I would be able to tip the odds back in my favour and steer a course to health.

---

12   'Benefits of daily aspirin outweigh risk to stomach, study suggests.' **Science Daily**, 30 November 2016.

13   Restivo A, Cocco IMF, Casula G, Scintu F, Cabras F, Scartozzi M, Zorcolo L (2015) Aspirin as a neoadjuvant agent during preoperative chemoradiation for rectal cancer. Br J Cancer 113(8): 1133–1139.

The early use of anti-inflammatory drugs and growth blockers, like the humble aspirin, made so much sense to me. Why was it that oncologists and surgeons who should know these facts still resisted? When faced with overwhelming odds of failure, why was it unreasonable to try a combination that might produce a synergistic and potent anti-cancer formula?

If 90 per cent of deaths from cancer are a direct result of the cancer spreading, stopping 20 per cent of metastases would improve survival statistics significantly. And that's just with aspirin. It is shocking that only in 2016 did Cancer Research UK begin a trial of aspirin – the 'AddAspirin trial' – but at dangerous levels of 100mg, 300mg and even 600mg! It's a double-blind trial, meaning neither the patient nor the doctor will know the dosage given. If and when patients end up with stomach bleeding as a direct result of these higher doses, will they then claim that the risk is too great, putting cancer patients off taking it and thereby keeping the pharmaceutical industry alive? Every other piece of research suggests the half dose of 75mg is enough and the evidence is there to see. Professor Peter Rothwell has run many trials on aspirin, all reported in the Lancet or Lancet Oncology. Simply, I believe the trial is not needed and is a waste of public money. It would be more productive for the cancer charity to lobby NICE to change their guidelines and list low-dose aspirin as an anti-cancer medication.

If you're one of the intended 11,000 participants in the AddAspirin trial, I urge you to check the literature and discuss with a doctor familiar with gastro-intestinal problems before taking what could be potentially harmful levels of anti-coagulants. Consider taking a smaller amount of aspirin, otherwise you may be putting yourself at unnecessary risk of harm. In the meantime, patients could needlessly die without that small preventative dose. As Benjamin Franklin said, 'An ounce of prevention is worth a pound of cure.' Ah, but there is no money to be made in prevention.

Many natural substances can help reduce inflammation. I had included quite a few of them in my pre-surgery regime: ginger, curcumin from turmeric and of course omega-3 fish oils, which are clinically proven to reduce inflammation and increasingly are used in lieu of drugs for conditions such as rheumatoid arthritis. All these supplements have well-researched anti- cancer effects. Even old-school oncologists know of curcumin! They don't suggest it though.

As I went about discovering more about cancer, I realised I needed to reduce something called vascular endothelial growth factor (VEGF). VEGF is a main stimulator of tumour growth, encouraging the development of new blood cells to feed itself – a process called angiogenesis. Aspirin, as well as reducing inflammation, also reduces angiogenesis.

At this point, my menu of supplements was as follows:

- Green tea with high levels of the catechin ECGC
- Ellagic acid (found in pomegranates, raspberries, walnuts, and very hard to source as a supplement at the time!)
- Resveratrol
- Silibinin (milk thistle)
- Pycnogenol
- B vitamins (sublingual methylated form of B12 and folate)
- Glucosamine sulphate
- Curcumin
- CLA

Pycnogenol, like aspirin, can increase the risk of bleeds so it needs to be taken with caution. It's a patented blend of several bark extracts (aspirin comes from bark too) but it can also lower blood sugar. I took it with aspirin even though I might have been doubling their risks, reasoning that cancer patients have far worse risk of blood clots. As instructed, I stopped all anti-coagulants several days (some surgeons suggest a week) before my operation. I had no intention of bleeding to death on the operating table!

The operation went well with no complications. One third of my lung was gone. Oh well. I could live with that. Pre-op I'd had exceptionally good lung volumes, above normal, so now I was about average. Damn. I didn't like being average.

After surgery, my blood antigen markers were taken again. Post-surgical metastatic spread is a common problem, and I knew that blocking VEGF with the aspirin peri-operatively would have helped. But waiting to hear the results made me feel sick with worry.

It took all day to summon the courage to phone up to find out. On the one hand, I wanted to stay in denial. But on the other, I knew I needed to plot and chart these markers. My head eventually won the argument. Sticking it in the sand was not going to help.

Andrew stood next to me as I received the news. I was gutted to learn my markers had surged to a new high, a reading of nearly 600, up from 190 despite my best efforts. Normal was anything under 150. This meant I now had tumour cells roaming around my body in my blood. I couldn't bear to think about it.

I was so dismayed. I told myself it was to be expected, surgery always did this, but I was incredibly disappointed. I felt I was failing already. My positive mood sunk again. Would I ever get back in the driving seat or did the cancer now control me? Medical interventions had made me worse, but I was hoping this was just a temporary problem. Had I tipped it to the point of no control? Was I powerless to defeat it? How could I get those markers down now? Had surgery been a mistake?

Andrew was far more practical. 'We knew that was going to happen, you told me the markers would go up. Try not to worry about it too much. It won't help. You always said there'd be a spillage of tumour cells and inflammation. Let's stick to the plan and keep those tumour cells whizzing around your system. You told me it was when they got stuck in the blood vessel wall that they can then metastasise.'

He was right. I had decided the best strategy would be to keep those pesky cells in my circulation and not allow them a chance to settle, to cling to the blood vessel linings (endothelium) and set up camp somewhere else in my body. It was the metastases, or secondary cancers, that caused death. If I kept the little blighters moving with aspirin, an anti-coagulant, maybe my army of cancer-killing white cells would be able to pick them off. Aspirin was also an anti-platelet drug. If the platelets were kept from forming little clumps that hid the tumour cells, would my Natural Killer cells, my white cell army, find it easier to win?

I now added nattokinase, an enzyme supplement that digests fibrin to reduce my tendency to excessive scarring. Combined with the aspirin, they would help keep my blood from becoming too sticky. With hindsight, some blood clotting tests (rather than just self-hacking) would have been useful. Clotting issues can be a tricky and very personalised area requiring professional advice. Getting this wrong could be dangerous.

After the operation, life was a daily ritual of green and apple/carrot/celery/beetroot juices, swallowing pills, meditating, and engaging in gentle exercise, such as a brisk walk or a bike ride. Then came the dilemma of chemotherapy.

I wasn't sure what to do, but now that my cancer markers had shot up so high, chemo seemed like the right choice. It would help mop up the potential of 'micro-metastases', any little clumps of cancer cells. However, it would also suppress my immunity.

What if I only had enough chemo to kill cancer but not enough to wreck the immune cells in my gut? Perhaps I could halve the normal dose but take it for twice as long? It might be less damaging. Why did I have to have the 'maximum tolerated dose' anyway? Was more really better? It seemed so brutal. And one-dimensional. Given that I was already attacking the cancer from so many angles, was it possible that chemotherapy could be equally effective at much smaller doses?

And were there drugs or supplements that might synergise with chemotherapy? I'd discovered green tea, resveratrol and curcumin all made it more effective and decided to carry on with these if the nausea would allow it. [14]

When I had raised the subject of taking supplements with chemotherapy to my oncologist, her response had been negative.

'You have to try and make this as effective as possible. Antioxidants can wreck chemotherapy's power. It's best if you avoid all of them.'

Green tea was an antioxidant. So was resveratrol. Both had well reported anti-cancer effects in combination with chemo. I deduced there were certain antioxidants that were synergistic with chemotherapy and others that might interfere. I was not convinced she was right. The articles I had read stated quite clearly that there were benefits. Perhaps their powerful anti-cancer properties outweighed their small antioxidant capacity.

Ultimately, I decided that chemo was something I probably had to undergo, despite my huge reservations. I was under a lot of pressure, not just from the oncologist but also from my family. I knew if I refused it would cause enormous stress for them. They would be terrified that I

---

14 Hydroxycitrate, fasting pre and post chemo, statins and metformin would have helped me but were yet to be written about.

was turning it down and 'doing nothing,' passively waiting for cancer to return. But to me, chemo felt like passive acceptance.

As I have come to realise, many patients die of politeness to their oncologist and fear of upsetting their loved ones. It happens far more than anyone would imagine. Relatives and friends wade in with their personal opinions on what you should do, pushing for high-dose toxic treatments because that's what the men and women in the white coats recommend. Conversely, some well-meaning relatives put patients off chemo altogether, when it could be so much more effective if used differently. Oncologists give either the maximum tolerated dose or a palliative dose. Often too much or too little. Neither will be curative. Where is the sensible middle ground? One that doesn't crucify the immune system. Perhaps a low 'metronomic' or regularly spaced dose of chemotherapy that is used in combination with other treatments?

Being ill is quite enough to contend with without the extra emotional baggage of tiptoeing around everyone to make sure all their wishes and wants are looked after. My family were of course gunning for me to survive and fortunately for me they didn't interfere with my decisions, though I was sure they didn't always approve. They were expecting the disease to return, expecting to watch the 'car crash' happen in slow motion. The medics among them had been told there was no cure, and that death was inevitable. They watched silently, not sure what to say, wondering whether I might be harming myself or making things worse, hastening my demise.

Chemotherapy reduced the size of tumours. Agreed. It was hard to argue against that. But did it get rid of cancer? I had read that chemotherapy given to stage IV patients encouraged the cancer to come back faster and more aggressively than before. This is because chemo and radiotherapy fail to touch the cancer stem cells. My oncologist agreed that it was a crude and blunt tool and that it caused much collateral damage, but she had little else to offer me. How to get those pesky cancer stem cells? Would they respond to being starved? Be that through cancer-starving supplements or an altered diet?

So my choice was either high dose or nothing. Low dose was not even an option in 1999 (and still isn't offered, despite good evidence that it's as effective and less damaging to the immune system). Cancer was an invincible foe requiring the most barbaric of treatments: a full onslaught which came with huge potential for personal suffering. How else could it be defeated? Anything less would surely not be enough.

But as much as I told myself that, another voice inside me whispered that there were options. Perhaps I could start with a high dose and taper it off? After a couple of months, maybe I could persuade my oncologist to gradually lower it if I was responding well. That seemed to be a good compromise. I might have to lay it on thick though and complain loudly about side effects to persuade her.

I knew boosting my immunity would be key to surviving. The immune system is ultimately the master controller, the final piece of the jigsaw, and it would be needed to wipe out the cancer cells naturally. In contrast, high dose chemo was an immune system destroyer and the statistics clearly showed it failed in every case at my stage of disease. Perhaps a reduced tumour load would make it easier for my body to cope? Even as I said it to myself, I was not convinced.

Reducing the stress hormone cortisol would be essential. Raised levels suppressed lymphocytes in the gut, in an area known as GALT, the central hub of my immune cells. Intermittent fasting or reducing food quantities, I'd read, also helped immunity. On the advice of Dr Callebout I dropped my food intake significantly. I finished eating for the day at 6 o'clock in the evening (although he suggested 3 o'clock) and ate a late breakfast. I added medicinal mushrooms, maitake-D-fraction, beta glucans, a rice bran extract called MGN3, DHEA, and I took melatonin at night. All would help boost the number of Natural Killer cells (NK cells) in my body to help counter the immune depleting effects of the chemotherapy.

Although I was outwardly positive and upbeat, I desperately needed to address my rocketing stress levels. My constant research was taking over my life and inevitably I'd regularly come across my deeply depressing survival statistics. No matter how hard I tried, the harsh reality of my situation would knock me back for days.

I knew making it to six months would be an achievement. The cloak of death could descend at any moment and smother me, striking me down when I was momentarily off-guard. Cancer demanded my full attention. Someone told me I would have to get through '180 dark days of the soul' until I could start to come to terms with the diagnosis. Would I even get that far? My soul felt pretty gloomy already as I peered over the edge into that fathomless abyss below.

These negative feelings needed banishment. I was tormenting myself with such morbid thoughts. Cancer was all-consuming; it allowed precious little time for joy, laughter, and fun.

I had read that hypnotherapy might be useful, so I sought out a brilliant hypnotherapist based in Putney. He was wonderful. After every session, he handed me a personalised tape of his treatment to play back at home. When I first started seeing him, my future timeline stopped at just six months. Eventually he talked me into believing I had a future that would last years. Yes! His sessions helped me improve my diet and encouraged me to drink more – I had been very dehydrated. He also focused on the white cell army roaming my system. Through visualisation, I could see those white cells as soldiers, picking off the nasty intruders one by one.

As well as hypnotherapy, I also received spiritual healing from a local healer, I learnt to meditate, went for walks in the park, and spent time connecting with nature. When everyone else was complaining about the wet, blustery weather, I'd wrap up warm and grin as I paced around the park, Mother Nature battering me with her awesome power. I saw beauty when everyone else saw the mundane. The twinkle of dew drops, the greenness of the leaves, the majesty of trees and the hills, the sparkle of the spray when I was sailing. Why did everyone complain so? Why didn't people rejoice every morning to be, well, alive? It was as if the rest of the world was too busy, wrapped up in day-to-day minutiae to realise what an incredible blessing it was to be part of creation.

I would lie down on the grass, stare up at the sky and feel my connection to the infinite universe. How small and insignificant I was. I felt reborn, like I was seeing life through the eyes of a child.

Just three months after finding the spot of bother in my lung, I'd made huge strides. My list of supplements was growing, even if it seemed to be never ending. I wanted the terrain, the area around the cancer cell, to be as inhospitable as possible and the rest of my body to be functioning as well as it could. My diet was becoming ever more extreme as I gradually added in more low-glycaemic foods and took out simple carbohydrates and inflammatory foods. To my surprise, I felt less hungry on this diet and my energy levels soared. I felt truly alive!

Shopping for health foods in 1999 was another nightmare. Choice was extremely limited. Even green tea was virtually unheard of in those days. Waitresses stared at me in confusion when I asked for it in a cafe. 'Do you mean peppermint?' they would ask. Aargh! I took to keeping a ready stock of teabags with me wherever I went, along with my little sachets of pills.

I was still on the hunt for supplements to lower blood glucose. It seemed increasingly clear that the medics were ignoring the obvious. Diabetic patients were a third more likely to contract cancer – they had higher insulin and higher glucose and both fueled cancer's growth. Was I oversimplifying the problem? I didn't think so. Inner wisdom told me that perhaps diabetes medications might help control blood glucose in cancer patients too.

I knew nothing about the wonder drug metformin at this point. I only associated diabetes with taking insulin. But insulin, I deduced, would fuel the fire by allowing the tumour to take up yet more glucose. This was not the answer. I wanted to pursue the natural route, supplements or a diet that might lower my blood glucose **without** raising insulin.

It was then that I stumbled on research in a Journal about an ancient Traditional Chinese medicinal extract that it seemed no-one else in the West was using for cancer. It would control my blood glucose and offer several other incredible anti-cancer properties. It would help with every aspect of my treatment.

Chapter Seven:

Summoning My Inner Dragon

My discovery of berberine, a herbal extract used for centuries in China to treat diarrhoea and other infections but almost unknown in the West, came out of left field. I had quizzed my oncologist extensively about my tumour. I needed to know not only the basics of the cancer biology but exactly how and what my tumour was made up of, the types of cells, how quickly they were dividing, my cancer's doubling time. All of this information helped me to determine that I had a keratinising tumour. Keratin is a protein found in hair, nails, and skin. It was also an epithelial cancer, in other words a surface tumour.

As I listened to my oncologist, I realised the description of my tumour had many striking parallels with psoriasis. They were both made up of squamous epithelial cells. Both involved inflammation, rapid cell turnover, and an over-production of keratin. That was interesting. Could any psoriasis treatments be useful for my cancer? I decided I'd look into it.

One afternoon, I was leafing through health journals when I came across an article on psoriasis. It had been published in the *Journal of Herbal Medicine* in February 1999 by Dr Maher Succar, who trained in the Ukraine and was teaching Traditional Chinese Herbal Medicine at the University of Westminster. He described how a particular extract from a plant was found to be effective in 80 per cent of patients with psoriasis. It was called **Mahonia aquifolium**, and its main ingredients were berberine and berbamine. He wrote:

*In recent years, scientists have discovered that the extract of the bark and root of **Mahonia aquifolium** contains alkaloids which have been shown to be strong **antimicrobial and antifungal** agents – berberine, protoberberine, berbamine and oxycanthine.*

*Cell culture studies have demonstrated that these alkaloids **inhibit the growth of various tumour cells** as well as induce powerful antioxidant activity which **inhibits keratinocyte (abnormal skin cell) growth** and alleviates inflammation. The action of these alkaloids explains why **Mahonia aquifolium** extract has been successfully used to treat a variety of skin disorders (e.g. psoriasis, dermatitis, eczema, fungal conditions) as well as digestive disorders and blood conditions.*

Even more interesting! So much in there to make me sit up. It didn't just focus on the inhibition of tumour cells, either. All cancer patients seemed to have problems with their guts, so anything that might kill the nasties in there sounded good too. Perhaps it helped kill fungi, parasites and other bugs? A healthy intestinal tract was of paramount importance to the immune system.

Dr Succar went on:

*'Tests by US and Canadian researchers have revealed that **Mahonia aquifolium** is one of the **top five most powerful herbal antifungal agents** and that it **promotes healthy fat metabolism**. Scientists at the National Cancer Institute, NIH, Bethesda, USA have demonstrated that **Mahonia aquifolium** inhibits lipoxygenase and lipid hydroperoxide, and that this effect may be a crucial factor in explaining why it seems to be so beneficial for psoriasis sufferers.'*

Wow. Clearly this was awesome stuff.

More hunting about berberine unearthed a report from 1995. With mounting excitement, I read that through serendipity, researchers in Changchun, China had discovered berberine also reduced blood sugar.

The research had been led by scientist Ni Yanxi who'd been treating diarrhoea in patients with diabetes.

So, it lowered blood glucose, reduced inflammation, promoted healthy fat metabolism, fought off bugs in the intestine – **and** fought cancer – amazing! Exactly what I needed.

The article reported the reduction in blood glucose was achieved with doses between 300 and 500mg, three times a day. There were no side effects at all, even with doses up to 2 grams! This was perfect. And it was good for diarrhoea too – it helped gut infections as well as diabetes. I knew my gut health was crucial for my immunity and although I didn't have diarrhoea, I wanted to kill off any pathogenic bacteria that might compromise me. I wanted my immune system focused on the cancer.

The full effect of *Mahonia aquifolium* and its berberine and oxyacanthine content is pretty inspiring stuff. It:

- Reduces inflammation.
- Reduces blood glucose.
- Is antimicrobial and antifungal.
- Has strong anti-cancer activity.
- Improves lipid profile and fat metabolism.
- Reduces keratinocytes and improved psoriasis.
- Improves gut health (and thereby reduces leaky gut).

What wasn't there about this supplement to love? If everyone took it then doctors might be out of a job! I simply had to have it.

If it helped the gut, inflammation and glucose levels, berberine might also help many cancers. I was bouncing with excitement as I told Andrew all about it that evening. He was delighted I was so happy but was concerned that no-one else was using it.

'Are you sure about this? It doesn't have any trials or research in the West at all.'

'What's the downside? Berberine had been used extensively in Chinese medicine for centuries. We're way too aloof and dismissive of Eastern concoctions in the West and far too reliant on Randomised Clinical Trials.'

'Why don't they just run those on natural botanicals?'

'Because there's no money in it. No new drugs to market. I've no doubt many of their medicines are very powerful and useful. Modern medicines mostly start from plant discoveries, which are reproduced synthetically, then patented. I'm going to hunt it down, take it and see how it goes,' I said.

I mentioned **Mahonia aquifolium** and berberine to Dr Callebout, my lovely integrative doctor, when I next saw him. On my first appointment I'd been armed with a long list of supplements, thinking he'd cut them right back, but to my horror, he suggested a whole lot more! This time he rubbed his beard thoughtfully and said berberine sounded 'very interesting.'

It sounded more than interesting to me. I felt like Alice in Wonderland at the bottom of the rabbit hole in a small room staring at a bottle with the words 'Drink Me' written on it. I had terminal cancer, I felt boxed in and berberine sounded like a magic potion. I didn't want it to shrink me though, but shrinking any little tumours lurking in my system would be great, thank you!

I found a website for psoriasis sufferers that sent it out by mail order, and into my regime it went.

Today, researchers are falling over themselves to explore berberine's amazing potential, not just against cancer but as a PPAR gamma agonist, antiviral, antimicrobial, antifungal, and anti-inflammatory. Many herbalists now describe it as the most powerful supplement in the world. There are moves afoot to make it prescription – which of course plays to Big Pharma's clampdown on our choices.

I began taking **Mahonia aquifolium** just before starting chemotherapy, unaware of how much it synergises and enhances the drug. I was facing six months of the maximum dose of gemcitabine, cisplatin and 5FU (affectionately known as 'five foot under'). Ugh. Was I going to be able to handle that? My body recoiled at the thought. I knew full well how I was going to feel, I'd been through chemo five years earlier and had been sick as a dog. This time it was going to be a much heavier dose and for much longer.

Little did I know (and to be fair to my inner Sherlock Holmes, neither did the scientists at the time) that berberine is also a calcium channel blocker, which meant that when I was given chemo, the cytotoxic drug was held inside my cancer cells for longer. Chemo must 'catch' a cancer cell when It's actively dividing or else it doesn't work. Balancing toxicity with effectiveness is why the maximum tolerated dose is favoured by medics, even though this high dose destroys the immune system.

Every cell in the body goes through a period of rest before dividing. Chemo cocktails are made up of different cytotoxic drugs that work by catching cancer at different stages of its division. So, the longer you can keep the chemo in the cell, the better the chance of catching it during its active dividing phase and killing it. Cancer cells have far less rest and lots more action than healthy cells. But other cells are fast dividers too, which is why healthy cells in the gut (the centre of our immunity) and hair are the losers by collateral damage.[15]

High-dose chemo only reduces the size of a tumour. It does nothing to reduce stem cells at the heart of the cancer. Conventional treatments using both radiotherapy and chemotherapy leave behind these disparate cancer cells, they act and behave differently to the rapidly dividing and obvious tumour cells. In the vast majority of cases, chemotherapy does not offer a cure[16] (the real reason it works with Acute Lymphoblastic Leukaemia, I describe later in Part 2) and the percentage of positive outcomes at stage IV are zero. There was no benefit, when you examined the statistics. Was it worth it? How could I make it more effective without crippling my immune system, destroying my gut, developing neuropathy, hearing issues, cardiac damage and other horrid side effects, not to mention the risk of death by toxic lysis syndrome?

I was also concerned by the medical profession's unhealthy obsession with a tumour's size which often had little correlation to survival. Perhaps I could put cancer's future growth (as I was assured would happen, it

---

15   In our bodies the gut, hair follicles and the cells inside bone marrow making red blood cells all divide much faster than other cells in the body. Immune cells in the gut have a rapid turnover of every four or five days, hence the collateral damage to the lining of the gut. So, holding the chemo inside the cells until it begins dividing makes it much more effective. Professor Ben Williams, a long-term survivor of Glioblastoma (brain cancer) used verapamil, a calcium channel blocker during chemotherapy, as an off-label drug.

16   A 2016 study in the BMJ, looking at five-year survival, agrees. Dr Peter Wise reported: 'An important effect [of chemotherapy] was shown on five-year survival only in testicular cancer (40%), Hodgkin's disease (37%), cancer of the cervix (12%), lymphoma (10.5%), and ovarian cancer (8.8%). Together, these represented less than 10% of all cases. In the remaining 90% of patients – including those with the commonest tumours of the lung, prostate, colorectum, and breast – drug therapy increased five-year survival by less than 2.5% – an overall survival benefit of around three months.' The 12% survival figure for cervical cancer was for primary cancer with lymphatic spread. *http://www. bmj.com/content/355/bmj. i60*

would inevitably return) on pause with my cancer-starving diet and supplements.

Could I push the cancer cells to die off by depriving it of key nutrients it needed to grow, without subjecting myself to chemo? Why was there no interest in any of the other areas of my health, like exploring the reasons cancer had begun in the first place? Why didn't they even bother to take serum vitamin levels, like vitamin D?

Starving the cancer cell seemed to be a perfectly logical intervention to me. And recent research proves that fasting prior to chemo will one day be standard practice. But the medical profession will only learn of this when the cancer charities have somehow patented their own approved diet sachets (they are working on this as I write, despite telling patients that diets don't work). The correct diet protects normal cells, leaves the immune cells more active, and decreases side effects. Professor Valter Longo, a Professor of Gerontology in Southern California, had initially been studying reducing food intake for its known anti-ageing effects, then began investigating a three-day starvation diet before chemotherapy. The results were so impressive, he now advocates a fasting-mimicking diet.[17] Professor Thomas Seyfried, a lead researcher in the field of metabolic cancer therapy, is also an advocate of starving cancer with the ketogenic diet. Dr Callebout suggested in 1999 that I stop eating at 3pm, which I did for a few weeks. His reasoning was that the liver was more efficient in the mornings and digesting food was harder in the evenings. Also, slouching on the sofa after an evening meal, watching telly and not burning off the food, seemed a bad idea.

I hadn't heard the term ketogenic in 1999, and creating ketones was not something I had focused on. My diet had been what would be described as 'Paleo' nowadays, a diet that perhaps our ancestors would have eaten,

---

17   He has also been helping to formulate a product called Chemolieve, which is to be launched soon, in which he apparently has no commercial interest.

with a focus on removing inflammatory foods as well as reducing simple carbohydrates and lowering IGF-1. My number one priority was to reduce the dangerous insulin spike after meals and lower any glucose in my blood that might feed any little seedlings of cancer.

My tumour load at this stage was low. I had witnessed others, persuaded by well-meaning doctors that they had 'got it all,' do little until cancer returned. Instead, I was proactive. I knew the statistics. I would kick it hard while it was weak and vulnerable. I was convinced there was much I could do to change the rate of its inevitable return. Changing the chemotherapy type, perhaps to a less aggressive drug, lowering the dose, but give it in more regular pulsed intervals would allow me more time to starve the cancer and give my immune system a chance to be maintained. I was desperate to have a lower dose. It would mean less nausea, so in theory it would be easier to combine chemo with other treatments and boost its efficacy and attack from different directions. Sadly for me, this was not offered.

Green tea's properties seemed almost magical to me. Not only did it boost the effectiveness of chemotherapy, but it is a growth inhibitor, its two extracts epigallocatechin gallate (EGCG) and catechin gallate (CG) blocking vascular VEGF. But its effects seemed to go beyond merely blocking new blood vessel growth (angiogenesis). I later discovered both EGCG and CG are inhibitors of glutamate dehydrogenase (GHD), a precursor of glutamine (an amino acid), the other key nutrient cancer uses with glucose to fuel its growth.[18]

---

18 Some cancers use as much or more glutamine than glucose, including triple negative breast cancer, ovarian or pancreatic cancer, glioblastomas and the more aggressive prostate cancers. Malignant cells create lots of ammonia as a by-product of their excessive metabolism and they need glutathione (an antioxidant) to neutralise it. Without this they're very vulnerable to being tipped into cell death by the presence of enough free radicals.

Even though I knew nothing about 'mTOR' or other metabolic pathways that are abnormal in cancer, I was taking many supplements that inhibited these during chemo: berberine, hydroxycitrate, gymnema, and pycnogenol. My oncologist was interested in what I was doing, intrigued to know why I wasn't deteriorating as she expected, but I was worried about telling her. I expected only negativity, which seems to be the default position of many oncologists to supplements. I didn't want that. I was confident with my choices and I'd double-checked everything with Dr Callebout. But I was tiptoeing around my oncologist. It didn't feel good to mislead her and lie. That made me extremely uncomfortable.

With hindsight (an especially wonderful thing – I never thought I'd be looking back at all) so much research has been published in the last three or four years about berberine, the natural equivalent to metformin, that I can honestly say this may have had the single biggest effect on chemotherapy. But of course, it would have been a combination of everything I was taking, the synergistic effect.

I became ever more convinced that starving the cancer, stressing it by making access to nutrients more difficult or impossible, then adding the killer blow of chemotherapy, was the way forward. Why waste energy and resources on a foe without shutting off its supply system first, weakening its heavy defences?

Historically, the thinking has been that patients should be given as much chemotherapy as they can tolerate without dying. Expert opinion is now that a reduction by 50-70 per cent in the amount of chemo, taken for a longer period, metronomically (with rest periods), may be equally effective and far less toxic, especially if used in combination with other drugs or modalities.[19] But high-dose chemo is so ingrained as the only

19   Nars, M. S. and Kaneno, R. (2013), Immunomodulatory effects of low dose chemotherapy and perspectives of its combination with immunotherapy. Int. J. Cancer, 132: 2471-2478. doi:10.1002/ijc.27801

method of administration, oncologists are fearful of offering anything less, even though the evidence has been out there for some time. If they chose this different path, not only would they risk the scorn and derision of their colleagues, they could risk the loss of their license to practice if the patient sues or a fellow oncologist claims they're not following protocol. This is exactly what happened to a doctor in Australia. It's no wonder cancer treatment has changed so little in 50 years.

If I dropped the chemotherapy, I would be directly disobeying doctor's orders. High-dose chemotherapy felt wrong. I feared I was letting my body down by agreeing to it. But I also had great respect for my oncologist. She was very persuasive.

'See it like a course of antibiotics – you have to finish the course,' she told me. This line of argument was repeated by my obviously worried relatives and my husband every time I mentioned giving it up.

'But it might kill me! What if it destroys my immune system and I never recover?'

'Yes, I'm afraid I might kill you with it too, but it's the best option we can offer,' she said, trying to keep things light.

Jesus. It's not like I didn't know this already. Was this really the only option? It was now 2000, the millennium. Chemotherapy felt like a torture from the Dark Ages.

So, still reluctant, I caved in and went ahead. And despite all I was doing to help mitigate the side effects, I felt dreadful. I had not yet come across the research suggesting that a fast for three days before chemotherapy would help maintain the immune system and reduce side effects.

I tried to continue with supplements when I wasn't feeling ill, keeping as fit as possible with regular walks, cycling and bouncing on a mini trampoline to boost my oxygen, energy, and wellbeing. If I felt up to it, I'd go sailing at weekends and try to keep my wig on!

Berberine will help heal a chemotherapy-damaged leaky gut, an inevitable side effect of treatment. Glutamine is also a useful supplement during the chemotherapy in small doses, it is pretty much all absorbed into the gut wall, and although some cancers use glutamine as fuel, it doesn't 'feed' the cancer in the same way as glucose.[20] By helping to salvage my gut lining and maintain a better microbiome, it would help maintain my precious immune system, which was vital for my long-term survival.

The effects of my cancer-starving supplements (berberine, EGCG, gymnema sylvestre, hydroxycitrate, pycnogenol, silibinin, niacin) and a low- glycaemic diet made the chemo far more effective than anyone had hoped for. To my absolute joy, after my first round of chemo my blood markers plummeted from nearly 600 to 130, below the normal range of 150. The relief of being in that 'normal' bracket again was huge, although I knew it was quite possibly false hope and a temporary reprieve.

Chemo on its own never cures my type of cancer at stage IV, it merely puts it on the back burner for a while. But it was time to celebrate, because I had won a small battle. Andrew and I went out that night for a quiet meal in a local Italian restaurant. Perhaps high-dose chemotherapy was OK after all.

Tempting though it was to think otherwise, I knew it was unlikely that I had won the war. And after another two months of the toxic infusions, I was steadily feeling worse and worse. By now I was completely bald and the nausea was unbearable. Would this maximum-tolerated dose kill me, as my oncologist and I feared?

---

20 An exception may be gastrointestinal tumours that may be able to use glutamine directly. Glutamine can be made from scratch in the body or shunted from one place to another to provide nutrients that cancer needs.

Enough was enough. I was being dragged down and no longer felt empowered and in control. I was feeling frail and weak, yet again becoming a passive and submissive patient. I had to find the strength to stand up for my rights and have chemotherapy on my own terms.

I was in a tough spot. I realised that the wrong decision might mean the difference between survival, permanently disabling side effects, or worse, death. But I was comfortable with my choice. I was sure a lower dose at this point would be equally effective and less damaging.[21]

Somehow, I had to persuade my oncologist to drop the dose. But she had been so insistent I knew it wasn't going to be an easy debate to win. Exhausted, my willpower and my energy drained, my spirit quashed, how would I persuade her? After a lengthy discussion with my hypnotherapist, I decided I'd try the bolshie patient tactic. I was going to be an obstinate, difficult and bloody-minded. Passive patients die. Noisy ones survive. Known fact.

'It is **your** body, don't forget that. You have every right to refuse chemotherapy if you want,' he'd said. I knew that, but it was so hard to break the 'doctor's always right' mentality. It's hardwired into our psyche. We are conditioned from a young age to listen and follow every suggestion that leaves their mouths.

Oncologists seemed to dismiss the Warburg Effect,[22] the differing metabolism of cancer cells. Was I now becoming just as much of an expert in my own cancer as the oncologist? Did much of what they suggested stem from the NICE guidelines, from following the recommendations

---

21 Recent research shows an initial high dose followed by decreasing amounts show far better results. Instinctively I had felt this too. *https://www.independent.co.uk/life-style/health-and-families/health-news/cancer-low-doses-chemotherapy-may-control-disease-more-effectively-a6893701.html*

22 Nobel prize winning German scientist Otto Warburg noticed the abnormal fermentation of glucose (glycolysis) in cancer cells in the 1920s.

of (biased) pharmaceutical companies, or from a fear of being sued? Rather than take a risk and try something different, do most just follow the herd? I refused to be a sheep. I was a 1964 baby, the Chinese year of the Dragon. Time to summon my inner Dragon and exhale some fire.

My therapist made me repeat the phrase, 'I am in control. My body can heal', several times a day. The more I said it, the more I began to believe it, and regain the feeling of being in the driving seat. Yes, I could steer the treatment direction back down my path. Yes, I knew I needed lower dose chemotherapy. I could fight the disease on my own terms. The positive affirmations helped me switch off my defeatist attitude and empowered me enormously.

When I next saw my oncologist, I begged her to stop the chemo. I knew she was unlikely to, but I told her I felt dreadful, that it was intolerable. I laid it on thick, describing terrible stomach pains, telling her that I had been sick for a week. Of course, it was not all true, but I called on my best drama skills, gave an Oscar-worthy performance and gave her no choice.

It worked. She promised to lower the dose right down for my last three months. 'As your blood markers have remained steady, below normal ranges, I'll drop the dose,' she said. 'And we'll keep the remainder in reserve if you ever need more.'

I nearly hugged her! I was so relieved. I believe she saved my life that day.

Despite the lower dose, my six-month chemotherapy was still a gruelling endurance event, like competing in the Round the World Yacht Race with no stop-overs. I was also vaguely aware that another consequence of all the prior treatments I'd already received, alongside a second wave of chemo, might encourage another type of cancer in the bone marrow called leukaemia. I shrugged that off. No, I was strong and fit enough not to succumb to that, wasn't I?

Chapter Eight:

Keeping the Beast in its Box

By the summer of 2000, I had finally finished my chemotherapy. I had survived nine months, far longer than my predicted expiry date of weeks, and my cancer blood markers were good. Now I just needed to keep them there, or better yet, push them further down, as far as possible. How low could I go?

I was bald, exhausted and full of toxic chemical garbage, but I was alive. I was wary that after high-dose chemotherapy cancer tends to return with a vengeance, harder and faster than ever because of the lack of any immune control, but I did not yet understand the significance of the stem cell. My body felt wracked and ruined by the treatment. It's at this point, looking at a reduced or absent tumour, that most patients take their foot off the gas, switch to cruise control, breathe a sigh of relief and assume they're cured, eager to return to some sense of normality. Some return to their former less than perfect lifestyle from before their diagnosis. This is a common and fatal mistake.

There was so much more I needed to do. I was confident I was starving the cancer of glucose, but not confident that the diet and the berberine would be enough. I needed to detox, get rid of any remnants of the chemotherapy and rebuild my gut, which I assumed would be badly damaged. My bone marrow, if that too had been hit, I hoped would heal on its own. My hair would eventually regrow – that was the least of my worries. I would just have to keep my fingers crossed about the possibility of future leukaemia and hope it wouldn't happen to me.

There were no statistics on this as women with my type and stage of cancer died in weeks. According to the research I was apparently a goner already.

Post chemo, my plan was to:

1. Detox with a hard-core macrobiotic, low GI, pescatarian, anti-inflammatory, low saturated fat diet for three months (must think up a name for it)
2. Check my gut microbes at Great Smokies Laboratory (now Genova Diagnostics)
3. Check my micronutrient status (minerals, vitamins, fatty acid profile
4. Take intravenous vitamin C and have UVBI (ultraviolet blood irradiation) as soon as possible.
5. Exercise more, go sailing, and enjoy life!
6. Launch a new business (hmm… perhaps not one of my better ideas).

By this stage, I had become a supplement junkie. Relaxing my rigid self-imposed timetable for even a day was a luxury I felt I couldn't afford. I wanted to control glucose release at every meal. I got stressed out when I forgot and missed taking them. Would the cancer get the upper hand? Every meal seemed like a life-or-death decision; would the meal feed the cancer, or would it starve it, help heal my body and boost recovery?

For now, I seemed to be keeping cancer under control. My blood tests showed I was still in remission. But how long could I sustain this lifestyle? Did I really need to be so tough on myself? On the other hand, I wondered whether I was doing enough. Would the supplements and diet really protect me? Would the cancer mutate and come back with a rage and force I wouldn't be able to contain? The only way to keep track of my progress was to take regular blood markers, that way I could be on the case immediately if it made an unwelcome return visit.

If diabetic patients needed to control glucose and insulin release every mealtime then so did I. Both levels spike after meals and this seemed to be the critical time to control it. I didn't know anyone else approaching cancer in this way but to me it seemed like common sense. I had felt too ill after chemotherapy sessions to be able to take much of anything let alone supplements, however in the preceding days before each session I would hoof lots of cancer-starving compounds to carry me through. Now I was feeling better I was making up for that.

If berberine controlled glucose release into the blood, then I concluded the best time to take it would probably be just before a meal. This was not easy going, but eventually it became a habit, religiously pill popping at breakfast, lunchtime and supper. The downsides were that taking as many as I did, washed down with green tea and sometimes even olive oil, I could end up feeling nauseous again.

Sleep had been an issue for years, ever since the first diagnosis. To help that, I took melatonin at night an hour before bedtime. It has immune-boosting effects, such as IL2 and IL12 (good cytokines), which are controlled by the pineal gland. But I now wondered whether I needed to take as much. I was afraid I had switched off my own endogenous supply and suspected I would have to stay on melatonin for life.

Fear and worry were my bed pals. Racing thoughts were hard to push aside. There seemed to be no escape from the nightmare. If I stopped the supplements, the cancer might return. That was not a risk I wanted to take. There was to be no denial of cancer, no going back to the carefree life I had before.

Organisation was going to be paramount. Nothing could be left to chance if I wanted to keep the beast in its box. I made a chart of everything I was taking; I wrote a list of where I was obtaining each supplement and made note of phone numbers and websites for re-ordering. Every

Friday, I would dedicate an hour in the afternoon to preparing for the week ahead, filling sachets and ordering up any supplement running low. Normal pill boxes just weren't big enough! 'Maracas' indeed. It was an effort, but the choice was this or quite possibly death. To my mind, it was no choice at all.

I became exceptionally strict with myself. Cancer was lifestyle related, wasn't it? If I believed the media stories, I would never have got cancer if I'd looked after myself better. But others lived far worse lifestyles than I did. I knew that blaming myself for my situation was not constructive. Instead, I harnessed the strength of my feelings, the anger, guilt, grief, sadness, fear and worry about my diagnosis to spur me on.

My expanding list of supplements, visits to integrative doctors, tests, and organic food was costing a small fortune but I needed this lifeline. We weren't poor but even so, it was a struggle. How could every cancer patient afford all this? And now I decided I needed intravenous vitamin. C. Yet another expense.

Andrew never mentioned the drain on our finances again. He was 100 per cent supportive. Even so, I felt terribly guilty that I was denying us both a much-needed holiday and digging into pensions and reserves. There can be so many unspoken factors weighing down on the subconscious of the patient, sapping precious energy, piling yet more stress onto the already overburdened psyche. But if the boot were on the other foot, I would do the same in a heartbeat.

Under the care of the medical profession, there is a sense of security, a safety net to catch you, that something is being done. When I came to the end of my six months of chemotherapy, I was going it alone. I had been cut loose and like many patients in this situation I felt vulnerable. But I'd already found my integrative doctors and alternative treatments.

I was also empowered with knowledge. I didn't wait around in limbo waiting for it to come back. There was so much more I could do.

I couldn't rest on my laurels, keeping my fingers crossed, hoping time would erase the memory of the dreadful treatments and the diagnosis, believing everything would be OK. I'd already been down that road and it had only led to more cancer. This time I wouldn't be complacent. While my tumour load was low and I was still in relatively good shape, I felt it was a good time to be proactive, to be taking control, not waiting for the axe to fall yet again, knowing each time the cancer would become more and more difficult to treat.

Top of my list was a detox diet for my damaged gut. And a series of intravenous vitamin C infusions, given twice a week with integrative physician Dr Kingsley in Leicestershire. The mere mention of high-dose intravenous vitamin C causes many to shout, 'This has been disproved! Linus Pauling was discredited!' I stood in a meeting with several health editors recently and this was indeed the response. Next time I'll be more prepared. I'll have the recent medical literature to hand, which definitely proves its worth. Many patients are put off this valuable therapy by angry doctors, convinced it will only hasten their demise.

In fact, this forgotten and maligned treatment is rightly making a comeback, this time in combination with drugs and supplements to create a new form of cell death called 'ferroptosis', using iron to create even more free radicals. Big Pharma have, yet again, been hard at work quashing this cheaper alternative to chemo, but its great results are hard to counter.

Linus Pauling was a Nobel Laureate for chemistry in 1954, then discredited because he made a hypothesis about the action of vitamin C that was proven to be incorrect. However, his assumption that higher doses might be useful for cancer were indeed correct, just not in the way he thought. He and Dr Ewan Cameron were both convinced it had something to do with lowering hyaluronidase, an enzyme that caused the extra cellular matrix (the ground substance surrounding cancer cells) to soften, allowing cells to move apart and the cancer to spread. Pauling was so in favour of vitamin C that anything seeming to disprove his theories led to fierce debate. He was angry with how the studies were carried out and made many enemies defending it, but his anger was mainly frustration. Others were not investigating it in the way he had suggested: intravenously.

The two-time Nobel Prize winner was a genius, dragged through the mire only to be proved right decades later.[23] If you look at recent trials using intravenous ascorbate vitamin C, they show he was correct. So, before you throw this book into the bin, it's important to note that the early trials failed because they were performed using low **oral** doses. And later intravenous vitamin C was combined with glutathione, an antioxidant, which totally negated its pro-oxidant effect, another reason why many believe it is not useful.

Cameron and Pauling published the results of a clinical study in 1978, which showed survival of ascorbate treated individuals was 20 times greater than non-treated subjects. Another study in 1991 showed survival was 343 days for treated subjects compared to 180 for controls who did not received ascorbate. Crucially, these tests were performed using intravenous combined with oral vitamin C, not oral route alone.

Two clinical trials followed in the late '70s and early '80s, conducted by Moertel at the Mayo Clinic in Rochester, Minnesota. They showed that using vitamin C orally produced no such results. Moertel and Mayo concluded that there was no significant difference in survival between

---

23   Sadly, Pauling now has a page on Quackwatch, a site written by Pharma-indoctrinated individuals. The ignominy persists, perpetuating the idea that vitamin C is useless.

ascorbate-treated and untreated groups, whereas Cameron and Pauling had administered ascorbate orally and intravenously together.

Any good oncologist will tell you that free radicals, given the name 'reactive oxygen species', kill cancer. This is exactly how intravenous vitamin C works. At high doses it turns from an antioxidant into a pro-oxidant, giving off free oxygen to the area around a tumour.

In this case, the reactive oxygen species (ROS) is hydrogen peroxide (H_2O_2). This oxygen production near the cell causes a kind of 'rusting' and allows the cell to be attacked and killed. The balance of ROS production and the antioxidant status of cells is crucial to the survival or death of tumour cells. The judicious use of antioxidants is something I have seen patients continue to get wrong. Many patients take antioxidants that counter the effects of the intravenous vitamin C and then are disappointed it hasn't worked.

As is the case with any drug or supplement, the dosage determines whether it is effective, ineffective, or toxic. Using it in the right combination is also key. In the case of vitamin C, the sweet spot for its cancer-busting properties is a high dose. Unlike the situation with chemotherapy, more is most definitely more, and the higher the amount (up to 75g or in males 100g) the more it becomes selectively toxic to cancer cells by producing more H_2O_2. Patients often fail to understand the need to avoid specific antioxidant supplements like CoQ10, vitamin E, cysteine, and N-Acetyl Cysteine (including whey protein). However, ALA – alpha lipoic acid – in its reduced form as dihydrolipoic acid, with or immediately after intravenous vitamin C infusions recycles the vitamin C and helps maintain levels in the tissues, synergistically increasing its effects.[24] At lower oral doses ALA scavenges free radicals and in so doing

24   Scott BC, Aruoma OI, Evans PJ, O'Neill C, Van der Vliet A, Cross CE, Tritschler H, Halliwell B. Lipoic and dihydrolipoic acids as antioxidants. A critical evaluation. Free Radic Res. 1994 Feb;20(2):119-33. doi: 10.3109/10715769409147509. PMID: 7516789

can help prevent some of the common side effects of chemotherapy such as hearing loss with cisplatin or neuropathy symptoms such as pain, tingling or numbness with oxaliplatin.[25]

The hydrogen peroxide created by intravenous vitamin C treatment releases one of its oxygen molecules into the cancer microenvironment. The cancer cell must deal with the extra free radicals. Because cancer cells are unable to neutralise them – they lack the enzyme catalase – they die. Best of all, for such a potentially useful therapy, normal cells remain completely unharmed as the extracellular spaces adjacent healthy cells contain the catalase enzyme. In fact, intravenous vitamin C stops a key step in the process of glycolysis, effectively starving the cancer as well as triggering apoptosis or cell death. It helps block off one of cancer's main energy supply lines. This makes it 100 times more effective than chemotherapy for ridding the cancer stem cell which divides at a much slower rate than the bulk of tumour cells. Without getting rid of the stem cell, chemotherapy is doomed to fail.

It also makes it significantly safer than chemo. After coming into contact with the tumour, vitamin C releases one of its oxygen molecules, kills the cancer and then the H202 (hydrogen peroxide) turns into plain old water (H2O), which is then excreted safely by the kidneys. Simple chemistry that even a six-year-old could understand.

For a short time, I was fooled into thinking that oral levels of vitamin C could be taken up to 'bowel tolerance', but this is a dangerous strategy. It is my view that it is unlikely to raise blood plasma vitamin C to the pro-oxidant levels necessary to create hydrogen peroxide by oral route alone.

25   Guo Y, Jones D, Palmer JL, *et al.* Oral alpha-lipoic acid to prevent chemotherapy-induced peripheral neuropathy: a randomized, double-blind, placebo-controlled trial. *Support Care Cancer*. 2014;22(5):1223-1231. doi:10.1007/s00520-013-2075-1

If you go the liposomal vitamin C route, it **must** be ascorbate and **no less** than 5000mg should be taken in one go – possibly, to be safe, a little more – to block glycolysis.[26] There are alternative methods to block glycolysis which we will discuss in Part 2, but this is an important point because there are still many advocators of the bowel tolerance method. It may instead help immortalise the cancer and fuel its growth. The research is not clear on this yet and I may revise my thoughts as more information is made available as I predict vitamin C, especially given IV, will become more important in the future.

An infusion dose of vitamin C is typically from 25g up to 75g, depending on the tumour size and the weight of the patient. It is given three times a week or even daily for several weeks. The infusion of IV vitamin C increases plasma levels until it changes from being an antioxidant (neutralising oxygen) to a pro-oxidant by accumulating and creating hydrogen peroxide (H2O2) in the connective tissues around the tumour, but not in the blood. Perhaps because of this, intravenous vitamin C has been found to be more effective in solid tumours than in blood or lymph cancers, but more recent research is showing it is useful for these cancers too, probably because of its normalising effect on aerobic glycolysis, the abnormal cancer metabolism.

While on chemotherapy, I had seriously considered adding the high-dose intravenous vitamin C between sessions, but I didn't have the confidence to go through with it. Now, with hindsight and new research carried out at the University of Iowa by Levine and Buettner, I wish I had taken it between sessions of 'metronomic' (regularly spaced apart) low doses of chemotherapy.[27]

---

26 A 'liposomal' formulation means the molecule is encapsulated in a lipid so that it passes through the digestive tract in the small intestine and is taken directly into the blood stream.

27 https://now.uiowa.edu/2017/01/why-high-dose-vitamin-c-kills-cancer-cells

Integrative and alternative doctors have stood by and watched the misrepresentation and skewed results of the promising early data. Integrative doctors knew it worked and have been successfully using intravenous vitamin C as part of an overall strategy to treat cancer for decades. They witnessed with their own eyes its beneficial effects. But mistakes were also made by some integrative doctors, who tried adding glutathione to the infusions. This is the most important antioxidant in the body. It rendered the intravenous vitamin C useless by neutralising the pro-oxidant effect and may have made cancer patients worse by helping the malignant cells remain immortal, able to resist normal apoptosis mechanisms.

Doubt, disbelief and discreditation of doctors using natural, cheaper alternatives are recurring themes in complementary therapy. It takes a brave soul in the medical establishment to step outside the box, research a publicly discredited treatment and claim it does indeed work. A small trial on nine patients with pancreatic cancer using twice-weekly intravenous ascorbate infusions of 15-125g showed some efficacy.[28] Another trial on ovarian cancer showed that combining intravenous vitamin C with chemotherapy extended cancer survival and reduced toxicity. Mark Levine and Gary Buettner, authors of the latter trial, note that 'the atmosphere was poisoned' by the earlier failures with oral vitamin C.[29]

Few doctors feel ready to take the risk of scorn and derision by colleagues, so hats off to Buettner and Levine. Public criticism and humiliation on sites like Quackwatch provide the ultimate deterrent to doctors trying anything new or innovative. Thanks to their bravery this treatment is

---

28 Welsh, JL, Wagner, BA, van't Erve, TJ. Pharmacological ascorbate with gemcitabine for the control of metastatic and node-positive pancreatic cancer (PACMAN): results from a phase I clinical trial. Cancer Chemother Pharmacol. 2013;71:765-775.

29 Cieslak JA, Cullen JJ. Treatment of Pancreatic Cancer with Pharmacological Ascorbate. *Current pharmaceutical biotechnology*. 2015;16(9): 759-770.

now about to return, not as a miracle cure, but as an adjunct to other treatments.[30]

I wanted to start having intravenous vitamin C immediately after finishing chemo, so I hopped on a train up to see Dr Patrick Kingsley in Leicestershire a week later. I had asked the medics if I could keep my 'PICC line' in, a small tube that passed through a vein in my arm up into my chest for administering the chemotherapy. It would be useful for the vitamin C too.

When I arrived at Dr Kingsley's house (which was also his clinic) I saw why patients travelled from all over the country to see him. He was so reassuring that I immediately felt at ease.

My friend Cathy kindly offered to accompany me on my first trip. When I sat in the consulting room, I suddenly found I couldn't help crying. To my surprise tears just began rolling down my cheeks. It was a kind of emotional release I think, and relief that there **were** amazing doctors out there willing to administer these treatments and keep hope alive. These doctors were thinking and researching for themselves rather than blindly following protocols laid down by Big Pharma, the General Medical Council and NICE.

Cathy was a huge support, although slightly taken aback by the tears. I'd been laughing and joking on the train there. Dr Kingsley didn't try and make me stop. He let my cry, handed me tissues and instead talked me back to positivity.

'If there is any cancer left, we have to make sure we've stopped it growing, then we destroy it. Finally, we flush anything left out of your system.

30   Levine M et al Ascorbate in pharmacologic concentrations selectively generates ascorbate radical and hydrogen peroxide in extracellular fluid *in vivo* Proceedings of the National Academy of Sciences May 2007, 104 (21) 8749-8754

Only once we've done all of that can we get you back to full health. Intravenous vitamin C will help.'

Dr Kingsley didn't offer any guarantees but assured me he'd seen some great successes. I was keen to get going as soon as possible and blitz any remaining tumour cells. It only took a few of these little buggers to seed a new tumour and given there can be billions of tumour cells in an area the size of the end of a pencil, I wanted to get started immediately. I might have little time left to fight it. Effort now might pay huge dividends later.

I relaxed in one of the comfy armchairs in his sitting room to read a paper while the vitamin slowly infused into me over a period of a few hours. It was nothing like the clinical, sterile atmosphere of a medical setting. The Hammersmith Hospital instead screamed, 'You are a patient, you are ILL!'

At first, I was a little nervous about how it would feel. Other patients report an occasional mild stinging. But with the PICC line in place, I felt nothing.

After each intravenous infusion he would give me a treatment called Ultraviolet Blood Irradiation (UBI) to kill bacteria and viruses.[31] Cervical cancer (along with head and neck cancer) is linked to the HPV virus, so this made perfect sense to me.[32] An altered 'microbiome' (the mix of bacteria, fungi, parasites surrounding tumours) is slowly being recognised as a cause of the disease. It is this tumour microenvironment or terrain surrounding the cancer cells that is now the focus of research.

---

31   Wu X, Hu X, Hamblin MR. Ultraviolet blood irradiation: Is it time to remember "the cure that time forgot"?*J Photochem Photobiol B.* 2016;157:89-96. doi:10.1016/j.jphotobiol.2016.02.007

32   In fact scientists have now discovered at least seven cancer causing viruses and I suspect more will be found in the future. Also the tumour microenvironment can host many pathogens that might be parasites, bacteria, protozoa or fungi.

UBI was achieved by withdrawing a large syringe of blood from my arm through a line that was then passed under a UV lamp. This simple but effective technique (the Knott Technique) was regularly and successfully used back in the 1940s for polio and other viruses. With the introduction of mass vaccination programmes, it was side-lined and eventually phased out, except by a few holistic doctors. Nowadays, it's still used by the famous Riordan Clinic in Kansas but most people I talk to have never heard of it. There are clinics that now offer a more modern version of this treatment.[33]

UBI works its magic by acting as a natural antibiotic and stimulating an immune response. There is no question that UV kills pathogens – that's how city water supplies are sterilised, as well as some spas or pools. But how might it work if you can't treat the entire blood system, but only a few syringes of blood?

The difference between us and a swimming pool (well okay, not the only difference) is that we have an immune system, an army that normally does the job of cleaning up infections very efficiently. In cancer this immune army is suppressed, but UBI triggers a vaccine-like response, up-regulating it again. When pathogens die, they're left in a broken-down state in the blood. The remnants can then be recognised by the immune system. These become antigens that then stimulate your white cells to mount a more efficient attack on the pathogens, viral, bacterial or otherwise, that may be at the heart of your cancer.

Even when treatments use a very small amount of blood, UBI seems to have a beneficial effect. Is this a much cheaper, simpler and more effective alternative to the emerging use of dendritic vaccines that work on stimulating a patient's immune response? Or would the addition of this therapy alongside a dendritic vaccine help them work better? UV blood irradiation has been shown to provide a beneficial systemic response

---

33   See resources online at *www.howtostarvecancer.com*

(throughout the body), improving the abnormal microenvironment around cancer cells.[34, 35]

It may sound counter-intuitive, but when you have cancer you want, you **need** some free radicals to kill your tumour cells. Free radical generation is exactly the method orthodox medicine employs with chemotherapy and ionising radiation to kill tumour cells and why intravenous vitamin C works. Each method produces so many free radicals that it pushes cancer into self-destruction. Yes, those things we're all told to steer clear of, those troublesome radicals that cause so much damage and allegedly age us (I fear ageing has been mainly excess glucose and insulin, not just free radicals). We are told we should avoid them at all costs, right?

Wrong. Not when you want to get rid of cancer cells. Tumours defend themselves by neutralising ammonia (a result of abnormal cancer metabolism) by producing more of the major antioxidant glutathione to stop too much internal damage from oxidation and ammonia. By being able to do this, the cancer cells become immortal, resisting normal cell death. Glutathione and cysteine, which creates glutathione, are to be avoided, especially during a kill phase.

Giving these tumour cells an excess of free radicals overwhelms their defences, giving them the push they need to die through a normal

---

34 Given the huge implications of superbugs, a looming crisis for which we currently have no pharmaceutical solutions, using UBI would be an easy and cheap trial to run on patients. As the Riordan Clinic website says: 'The net result is the induction of a secondary kill of these infecting agents throughout the entire body. Treating only 35 cc of blood with UBI induces a beneficial systemic response.'

35 The current trend with resistant bacteria – like MRSA or clostridium difficile – is faecal microbiota transfer (yes, poo transplants – don't throw up). MRSA now kills more people than AIDS, and TB now has a resistant strain. Both are gaining ground fast. Maybe in the future there will be UBI clinics in every surgery, walk-ins for a six-monthly zap! Will UBI work against these superbugs on its own or as an adjunct to antibiotics and FMT? Phage therapy (viruses that kill bacteria) is another option with specific phages being bred to fight specific infections, a therapy to fight bacteria that has been used for decades in Russia.

process (apoptosis) activated in the mitochondria when there is too much damage. Chemotherapy and radiotherapy do the same, they provide free radicals, but they're normally given in such a way that they damage healthy cells in the process. What is not generally known is that you can replicate this free radical effect efficiently, and more selectively than either chemotherapy or radiotherapy, with high dose intravenous vitamin C. Even more exciting is the potential of certain supplements (e.g., artemisinin, piperlongumine) and drugs (e.g., sulfasalazine) in combination with intravenous vitamin C to trigger a process called ferroptosis, which could be the answer for many resistant cancers (see Part 2 for my ferroptosis protocol).

Free radicals (Reactive Oxygen Species or 'ROS') are chemically unstable oxygen molecules. ROS are chemically **reactive** molecules containing oxygen, such as hydrogen peroxide and superoxide, normally produced in low numbers during normal cell metabolism. It has been known for almost a century that oxygen selectively kills tumour cells. Cancer cells mostly favour a process of fermentation to make their energy, an anaerobic (oxygen free) process unlike normal healthy cells. This alternative energy pathway (known as The Warburg Effect) keeps the production of ROS lower and so helps ensure the tumour's survival. When a normal cell is injured (in the mitochondria, for example), an increase of ROS signals the white cells to come and sort out a problem to either repair or destroy the defective cell. The aim of chemotherapy, radiotherapy, and indeed high-dose intravenous vitamin C 27 is to create an excess of ROS, unstable free radicals, because when this exceeds the tumour cell's ability to neutralise the damage caused by the free radicals with glutathione, the cell is earmarked for destruction.

If you're now scratching your head, let me summarise: in cancer, ROS (oxygen free radicals) in high enough levels are good as these kill the cancer cells. Glutathione (antioxidant) is bad as it keeps the cancer cells alive. If you're healthy, it is the opposite. Almost everyone seems to confuse this point. Compounds for cancer prevention are not equally beneficial for treating active cancer. They are two separate situations entirely. There are major natural cancer organisations out there who mean well but have yet to realise this fundamental flaw when they recommend patients take N-Acetyl Cysteine (NAC), a precursor to glutathione, to help treat their disease.

NAC, low dose **oral** vitamin C – at an antioxidant dose, tocopherol vitamin E and CoQ10 all recycle the master antioxidant glutathione. All are to be avoided during chemotherapy treatment unless you want to blunt the effects. NAC is also found in whey protein and bone broth. Bone broth is great for healing the gut but choosing the right time to take this becomes paramount so that treatments don't cancel each other out. Taking glutamine with glucosamine is in my view a better strategy to heal the gut during chemotherapy as it is cysteine that is more dangerous. However, if at some point you need to boost white cells, detoxify of harmful metals (NAC is good at this too), or detox the effects of too much chemotherapy, then seek advice. A short burst of NAC may be beneficial. It is contentious and there will be divided opinions. If in doubt, leave it out.

I have also come across differing opinions between complementary therapists and other health practitioners about whether you should take the amino acid glutamine during chemotherapy, which can also be used to make glutathione, but it cannot create this without the presence of cysteine. Lowering cysteine intake is a better strategy than reducing glutamine. Glutamine can indeed fuel cancer cells but it's also crucial for the defence of the body. It heals and maintains a good gut lining and is essential for the proper workings of the immune system. It is the most abundant amino acid in the body. It can be sequestered from anywhere in your system to feed cancer's insatiable appetite, so cutting it out from the diet may be a poor decision during chemotherapy. If your muscles are wasting away, it's a sign that your body has a high demand for glutamine.

It's best to starve glutamine indirectly, by working on the enzymes that break down glutamine for fuel (e.g., glutaminase or ketoglutarate dehydrogenase – see my 'Metro Map') or glutamine transport (EGCG). Although your cancer cells demand it, your body needs it too.[36] Cancer will grab glutamine from any of your tissues whether you starve it or not and replenishing it should not be feared. It is lowering cysteine levels thereby blocking the production of the antioxidant glutathione that is a more important strategy to weaken the cancer cell.

Researching diabetes treatments, I discovered that elevated circulating insulin also elevates insulin-like growth factor (IGF-1), which in turn stimulates cysteine and other amino acid uptake. This in turn then boosts glutathione levels, allowing the cancer cells' immortality and the ability to neutralise ROS.[37] This is one reason why diabetics have much higher rates of cancer and are much harder to treat.

Oxygen is known to attack and kill cancer cells. In fact, researchers use it to destroy cancer cells at the end of an experiment. Normal cells are aerobic – they can deal with an oxygen environment – whereas the stem cells in a tumour cannot. They metabolise their energy anaerobically, like primordial single cells did aeons ago, before the earth was oxygenated. With glutathione lowered, the cell is much more vulnerable to an increase in oxygenating substances, making it far easier to destroy (through the 'caspase cascade'). I was to discover a way to trigger this apoptotic (cell death) process more easily using a better combination a few years later.

---

36 Glutamine is excellent for healing a leaky gut and for helping to arm your white blood cells, in particular your Natural Killer cells. It is also vital to the peyers patches, which is where a large part of your immune system lies. I'd use alongside arginine (unless you have an arginine-fuelled cancer like sarcoma). Both are vital in this battle.

37 I would find out later that this is one reason why metformin is useful for cancer treatment – it lowers IGF-1, which in turn reduces the cysteine uptake and therefore lowers glutathione.

Most cancer patients, when they think of oxygenating the body, immediately think of hyperbaric oxygen therapy (HBOT), a chamber used initially for deep-sea divers to stop the bends and now used for MS sufferers. Or they think of ozone or DMSO, both useful too. But patients need to seriously consider using intravenous vitamin C as a powerful oxygenating method to kill cancer alongside chemotherapy.

Chemotherapy at high doses wrecks the gut. No question. Many patients are so severely affected it means they can no longer eat normally afterwards. My gut, I felt sure, had suffered damage too, but because I'd insisted on the lower dose I hoped I'd fared better than most. I was confident I could repair it.

By now my head was swimming with a lot of information which was hard to compute with 'chemo-brain'. I was learning and assimilating so much. There was no doubt the medical profession was failing to realise that whatever they were prescribing, it was nowhere near enough to fight the disease. It was hard to take everything I wanted to take during treatment. Worried for my stomach, I had dropped taking aspirin and instead I took pycnogenol, a natural but not necessarily equal alternative. I tried curcumin for its anti-inflammatory benefits, but it often made me feel nauseous. Instead, I kept inflammation down by taking more fish oils.

After my chemotherapy treatment finished, I came across another fish oil, shark liver oil (SLO), which would not only help control inflammation with its omega-3 content, but also contained high levels of other beneficial substances. Sharks rarely get cancer although a few solid tumours have been detected. But there have been no cases of blood cancers that I can find. A Scandinavian oncologist called Dr Astrid Brohult decided to study shark liver oil after first noting the beneficial effects of calves' marrow on children with Leukaemia (a blood cancer). She discovered that the calves' marrow had immune stimulating effects because of compounds called alkylglycerols (AKGs). Dr Brohult then realised these compounds were found in significantly higher levels in shark liver oil.

The AKGs occur in humans in our bone marrow and spleen (in very small amounts) and are involved in making our white and red blood cells. These compounds are also found in human breast milk (there are ten times more AKG compounds in breast than in cow's milk) and these are thought to make a significant contribution to an infant's immune system.

Dr Brohult discovered that shark liver oil stopped cancer proliferation and radiation sickness. A study on cervical cancer patients taking SLO before, during and after radiotherapy found that it reduced radiation-induced injuries by a very significant 50%.[38] Dr Brohult suggests that a dose of 0.3-2.6g will help minimise the associated decrease in platelets and white blood cells that accompany radiation treatment.

The mighty shark's resistance to cancer was mistakenly thought to be attributed to shark cartilage after William Lane published his book *Sharks Don't Get Cancer* in 1992 reporting that this was the secret ingredient. The medical profession was quick to damn this suggestion after repeated experiments with shark cartilage failed to show any direct cancer killing effects. After that anything 'shark' related was tainted and it caused much uproar when it was discovered that William Lane's son was selling shark cartilage products.

Shark liver oil contains four anti-cancer substances: squalene, omega-3, alkylglycerol and squalamine.

The substance squalene has a partial inhibitory feedback loop on the mevolonate pathway, the same growth pathway used by cancer cells to

---

38   Iannitti T, Palmieri B. An Update on the Therapeutic Role of Alkylglycerols. *Marine Drugs*. 2010;8(8): 2267-2300. doi: 10.3390/md8082267.

make cholesterol that's blocked by statin drugs, as I would learn later. (Statins are particularly effective for blood cancers). The alkylglycerol component of shark liver oil has an immune stimulating effect, improving the production of all the blood components (haematopoiesis) so it reduces side effects of radiotherapy, also boosting white cell counts and improving platelet counts during chemotherapy.[39] There was a suggestion that taking shark liver for several months might 'thicken' the blood too much. But most patient's blood counts suffer horribly with the traditional treatments, as mine did. I wish I had discovered it earlier.

The alkylglycerols also perform another important function alongside their immune-boosting effects – they reduce a key growth factor that promotes angiogenesis called basic Fibroblast Growth Factor.[40] And the squalamine content is causing much excitement amongst researchers for its antiviral effects. Sharks have a rudimentary immune system but are surprisingly resistant to viral infections. Viruses are known co-factors associated with many cancers. Rather than fighting the virus directly, it makes the blood and liver resistant to infection by 'kicking off' proteins that stick to the inside of blood vessels. These proteins are a source of food for some viruses and without them the viruses are starved to death.[41]

Squalene is also found at lower levels in olive oil (0.7% versus circa 40% in SLO) and amaranth oil (6-8%), which of course are more

39   Mitre, R., Etienne, M., Martinais, S., Salmon, H., Allaume, P., Legrand, P., & Legrand, A. (2005). Humoral defence improvement and haematopoiesis stimulation in sows and offspring by oral supply of shark-liver oil to mothers during gestation and lactation. British Journal of Nutrition, 94(5), 753-762.

40   **-O-Alkylglycerols reduce the stimulating effects of bFGF on endothelial cell proliferation in vitro. Pédrono**, Frédérique *et al.* Cancer Letters, Volume 251, Issue 2, 317-32

41   Michael Zasloff, A. Paige Adams, Bernard Beckerman, Ann Campbell, Ziying Han, Erik Luijten, Isaura Meza, Justin Julander, Abhijit Mishra, Wei Qu, John M. Taylor, Scott C. Weaver, Gerard C. L. Wong. **Squalamine as a broad-spectrum systemic antiviral agent with therapeutic potential.** *Proceedings of the National Academy of Sciences*, 2011; DOI: 10.1073/pnas.1108558108

environmentally friendly (I blush with shame at my use of shark liver oil, but it was the only option I knew about). It's one component that may make extra virgin olive oil (EVOO) especially good at fighting cancer (hydroxytyrosol and oleocanthol are others, found in high enough levels in quality oil only though). I used lashings of it on my food – I still have a couple of spoonfuls first thing every day even now – along with cod liver oil for its omega-3 DHA and EPA anti-inflammatory effect. I also add danshen (red sage) to mitigate any downsides of oleic oil. Fish liver oils are also a natural and balanced source of vitamins A and D, both essential for the correct functioning of the PPAR gamma pathway, which monitors inflammation and metabolism homeostasis.

I am hoping that alkylglycerols are now available without damaging the populations of those majestic sea creatures. If you do decide to take shark liver oil, perhaps take for three months only as I did as this may be enough to have a long-lasting effect on your immunity.

Was I winning? I couldn't be sure, but regular blood tests helped confirm that for now I was doing all right. I was staying within 'normal' limits. I had to keep blind faith that I was on the right track.

The diet was especially hard to maintain. I no longer craved the sweet foods, but could I never let my hair down again? Was my future to be lived on a knife edge, checking foods all the time, unable to go out and allow myself a couple of cheeky drinks? Was there no easier way?

Chapter Nine:

Beating the Odds

Each month I tracked my blood markers. Even as a physiotherapist I had been taught that stage IV meant certain death. It was unavoidable. The cancer would come back.

I tried hard to block out the negative thoughts. I refused to believe it. I knew starving the cancer and halting its growth was key to preventing an unwelcome return. It was tough going, sticking to the diet, but I learnt to adapt, and soon realised that I really didn't miss all those unhealthy foods I'd eaten in the past. Well, maybe watching others tucking into a bacon sandwich on a Sunday morning still made me yearn wistfully for a bite – but mostly, I didn't feel like I was missing out.

As my blood markers remained within normal levels, my faith in my own abilities was slowly growing. And as self-doubt faded, I began to feel so confident in my progress that I threw myself back into the toiletries business I'd started just before the diagnosis of secondary cancer in my lungs. It was certainly a welcome distraction from the dreary hospital appointments, the nail-biting wait for results and the sad and sorry looks from the medical staff. I could see what they were thinking. They'd all been taught the same dogma. 'Stage IV. I wonder how long she's got?'

In the hospital, I was constantly putting up barriers to the undercurrent of negativity I knew was lurking just below the surface. I was not immune to thoughtless off-cuff remarks from the staff. My inner equilibrium could be knocked off balance by the slightest hint of pessimism.

'I am really pleased with my progress,' I said to a nurse taking my blood pressure. 'Let's hope I can keep it at bay now.'

'When it comes back, I'm sure there'll be many new therapies to consider.'

'Don't you mean if?' I replied, shocked at her lack of empathy. I bet I knew more about how to control my cancer than she did. How dare she assume progression was inevitable? It made my resolve even stronger.

At home I was juggling sales meetings, new toiletries formulations, creating designs for bottles, tubes and gift boxes, and sourcing production from all over the world. Creating a brand-new product range was exciting. It was also a kind of organised chaos, an antidote to my structured and scheduled medical regime.

A period of 'extreme multi-tasking' is how I would describe these years. But I always put aside twenty minutes for daily meditation. I did this immediately after my morning supplements. I made time for a bike ride or a brisk walk to the park after lunch. This was surely boosting my immunity, oxygenating my blood and allowing my body to soak up any glucose released from my food.

Starve cancer. It became my mantra. I would chant it as I marched briskly around the block or the park, squeezing each buttock in turn with every step as I did so, hoping no-one noticed my bizarre bottom-clenching gait! I would stop occasionally to do a few knee squats by a bench. I wanted to make sure my gluteus maximus, the biggest muscle in our bodies, was getting a decent workout. It didn't take a genius to work out it'd be the ideal one to target (along with the quads in the thighs). Muscles make up 40% of our body mass and provide a valuable sink to soak up excess glucose, the bigger the muscles, the better you responded to treatment.[42] Exercise also increases insulin sensitivity in the tissues, so it becomes ever more efficient at taking up the glucose and using it.

Even with the distraction of starting a business, I was still learning and assimilating new cancer information and trying to formulate a new anti-cancer strategy. If, after everything I'd done, the cancer made its return, I would need a contingency plan. I continued to buy survivor stories, huge tomes on alternative medicine and many other books and journals. My home cancer library now filled several shelves.

I still felt sure there were other 'big guns' I might have missed. Green tea, with its powerful ingredient epigallocatechin gallate (EGCG) was at the top of the list. But it only had a short half-life, so I would need to drink it constantly through the day, sometimes as many as ten cups per day! Other natural compounds were also big guns. Curcumin targeted inflammatory pathways, while genistein, silibinin (milk thistle), quercetin and resveratrol all seemed to stop cancer growing and spreading.[43] All became constants in my routine, alongside my supplement cocktail and morning juice of beetroot, celery, carrot and apple. Quite how they might starve cancer I had yet to find out, but each seemed to be very effective from the research I'd seen on their cancer-killing and angiogenesis-blocking activity. All were taken at every mealtime.

There seemed to be no 'one size fits all' for diet. Each complementary doctor had an individual style of treatment, yet all focused on rectifying

---

42　Osaka University. "Increased muscle mass improves response to cancer treatment." ScienceDaily. ScienceDaily, 4 March 2019. <*www.sciencedaily.com/releases/2019/03/190304100040.htm*>.

43　Genistein may promote oestrogen-driven breast cancer. However genistein levels in fermented soy products such as tempeh, tamari and tofu are low. These foods appear to be beneficial for every cancer, including breast cancer. Young H. Ju, Kimberly F. Allred, Clinton D. Allred, William G. Helferich, Genistein stimulates growth of human breast cancer cells in a novel, postmenopausal animal model, with low plasma estradiol concentrations, Carcinogenesis, Volume 27, Issue 6, June 2006, Pages 1292–1299, https://doi.org/10.1093/carcin/bgi370

deficiencies of vitamins and minerals (e.g. magnesium and A, B, D, K vitamins) or adding supplements that would enhance other treatments. But more than anything, they were all completely against sugar.

Making vegetable juices, exercising, home cooking, sourcing healthy food, exploring new ones, researching, meditating, hospital appointments, the business, it all took time. This was hardly the kind of lifestyle I would recommend to anyone just out of a terminal diagnosis. It was exhausting. In the evenings I would slide into a warm naturally fragranced bath, light candles, play music and relax for half an hour. Shutting out the hustle and bustle of the day was important. I needed my own little sanctuary just for thinking. Or not thinking. It became my nightly refuge.

In the end I created my own Tranquillity Spa CD, a relaxation ritual with a bit of reflexology, affirmations and visualisations all included, designed primarily for myself – but later I packaged it up as a gift pack with candles, mineral-rich bath salts and a bath pillow. When I launched, the pack was shortlisted for Gift of the Year.

Bath time was a great place to ponder life, business, my cancer and all its complexities. Once I had calmed my racing thoughts, I would think about how my cancer was behaving and try and see the bigger picture. I had no detectable cancer in my body, but I was not about to sit back and rest. It could pounce at any time. 'When it comes back', were the words that always haunted me. The wily cancer cell had been able to divert and steal my body's nutrients, rewire its blood supply and switch off my own immunity. How could I outwit this parasite?

Parasites thrive and reproduce unabated until either their food source runs out or, in the case of cancer, the host dies. I was determined to work out how I could starve my cancer without also starving and damaging myself. On the outside, it appeared to be super powerful, able to resist the most toxic of treatments, to mutate and create drug resistance just when you thought you were getting the upper hand. A cunning little beast. But was it really powerful, or did it just reroute itself down whichever path was left unblocked? What if you blocked all the routes? How many were there? Was it an impossible task to find out? Was it just IGF-1 and aerobic glycolysis, the Warburg Effect? If so, then why was it so hard to treat? There must be other metabolic pathways that needed blocking.

Cancer research was becoming more reductive, with scientists examining smaller and smaller parts of the cancer genome and then turning their attention to the immune system when the genomic treatments failed them. What had gone wrong with the patient's immunity to allow the cancer to thrive?

What had come first, the altered immunity or the cancer? What if the altered immunity was a result of an altered metabolism and inflammation? If so, targeting the immune system would be futile unless you shut down the altered metabolism and switched off the inflammation first.[44] Moreover, how had cancer started? Had researchers and orthodox doctors lost sight of the bigger picture?

I lay there thinking about how the cancer cell was different to a normal cell. It had been reprogrammed to endlessly divide and make two 'daughter' cells and to do this it used huge amounts of nutrients. On a very basic level, cells are made up of various proteins (enzymes, organelles, nucleic acids, etc.) encapsulated by a fatty membrane. Each cancer cell would need both the fat required for new cell membranes as well as protein for building new internal cell structures. Like building a house, you need a workforce (the energy to build it) and bricks and mortar. With cancer the main energy source seemed to be glucose, but it needed access to fat and protein too to build its cell structure.

---

44 This was a correct assumption. Cerezo, M., Rocchi, S. Cancer cell metabolic reprogramming: a keystone for the response to immunotherapy. *Cell Death Dis* **11**, 964 (2020). https://doi.org/10.1038/s41419-020-03175-5

The process was essentially the same no matter what type of cancer it was; pancreatic, lymphoma or breast. Starving these cells of fat and the protein they needed was surely important, as well as blocking the glucose they used for the cell division. Did that mean a starvation diet might work? But even when patients had cachexia, when the body began wasting away, the cancer often continued to thrive, stealing nutrients from other parts of the body. It certainly seemed to be a systemic problem, affecting the whole person, not just a zone or specific area in the body.

I gleaned information from every doctor I saw and read as many journals as I could find to try and work out the best diet. I had cut out potatoes, aubergines, tomatoes, rhubarb, strawberries and all citrus foods.

Grapefruit was the worst. They were all too acidic or inflammatory for me. I ate no dairy apart from a little parmesan as a treat (it contains butyric acid, or sodium butyrate, which stops the loosening and instability of DNA – an HDAC inhibitor)[45] and occasionally a little bioactive yoghurt. It was more about how my body was able to digest the food, the glycaemic index and how it reacted to different food types. We all have different gut microbiomes, and my body was sending me signals to avoid certain foods. If I bloated after a meal, then I must have triggered an inflammatory reaction in my gut and inflammation needed to be avoided at all costs.

Meals were no longer a source of comfort as they had been in the past and cooking was an added burden to my already jam-packed day, so my meals were very basic. I would have simple salads with a bit of short grain brown rice doused with olive oil at lunchtimes. I wondered if this intense level of commitment was necessary, there was really no way of knowing, but when I remembered the statistics, I knew I had little choice. I would never be able to return to my pre-cancer diet.

---

45   Steliou, Kosta *et al.* "Butyrate histone deacetylase inhibitors." *BioResearch open access* vol. 1,4 (2012): 192-8. doi:10.1089/biores.2012.0223

If cancer needed both fat and protein for creating two identical new progenies, as well as glucose for energy to create them, then starving the cancer was going to be tricky. I needed to cut all three food sources, the 'macros' in my diet — fat, carb and protein — and just starving myself might kill me in the process. It didn't seem to be a long-term solution. I wondered if there were some foods I could eat safely that cancer didn't like.

Cutting back on volume came first. The benefits of caloric restriction for cancer were reported as early as 1914 by Peyton Rous,[46] who also discovered that viruses could trigger the disease. His work on a viral cause for cancer was not given proper recognition until much later – he was finally awarded a Nobel Prize in 1966. No-one has yet acknowledged his observations on diet restriction in mice or his suggestion that it could be useful for many cancers. The effects of underfeeding gained attention again in 1940,[47] but it lost momentum with the advent of chemotherapy and the scramble for new 'game changers'. The latest drugs were supposedly magic bullets.

A reduction in volume seemed like an obvious approach to try, even without sight of this research. I gradually ate smaller and smaller portions. Perhaps this alone would be enough to tip the balance, weaken the cancer and allow my immune system to regain the upper hand.[48]

Reducing protein was relatively easy, but were beans and lentils a healthier substitute? I couldn't be sure.[49]

---

46 The Influence of Diet on Transplanted and Spontaneous Mouse Tumours. By Peyton Rous, M.D. 1914 Rockefeller Institute Laboratories

47 A. Tannenbaum, and Silverstone. The initiation and growth of tumors. Introduction. I. Effects of underfeeding. **Am. J. Cancer. 38: 335-350 (1940).**

48 If you have cachexia, then intermittent fasting may be more appropriate.

49 Some beans are indeed very high in glutamate, a fuel for cancer but great for ferroptosis.

In my quest to lower unwanted fat and simple carbohydrates, several supplements piqued my interest. Gymnema sylvestre is an Indian Ayurvedic herb and a trial on diabetic patients (Type 1 and 2) showed it reduced glucose. It also seemed to raise insulin levels, but this was in response to food, so it made insulin work more efficiently, improving sensitivity. I was still taking **Mahonia aquifolium** tincture but no-one else had written about berberine, the main constituent of **Mahonia aquifolium** for cancer. There was no trace of it in any of the literature.

If no one was using berberine for cancer maybe I was wrong, perhaps it wasn't as good as I thought. In 2002, I decided to swap berberine and try Gymnema instead as the article on Mahonia (which had mentioned its anti-tumoural, antimicrobial, anti-inflammatory as well as glucose-lowering effects) in the 1999 *Journal of Herbal Medicine* was fading from my memory, crowded out by the clutter of additional information. This swap was a mistake in hindsight. The combination may have worked synergistically.

Hydroxycitrate, from a plant called Garcinia Cambogia found in India, was able to modify and reduce fat in the body. My instincts were fortunately correct as I later discovered this compound could block ATP citrate lyase which converts the excess pyruvate produced by cancer cells into fatty acids for making new cell membranes.[50] But would it then just push the cancer to use more glycolytic or other fat driven metabolic pathways? Research relating to cancer was non-existent for both gymnema and hydroxycitrate – it was all about diabetes and weight loss. But in they went, into my cancer-starving regime. Blocking each cancer fuel supply was imperative.

But how many were there? Was I blocking enough?

---

50   Hatzivassiliou G., Zhao F., Bauer D.E., Andreadis C., Shaw A.N., Dhanak D., Hingorani S.R.,Thompson C.B. ATP citrate lyase inhibition can suppress tumor cell growth. (2005) *Cancer Cell*, 8 (4), pp. 311-321.

Chromium Picolinate was shown to improve insulin sensitivity and improve glycaemic control, so perhaps it would make the Gymnema work better and reduce the insulin. Taking the two together might work synergistically. Sure enough, a later review of both treatments by physician Richard Nahas in 2009 showed that both gymnema and chromium picolinate to be effective for glycaemic control.[51]

Niacin-B3. This precursor of the coenzyme NAD (nicotinamide adenine dinucleotide) has fat reducing properties too. It also has a beneficial effect on insulin although the mechanism for this is less clear. Niacin is important in not just the breakdown of fat, but also carbohydrate, protein and alcohol breakdown and storage, as well as cell signalling and DNA repair. It may be very useful in the post treatment period as well, when the body needs to rebuild cells with normal mitochondria.[52]

A higher caloric intake is associated with more aggressive and worse survival cancer rates, but was this a result of too much sugar, too much fat, too much protein, or just too much of everything? Omega-6 oils promoted cancer growth, this was very clear. I completely avoided sunflower oil and other processed vegetable oils as they made inflammation worse. In contrast, the Mediterranean diet had a much lower incidence of cancer. Perhaps olive oil was a 'safe' fat to use despite containing omega 6. Its high omega-9 content I learned neutralised the omega-6, which could be further reduced by taking a supplement called Danshen. I used butter sparingly, even though it contained the vitamins A, D and K and something called Conjugated Linoleic Acid (CLA).

CLA was reported to have huge beneficial effects for both prevention and treatment of cancer. Many natural substances contain this fatty acid (butter, cheese, saturated fat in red meat) but I wanted to avoid saturated

51 Nahas R, Moher M. Complementary and alternative medicine for the treatment of type 2 diabetes. **Canadian Family Physician**. 2009;55(6): 591-596.
52 Niacin is sometimes used in combination with statins to lower LDL cholesterol, but this can increase the risk of muscle problems. A slow-release version may be safer.

fat, so taking a supplement was the safer option. It was the omega-7 part of CLA, the palmitoleic acid, which I have since discovered was the beneficial part. Not to be confused with palmitic acid, a bad oil, (although this can be neutralised by omega 9), palmitoleic acid can be found in both olive oil and sea buckthorn oil. And the most beneficial part of palmitoleic acid is vaccenic (aka rumenic) acid. A natural trans-fat! This has beneficial effects on high blood sugar, elevated lipid levels, inflammation and excess fat gain, and it enhances insulin sensitivity. It is a super nutrient.

Instead of taking CLA as a supplement as I did in those days, I now take a daily Sea Buckthorn oil capsule, which contains omega 7. But it only really works efficiently in the presence of bifidobacteria in the gut. Hence the need for checking your gut has adequate amounts and no 'dysbiosis', or abnormal levels of pathogenic bacteria. For metabolic health, I believe everyone should include omega-7 alongside adequate omega-3 (fish oils) and omega-9 to help prevent all the major metabolic diseases: Alzheimer's, cancer, stroke, metabolic syndrome and heart disease. As a follower of both medical trends and the latest trends in cosmetics and toiletries, I always see the cosmetics industry taking on board these beneficial nutrients much faster. Sea Buckthorn oil has been big news for a while in toiletries, and yet is still virtually unheard of as a supplement. It should be big news in cancer and cardiovascular treatment too!

Periodically, Dr Callebout reviewed my supplements and to my horror he would prescribe yet more. He prescribed Vitamin K3 and maitake-D-fraction (a mushroom extract), which has been shown to both boost immunity and enhance the effects of intravenous vitamin C. He also prescribed DHEA (not recommended for hormone-related cancers) which enhanced my wellbeing and immunity and it also 'starves cancer' by blocking the pentose phosphate pathway, part of the process of building new DNA molecules.

All cancer patients researching their disease will come across articles that link cancer to sugar, poor diets or lifestyle habits. The result is that on top of feeling unwell there is an unspoken sense of guilt and shame that somehow you had played a part in causing your illness. This may not in fact be the case, despite reports that lifestyle and environmental factors (like pathogens) and carcinogens are thought to be up to 90% responsible for cancer.[53] Avoiding pathogens can be impossible unless you live like a hermit at the North Pole. Parasites, bacteria and fungi are all linked as well as the well-known association of viruses. Many viruses are linked to cancer such as Epstein Barr, HPV,[54] hepatitis B and C, CMV,[55] human T-lymphotropic virus, Kaposi's sarcoma-associated herpes virus (KSHV) and Merkel cell polyomavirus. More are being discovered as scientists actively search for a link; the bovine leukaemia virus (a virus highly prevalent in milk worldwide) was added in 2015 as a risk for breast cancer. I suspect many more cancers will be linked to viruses in the future.

Many people eat appalling diets and have shocking lifestyles yet remain immune to cancer, while vegans who pride themselves on their healthy lifestyle can be afflicted too. But the media propagates this blame culture. This victimisation of the patient is unwelcome and unhelpful baggage; those with the disease stoically submit themselves to tortuous and barbaric treatments with little complaint, a punishment they feel they deserve for failing to be a paragon of health before. With cancer shouldn't you expect to suffer horribly to get well? If a medical treatment

---

53   Genetics are responsible for just 5-10% of cancers.

54   HPV infection is thought to be the most common sexually transmitted infection, but like all viruses is only 'contagious' for a short duration when it is active. These retroviruses access the human DNA and when the DNA is 'loosened' (histones lose their polarity) and mutated they trigger further mutagenic changes, triggering faster cell division. Hence why they are often thought of as the 'cause' (another incorrect dogma) although they are 'downstream' to metabolic changes (acetylation of the histones/DNA).

55   40-100% of the world's population have CMV antibody present in blood as evidence of infection, the highest prevalence being in countries in the developing world.

doesn't make you feel violently ill and have terrible side effects, then it can't possibly be killing or controlling all those pesky cancer cells, can it? Isn't cancer virtually impossible to rid unless you load yourself up with large doses of toxic chemicals? After decades of burning and poisoning ourselves with these destructive treatments, the 'standard of care', we are programmed to believe this nonsense.

I felt the self-blame too. I had abused my insides all my life, thoughtlessly downing foods and drinks that disagreed with me and made me bloated or tired. I too felt I had to be strict and hard on myself with a punishing and gruelling diet. Had I in some way been remiss and allowed cancer to develop?

Dr Callebout pressed upon me the need to sort out whatever might be wrong with my intestinal health and to check the nutrient levels in my blood. Now I was through chemotherapy, I knew it was essential to be properly assessed and have my stools checked and my micronutrient, fatty acid, vitamin and mineral profiling examined. My medical training had done me a disservice in this department. Diet and my intestines had always taken a back seat, never receiving the attention they desperately needed, as the focus or the reason why other systems in the body go wrong.

Many cancer patients will be able to tell you about infection in the gut or in the site where cancer developed. Why these prior infections are treated as irrelevant and unacknowledged in oncology is truly astonishing. Oncologists see cancer as a totally organic disease that somehow developed out of nowhere, ignoring all the other infections that came before. There are many different causes of cancer, many from infectious diseases, but most integrative doctors will tell you that every cancer patient, at some point, has had a problem with their intestinal health.

Today, much emerging research is focused on the 'microbiome', the collection of organisms that live on and in us, and the nature of our symbiotic relationship. Scientists are trying to establish why correcting the microbiome has such a big impact on the health of the cancer patient, no matter where the cancer has developed.[56] Every little crevice on every surface in our bodies is home to legions of tiny microorganisms and the gut has by far the most.

I am not alone in my assumption that my intestines would just deal with dietary abuse, whilst accepting that fatigue, bloating and irregular bowel movements were perfectly normal. I had not appreciated how easily our gut linings are damaged, particularly in early life with the use of antibiotics, or other supposedly 'safe' drugs. How they might lead to later damage and longer term systemic effects and disease is only just beginning to be appreciated.

My own gut woes may have stemmed from an infection in my early twenties. I'd been on holiday with my family, windsurfing off a popular tourist beach in Turkey. After a series of failed 'carve gybes' and subsequent 'face plants', I drank far more seawater than I had intended and a couple of days later had developed lobar pneumonia in my lungs. The mere act of breathing brought out the searing pain of pleuritis (inflammation of the lung membranes) and if this wasn't torture enough, I had a dose of pericarditis (inflammation of the membranes around the heart) thrown in, which caused severe pain to radiate down from my neck and shoulder into my left arm. I couldn't lie down, so nights were spent sitting up on deck unable to sleep, watching the stars. I really should have been in hospital.

---

56 They need to look at the PPAR gamma pathway – in my view the most important for regulation of our metabolism, needed for prevention and critical for treatment too. This pathway begins in the gut

A local doctor prescribed a course of crude, uncoated and strong antibiotics, after which nothing stayed down, not even water. I have never been so thin! I dropped a stone in weight within a week to just over seven and a half stone. All of this in forty degrees of heat and on a boat. I became completely dehydrated, and felt so terrible I remember thinking that if I fell over the side I had no intention of saving myself. I would have quite happily slipped beneath the waves never to return.

Those antibiotics must have totally wrecked my gut and upset my microbial ecosystem. I had no clue about probiotic use in those days. No-one did. With both good and bad bacteria wiped out, my defences were at an all-time low. It may well have been at this time that I picked up a parasite.

Now I was fighting the spectre of cancer, years later, I was aware that the gut was the centre of my immunity and I would not be well until I had fixed it. Re-establishing a good 'gut balance' was a critical part of the jigsaw as well as mending my damaged insides.

I decided periods of intermittent fasting might allow my gut to rest, heal and reduce any inflammation. As a physiotherapist it was usual to advise rest and anti-inflammatory treatments (such as ice and ultrasound) for a damaged body part, before the process of rehab. Dr Callebout was in favour of intermittent fasting, or time-restricted feeding, allowing the intestines to rest after three p.m. until the following morning. The rationale being that the liver is more active in the morning and better able to process food. This would also starve the cancer of course.

He explained about the constant turf war going on in our intestines, the balance of our beneficial (commensal) versus bad (pathogenic) bacteria constantly shifting, particularly when we take antibiotics or eat and drink unhealthy foods. Doctors rarely suggest a course of probiotics after antibiotics or advise staying off sugary foods during treatment. But if the balance shifts the wrong way and pathogenic bacteria become more dominant, they may eventually secrete enough 'exotoxins' to cause a break down in the single cell gut lining. This single-cell thickness in our intestinal walls is all that protects us from infection entering our bodies from the outside. When those cells lining the gut are damaged by exotoxins, inflammation occurs and loosens the tight junctions between the cells. Once these junctions are disrupted, it creates the condition known as 'leaky gut' or Intestinal Hyperpermeability Syndrome, which if you mention it, elicits much eye-rolling in the medical community.

Because it's not taught in medical schools and the pharmaceutical companies have yet to develop a drug for it, to many doctors leaky gut is a condition that doesn't exist. But it is very real indeed and leaves us easy prey to opportunistic infections and it can also trigger autoimmune disease.[57] As luck would have it, I was already taking one of the best gut healing compounds as part of my self-treatment, I just didn't know it at the time. Hurrah for berberine!

While healthy levels of good bacteria make important nutrients like vitamin K and B, unhealthy levels of pathogenic bacteria create leaky gut, allowing other pathogens and their toxic by-products easy passage into our bodies. Once inside, they alter the microenvironment around normal stem cells, creating inflammation and thereby abnormal stem cells, which lie at the heart of every cancer. This, I believe, is the root cause of cancer, which coupled with other resident viruses, yeasts or other pathogens create a welcoming environment for the cancer stem cells to begin an abnormal metabolism and flourish.

'I have your test results,' Dr Callebout announced in the summer of 2000. 'You have really good levels of bifidobacteria and lactobacilli in

---

57   Qinghui Mu, Jay Kirby, Christopher M. Reilly, Xin M. Luo Leaky Gut As a Danger Signal for Autoimmune Diseases Front Immunol. 2017

your lower gut, but I'm afraid you have quite a number of parasites called *Blastocystis hominis*.'

'Blasted what?!' I said. 'Parasites? Gross! How do I get rid of them?'

'Parasites are far more common than you think,' he said. I was amazed to discover just how rife they are among humans: up to 100% in some poorer countries, with infection rates on the rise elsewhere. In the United States, 23% of the total population were infected with *Blastocystis hominis* in 2000.

'It won't be easy to get rid of it. You're going to have to follow a very strict regime,' he added.

Fine. I was following a pretty strict regime already, so in for a penny in for a pound. I knew a list of further supplements would be added to my growing compendium.

'This protozoal parasite might be the cause of your lowered thyroid results. The two are often connected,' he added.

I already had some of the classic symptoms associated with *Blastocystis hominis* infection, the main one being serious fatigue. I'd assumed it was the cervical cancer or my hectic lifestyle but perhaps this 'blasted' parasite was the real reason. Other common symptoms can include bloating, diarrhoea, nausea, flatulence, abdominal pain, hives and variable bowel habits.[58]

Parasites no longer just infect travellers abroad. With our increasingly migrant and urban communities, these little critters can be spread by poor food preparation hygiene, unwashed hands, even via our innocent-

---

[58] Some researchers reported being able to culture B. *hominis* from 46% of patients with irritable bowel syndrome.

looking cats and dogs. There is a strong link between prostate cancer and toxoplasmosis gondii found in our fluffy feline friends. We humans seem to believe we're immune to parasites, somehow superior, that anti-worming is unnecessary for all but our pets. But without paying attention to simple hygiene measures, we're at the mercy of these tiniest of creatures, be they bacteria, protozoa, mycoplasma, viruses, parasites, even calcifying nanoparticles, the smallest of the lot.

Izabella Wentz, pharmacist, sufferer of Hashimoto's Thyroiditis and bestselling author of *The Hashimoto's Protocol* also had **Blastocystis hominis**. She blames the infection in part for causing her thyroid condition and says she never felt completely well until she'd eradicated it.[59]

Wentz found 35% of her clients tested positive for **Blastocystis hominis**, making it the most common infection associated with Hashimoto's. But most medics consider it a commensal organism and do not see a need to treat it, despite new evidence pointing to its pathogenicity.[60]

Wentz has investigated the wee critter extensively. '[It's] known to cause multiple food sensitivities,' she writes. 'While true food sensitivities… will typically result in a resolution of symptoms once the food is removed, people infected with **Blastocystis hominis** will have the opposite: they develop multiple food sensitivities, and once they eliminate one food, they'll develop another sensitivity.'

---

59 Interestingly other co-infections she blames for a low thyroid function include *H. pylori*, SIBO (small intestinal bacterial overgrowth), yeast overgrowth, and reactivated Epstein-Barr virus. All of which I would also point to as being possible underlying conditions in many cancers.

60 The general drug of choice is metronidazole, but this may be enhanced by using a cocktail of drugs. The inclusion of both doxycycline and Mebendazole might be the best choice as both have anti-cancer effects. The probiotic *Saccharomyces boulardii* has shown to be efficacious if not better. It is a non-pathogenic yeast which interferes with the ability of pathogens to colonize the mucosal lining of the gut. It also improves immune response and stabilises the gastrointestinal barrier.

I too had discovered a sensitivity to wheat and eggs, but also dairy, tomatoes and citrus. I knew that cutting out inflammatory foods was imperative to my cancer-busting programme, and I'm certain now that every cancer patient should be routinely tested and treated to eradicate parasites.

Re-establishing a healthy gut and ridding myself of this intruder was not an easy job. It involved dedication to the cause, but I knew it was key. Without a properly functioning gut I would never hope to have a properly functioning thyroid or immune system. I was never going to get a complete recovery without fixing those.

If I had thought for a moment that the conventional medical profession would take the parasite infection seriously, I might have benefited from a short term hit of a combination of antibiotics alongside my supplements.[61] But I was concerned that taking these might have created further dysbiosis, although with hindsight it would have only been a temporary imbalance, easily rectified with the correct pre and probiotics. In the end what worked for me was several months of the following:

- An anti-parasitic supplement formula containing wormwood, black walnut, cloves, olive leaf, garlic, grapefruit extract and uva ursi
- Betain hydrochloride to increase acidity in my stomach.
- Proteolytic enzymes that digest protein, including bromelain (from pineapples) and papain (from papaya seeds) taken between meals
- Raw garlic cloves crushed in an avocado dip.
- Zinc
- *Mahonia aquifolium* (berberine)

---

61   In a randomized clinical trial in symptomatic children who had *Blastocystis* positive stools, both clinical and parasitological cure rates were 94.4% using *S. Boulardii* in comparison with 73.3% achieved in the metronidazole treated group. These findings challenge the existing treatment guidelines.

- Fish oils
- Freshly ground flaxseed.

The proteolytic enzymes are believed to digest the protein shell that makes up the bodies of parasites, making them less able to resist treatment.[62] The enzymes must be taken between meals otherwise they'll be used up digesting food instead. The flaxseed was in effect 'sweeping' my colon and helping to physically remove the burrowed parasites from the walls of my intestine, it also helps lower oestradiol levels. Psyllium husk is also used for this purpose. This was of course coupled with an exclusion diet that already no longer contained wheat and dairy, white rice, corn, carbonated drinks, black tea, coffee, alcohol or high glycaemic fruits.

With the discovery of my underactive thyroid (he had tested both my T3 and T4), I decided to try a macrobiotic diet for three months to really 'go for it' and detox. In this diet I included mackerel and sardines at least twice or three times a week for my protein, omega-3 oil and of course seaweed. Seaweed is rich in iodine which would help with the production of thyroid hormones, but it's rare that an iodine deficiency causes abnormal thyroid function. The root cause is almost always in the gut. Dr Callebout also prescribed half an 'Armour' tablet, a small amount of desiccated natural thyroid hormone.

I have to say the prospect of this diet was not exactly appealing. Information, recipes and inspiration were in short supply in 2000 and I'm not really a lover of miso soup or wakame. But I persevered.

If I slipped up, I became cross with myself. Did I not want to survive? Did I not care enough about myself to make the effort? The anger helped spur me on to do better next time. I learnt to pick myself up after a diet fail, forgive myself and carry on. Further cheating would only make the problem worse. I hoped my small transgressions would not have severe

---

62   Bromelain also assists Ferroptosis which we will discuss in Part 2

consequences, although I had no idea of the margin for error. I also had no information on how far I should take my diet. A glucometer would have been mighty useful for tracking the release of glucose into my blood and it would have given me some tangible data to work with, better feedback and motivation.

I became more obsessive about cutting out refined carbohydrates, but still ate slower-release carbs with high soluble fibre like sweet potatoes, all while knocking back the supplements and my 'primordial soup', a vegetable juice, green tea or olive oil. Ugh. But the feeling of regaining control over some part of my life was not to be underestimated. I was immersed in a world where it would have been easy to have felt helpless, at the mercy of the doctors and my disease. I needed to take back control.

Dr Callebout also told me my folate levels were very low. Folate and B12 are both essential for the 'methylation cycle', a biological pathway contributing to almost every important function in the body, like detoxification in the liver, cell repair and energy production. It also helps detoxify and rid the body of excess oestradiol; a strong hormone associated with stimulating the growth of cancer cells.

That I was low in these crucial vitamins was of no surprise. I'd been given methotrexate, a chemotherapy drug which acts by depleting folate so that the DNA, which relies on it, can't replicate. There had been no suggestion of supplementing afterwards – some doctors are sold on the idea that long-term folate depletion is good strategy. But depletion leads to further cancer, with a particularly strong link to cervical cancer.[63]

---

63 B vitamins support methylation, which is essential for the stability of the DNA, the epigenetic regulation of IGF-2 and to stop carcinogens causing further mutations. Many patients are low on this vitamin, and supplementing with folic acid rather than the folate version can make the situation worse if you have a common genetic mutation called MTHFR. Almost 25% of the population have MTHFR mutations, which means they are unable to process folic acid unless they receive the activated form as 5-methyltetrahydofolate. In the wrong form folic acid may even be toxic (sadly this is the form used in fortified cereals and bread).

B vitamins are also the natural victims of the stress hormone cortisol, and of course every cancer patient is stressed to a greater or lesser degree. Drinking alcohol is also linked to lower folate levels. One study showed that women taking folate supplements and partaking in an occasional drink had the same risk of breast cancer as teetotallers.[64]

With Dr Callebout's blessing, I took a mega sublingual supplement of 5g methylfolate a day for several months, alongside a mega methylcobalamin B12 sublingual vitamin. Both folate and B12 are normally made by gut bacteria, so while supplementing was a good idea, I also had to address the root cause. It is the lactobacillus colonies in our colons which are responsible for the manufacture of these vitamins and merely supplementing was not going to fix the problem long term. I learned that fermented foods would help boost my lactobacilli count. However, a common mistake with cancer patients is to focus heavily on boosting fermented foods, to the detriment of their bifidobacteria levels, which also need replenishing and may in fact be more important in fighting the disease.

Although I was told my cancer was not hormonally driven, I was of the view that the HRT I had been given, which contained the strong oestrogen oestradiol, was not healthy. I wanted to switch to the weaker form, oestriol. It took years of nagging and arguing with my doctors before I finally persuaded my GP to switch to Ovestin tablets, many times weaker than oestradiol but effective at reducing symptoms at a dose of only 2mg a day. Ovestin tablets later disappeared from public

64 'Any adverse effect of alcohol consumption [on breast cancer risk] may be reduced by sufficient dietary intake of folate,' Laura Baglietto, senior researcher at the Cancer Council Victoria, Australia. Baglietto, Laura & English, Dallas & Gertig, Dorota & Hopper, John & Giles, Graham. (2005). Does dietary folate intake modify effect of alcohol consumption on breast cancer risk? Prospective cohort study. BMJ (Clinical research ed.). 331. 807. 10.1136/bmj.38551.446470.06.

view,[65] not because it's ineffective but because the stronger oestradiol is much cheaper to manufacture. This has made getting hold of more biologically identical hormones difficult.[66]

I also took a natural progesterone for protection against breast cancer, at first in cream form, which I always felt wouldn't make a discernible difference. I spent six years arguing again with my GP, who insisted I did not need progesterone as I had no womb, to finally be prescribed a micronized natural oral form on prescription, a far cry from the synthetic, carcinogenic progestin my gynaecologist at that South London hospital had been pushing.

I had no idea what an extraordinary difference the oral progesterone would make – it was like sailing out of a fog bank! I hadn't realised what a muggy world I'd been living in.[67] Not only that, my sleep was suddenly deep and restful. Even with melatonin, I had been waking and struggling to go back off. Sleeping for a whole night was something I thought I'd never experience again. But that first night using melatonin and progesterone together came as a complete and very welcome surprise.

I believe in eating foods in the best bioavailable form possible to get maximal benefits. Broccoli needs a four-minute steam. Spinach I ate both raw and cooked. Fruit I kept to a minimum, mostly apples and berries. The basics of my diet for the first three months after chemo involved miso soup or hot porridge for breakfast with some berries. I would eat small portions of brown rice, fish, salads, broccoli and other cruciferous

---

65   It does still crop up in a cream for women to use you-know-where. I also use it on my face – oestriol is great for preventing wrinkles!

66   There are suggestions that the oestriol form (E3) of oestrogen may even be protective against cancer but there is no long-term data on this because of the dominance of the stronger oestradiol (E1) use instead. There is even a cancer busting oestrogen sitting in the lab for research that I doubt will ever make it from the lab bench to the patient, called 2-methoxyoestradiol.

67   Progesterone is a neuro-steroid. There are suggestions it might be useful for 'chemo brain'.

vegetables for lunch. I could have made it far more interesting had I used a bit of imagination, but I was too exhausted to make much effort and the thought of preparing meals was too taxing.

It was hard enough just shopping for food. Choices were poor all those years ago. Andrew was regularly subjected to a bland tasteless meal in the evening, no exotic sauces or flavours, and although he was welcome to make his own meals, he showed admirable solidarity by eating my barely palatable attempts with little complaint. There are now cookbooks and recipes that would have made my initial macrobiotic meals less of an endurance test, but not then. So I approached it like any other challenge. A mental test to see if I was a worthy adversary of my foe.

Eating out became impossible, not just because I could rarely find anything I felt I could safely eat (menus are far more diverse these days) but this was also pre-smoking ban. Within minutes of sitting in a smoky restaurant I'd have a sore throat, which made me stressed and anxious. Even a trip to the pub to meet friends was fraught with angst because of the smoke.[68] All of this meant I became somewhat of a recluse during the week, only emerging at weekends to breathe that clean sea air, not the smelly fumes of London.

I juiced daily. With hindsight, I may have overdone it on the beetroot and carrot! People would often ask if I'd been abroad because of my lovely tan…oops. My staple was a combination of celery, apple, beetroot and carrot. I wouldn't wash the organic carrots or beetroot perfectly. I'd read about soil-based organisms positively stimulating the immune system, but only if the soil had been properly tended, organic and from a trusted source (thank heavens for Riverford deliveries).

---

68 http://www.dailymail.co.uk/health/article-377742/Passive-smoking-killed – twice. html

'There's a name for this obsession,' said one of my friends as she watched me prepare a salad. 'It's called orthorexia.'

'What?' I asked, quite sure I had no eating disorder.

'I've been reading about it. It's an unremitting desire to eat only health food.'

'Well, it's not because I want to, it's because I have to! I hardly think I qualify for the tree-hugging hippie brigade just yet.'

I was cross that she didn't understand that for me it wasn't a fad, or an obsession borne of psychosis. I was astounded anyone could class healthy eating as a disorder, much less put me in that bracket.

My friend just raised her eyebrows. Obviously, she didn't understand the link between high glycaemic diets and cancer. Neither was she standing in my shoes or reading the research that I had. If people thought I was going too far and saw me as obsessive about my food choices, that was their problem. I was going to do what I thought was right for me. After all, I hadn't cut out carbs altogether and I wasn't obsessing over every gram.

On my next visit to Dr Callebout he questioned the wisdom of a mainly pescatarian diet, with only fish and nuts and pulses as sources of protein.

'You realise you need certain amino acids to build your white cells,' he said. 'And your test results show you're very low on arginine. That helps you detox nitrogen and build white cells too, particularly the natural killer cells.'

'And there's no arginine in fish?'

'It's found in game meats like venison and rabbit. These also have much better fat profiles, with far more omega-3 than farmed animals.'

And so a little arginine-rich grass-fed meat and arginine supplements came onto the menu, right at the end of my parasite flush. Recent research has backed this up, showing raised arginine levels help T cells fight tumours. They also make immunotherapy drugs work better although some specific cancers rely on arginine for growth and inhibition of this amino acid could be a useful starving approach.[69]

Meanwhile my oncologist was very pleased with my progress. She asked probing questions about what supplements I was taking but I thought it better not to say too much. The list was too long, for a start! There was no way I could tell her about the intravenous vitamin C, it was far too contentious an issue. And I'm not sure what she would have made of the Ultraviolet Blood Irradiation or my low glycaemic, iodine rich, high soluble fibre, parasite-flushing diet. So I kept my mouth firmly shut. I was sure she wouldn't approve, and I saw no reason to cause discord between us. Nowadays I would encourage a healthy dialogue, particularly as the Internet is awash with far more peer reviewed research to back you up.

She managed to get me enrolled for a trial dendritic vaccine. To this day I'm not sure whether it helped or not (I had a weak, 'partial' response) but I was sure it was the combination of modalities that helped. The UV blood irradiation is a natural vaccine, the intravenous vitamin C is fabulous for fighting pathogens and reigniting the immune system and I was improving my gut health with my immune-boosting diet, with herbs and supplements, probiotics, MGN3, the maitake mushrooms, the multi-faceted berberine. All of this must have had a direct effect on my response to the dendritic vaccine.

---

69 Ref. Sarcomas, melanomas, hepatocellular carcinomas and lymphomas may be an exception in the 'starving' phase of treatment when arginine needs to be depleted. Melissa M. Phillips, Michael T. Sheaff, Peter W. Szlosarek **Targeting Arginine-Dependent Cancers with Arginine-Degrading Enzymes: Opportunities and Challenges Cancer Res Treat**. 2013 Dec; 45(4): 251-262.

Still, from a medical point of view, my ongoing survival was seen as being purely down to the dendritic vaccine. They got very excited about it. I hated to break it to them that I'd more than likely improved my chances beforehand with intravenous vitamin C and improving my gut health. I was told not to expect any long-term effect. The vaccine would only help reduce the HPV component of my disease which was viewed as the instigator (although it is only part of a bigger equation), but it was not the reason the cancer continued to propagate. In fact, I discovered I was the only patient out of fourteen on the trial to survive longer than a few months.[70] I was sad that other women had died, and it made me realise once again just how lucky I was to wake up every day, to feel sunlight on my face, to be blessed with some medical training. Without that I was sure that I too would be five feet under.

I was beating the odds. I stayed upbeat and positive, blissfully unaware of the time bomb inside me.

---

70   This is why the vaccine was dropped for treating advanced cervical cancer – they now concur that it makes little difference to survival on its own, but no trials have been undertaken that treat the gut and immune system prior to vaccination. I feel the medical profession is missing a trick.

Chapter Ten:

Walking on Eggshells

'You are going to kill yourself if you carry on like this!' Andrew said as he watched me struggle up the stairs to my office. 'It's ten o'clock, you should be coming to bed! You are meant to be avoiding stress!'

'It's just one email. Won't take me long. I'll be back down in a sec.'

He thought I was crazy to be starting a business. He was right. Looking after my health was already a full-time job, running a business as well was nothing short of lunacy. But I couldn't see it. It was a primal need to have an encompassing task to take my focus off the cancer. I wanted to have something to show for my time on Earth, to create these toiletries and rituals.

Before the appearance of the lung secondary, I had already written and published two books entirely on my own. I had sold 10,000 and 5,000 of each (*Bathrobics* and *Bathrobics for Pregnancy*) through WHSmith, bookstores and the Innovations catalogue. Now I wanted toiletries to go with each spa ritual.

I had visited the head offices of Boots, The Body Shop and Virgin Vie and talked over my ideas with all of them. While they were all interested, none of them seemed willing to push the 'go' button and make it happen. The trouble with big companies is that such decisions become impossible, there is too much committee-think, too many hurdles to climb. I had found the same problem finding a publisher for my waterproof book years earlier. It was made of polypropylene and had a rubber sucker attached, a unique design that allowed it to turn inside out into a flip chart to hang over the bath. In the end I had given up and published on my own.

What the hell. I had published a book with no experience, I was sure I could create toiletries! None of the companies I'd talked to were producing the exact products I wanted for my rituals anyway. Finding a contract manufacturer and a chemist and then sourcing packaging and designs, selling into pharmacies and department stores, how hard could it be? Wow. It was exhausting.

With my illness and the growing awareness of the toxicity of our environment, I realised my initial formulations were nowhere near good enough to launch into the beauty market. My first creations had all contained parabens, oestrogen-mimicking preservatives, and some had sulphates and triethanolamine. I would have never been able to sell them with a clear conscience! I wanted to be proud of them, 100% happy they were top quality and non-toxic. So, at huge cost, the whole range was reformulated with clean, rich and natural ingredients. My toiletries weren't going to be just marketing gimmicks to accompany my waterproof books. They were stand-alone excellent products.

Between hospital visits and intravenous vitamin C infusions, I had managed to see the buyers from John Lewis, Debenhams and House of Fraser and they had all placed large orders. I was going to make this a success; I was sure of it. But after a few years of this hectic lifestyle the fatigue was overwhelming, and my blood markers were slowly rising again to the upper end of normal. I was worried.

I had kept up with all my supplements, my diet and exercise and for the first few years I'd seemed to be almost invincible, resistant to every cold that came my way. 'No self-respecting bug is going to live in me!' I would say, when all around people were succumbing to colds and flu.

I knew all was not well. Although I would describe myself as functioning, I was constantly exhausted. The kind of relentless lethargy that really drags you down. Getting out of bed and walking up a flight of stairs would leave me breathless. But sales, PR and orders needed to parallel production, so I could not afford to be tired. I knew I was taking on too much, but failure was not an option.

Steadily the fatigue grew worse. At night I was waking up drenched with sweat. Not just a little, but soaking. Was this a side effect of all the chemo? Perhaps my hormones were too low. My sixth sense told me I needed to investigate.

I had seen Dr Kingsley and Dr Callebout. Two opinions were good, three was better, so I decided to see Dr Kenyon too.

One of the tests Dr Kenyon performs is Live Blood Analysis, looking at your blood under a Darkfield microscope. There are many who scoff at this basic test (as usual there's a nice derogatory piece on Quackwatch) and right enough, it has been used by the likes of personal trainers and gyms to read blood. But with a qualified interpreter it is utterly fascinating: you can see in an instant what is going on inside your body in real-time.

It's also an easy test to perform. You prick your finger, then blood is collected on a series of slides and examined. 'Darkfield' just means it's set against a dark background, so that it's easier to see the red and white cells and any fungi.

Dr Kenyon and I sat there in silence. We looked at the slide for a minute or so while he moved the scope around. This is what we saw:

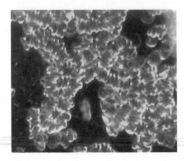

Live blood analysis

'Hmm. They're all stacked in rouleaux formations,' he said.

'Is that usual?'

'Well, it is common for a cancer patient to have some rouleaux formations. Cancer causes a release of abnormal clotting factors and inflammatory factors called cytokines, which causes sticky fibrinogen in the blood. You'll have to be careful to stop clots forming.'

'But that looks like a lot of rouleaux, throughout the whole of the blood! And surely I'm no longer a cancer patient? Are these rouleaux just a result of chemo? Is this worse or better than other patients?' I asked.

'We're going to have to monitor it,' he said.

No wonder I was exhausted! With these 'rouleaux', the stacks of red blood cells all piled on top of each other, abnormally covered in sticky fibrinogen caused by inflammation, how on earth would they be able to get through the capillaries, pick up oxygen efficiently in the lungs and then deliver it to the tissues? It's unsurprising that blood clots and heart attacks are common after a cancer diagnosis. And it would explain the extreme fatigue and shortness of breath. I had begun to wonder if I had become anaemic.

I had convinced myself I had to be improving, that as I got further away from the diagnosis, I must be getting healthier with my strict regime and lifestyle, despite the obvious symptoms that pointed to the opposite. I had been in denial.

A repeat Live Blood Analysis a few weeks later showed, to my dismay, that I was getting worse. 'Rouleaux' I have since read, are indicative of serious conditions, including cancer.

I wondered if perhaps I had another metastasis developing somewhere in my body, but my SCC (squamous cell carcinoma) marker was still in normal ranges, which pointed to a no. That was a relief. So what was going on? Inflammation and hypoxia – a lack of oxygen – are now known to promote cancer. Was I leaving myself open to further problems?

I needed to up my game. But I had been so good, 'orthorexic' as I had been told. But I realised I had lapsed with several of my supplements, aspirin included. Whatever I was doing, it was not enough. It was incredibly disheartening.

I headed home feeling low and hardly said a word to Andrew about my visit. I didn't want to let him know just how worried I was. I told him that all was fine. At the same time, I was relieved I had at least discovered a reason for my fatigue. If I'd relied on the NHS, I wouldn't have had a clue as no-one was making any connection to a possible blood disorder.

The first thing I did was take a little aspirin. That surgeon back in 1999 had sowed the seed of doubt about it, but I should have been more reliant on my own instincts. Now I wondered if I could have avoided this situation altogether if I had taken it every day.[71]

After a month of taking aspirin, more fish oils, nattokinase, pycnogenol and proteolytic enzymes, the rouleaux had started to break up a little.

---

71 A study in Hong Kong showed taking low dose aspirin for seven years can halve the risk of some cancers. 'Long-term use showed 24 to 47 per cent significant reduction on major cancers in the gastro-intestinal [GI] tract, including colorectal, liver, oesophagus, pancreas and stomach. Long-term aspirin use cut the risk of prostate cancer by 14 per cent, leukaemia by 24 per cent and lung cancer by 35 per cent.' Said Professor Kelvin Tsoi. *https://www.express.co.uk/life-style/health/873318/Aspirin-cancer-risk-study*

All these had anticoagulant effects, and the aspirin would break up any platelets which were threatening to stick together, too. I had improved the sticky fibrinogen and reduced the inflammation, but this did not ease the look of concern on Dr Kenyon's face.

He asked me if the night sweats were improving.

'No, they're still really bad. Is it a delayed post-chemo response?'

He paused, looked up from the Darkfield and said, 'It looks like you have some odd shaped red blood cells.'

He asked again about my treatment history, and the amount of chemo and radiotherapy I'd received. I was starting to feel uneasy.

He showed me the slide. When you looked closely you could see that many of my red blood cell membranes were deformed or broken.

'We need to run some further tests,' he said.

I began to panic. 'Do you think I might be getting leukaemia?' I remembered that patients run the risk of bone marrow damage from both chemo and radiotherapy, which only made my anxiety worse.

'I really can't be sure at this stage. You will need a formal diagnosis from your oncologist. Let's see what the blood tests say.'

The bone marrow is where red blood cells are formed. Together with white blood cells, they have a rapid turnover which makes them very vulnerable to chemotherapy and radiotherapy. Chromosomal damage to the DNA by treatments can lead to a reduced number of white cells and, if you're very unlucky, abnormally formed red blood cells. Instead of being nicely formed biconcave discs, my red blood cells now had odd spicules that stuck out of the sides. I knew leukaemia was more often seen in younger patients, but I was determined it wouldn't happen to me at thirty-nine.

When leukaemia was a result of prior treatment, the cancer was swift and fatal, usually within weeks. Would I live to see my fortieth birthday?

I groaned. I knew my poor pelvic bone marrow must have been hit very badly with chemo and radiotherapy. My oncologist had given me a huge dose of both in 1994, and then a larger dose of chemo in 1999, even though I had persuaded her to lower it after three rounds. The hope had been to give me a few extra months – to hell with the risk of further cancer. But instead, against every expectation, I had survived.

This was a mighty blow. I was four years from my secondary diagnosis and a full nine years from my primary diagnosis. Apparently, this was prime time for a treatment-related leukaemia to occur. I felt sick. Yet again time to find the answer might be in short supply. I decided to keep all of this to myself. Worrying Andrew at this stage without further information would mean both of us panicking. He hadn't accompanied me to these consultations as he was travelling a lot for work, so I didn't want to distract him. There was little he could do. But there had to be something I could do. When I got home it was back to research stations immediately.

I read that rouleaux are present in myelomas and acute myeloid leukaemia. 'Myelodysplastic' syndromes (abnormally shaped RBCs) after chemo or radiotherapy quickly progress to Acute Myeloid Leukaemia. Therapy related blood cancers have a poor prognosis, far worse than other blood cancers, and make up less than 10% of leukaemia cancers. Bugger, bugger, bugger. I thought I'd done everything I could. I had tried so hard. Was I going to die, not because of the original cancer, but because of the toxic treatment I'd received? Had I put myself under too much stress with my business and allowed this to develop? Almost certainly.

What was the treatment for myelodysplasia or AML? More chemotherapy. A treatment with retinoid (a strong type of vitamin A) was used for chronic myeloid leukaemia. The other option was a bone marrow transplant, but this was not offered to patients with prior cancer.[72]

Perhaps the situation wasn't that bad. I told myself not to panic, to 'stay in the present' until the test results came back.

When they came a couple of weeks later, I decided to take Andrew to the appointment with me this time.

Dr Kenyon handed me a piece of paper with the results.

<u>Neurotech Number:- 05/03/3936</u>

<u>Patient:- Ms. Jane McLelland</u>   H/S   <u>Date of Birth:- xx–xx–xx</u>
                                              Date of Sample:- 23–05–03

<u>Tumor Marker 2 Pyruvate Kinase</u>
Result:-   397 units/ml of plasma
Normal range:-   <15 units/ml of plasma

<u>Matrix Metallo Proteinase - 2</u>
Result:-   1,550 copies/ml of plasma
Normal range:-   >1 - <1,000 units/ml of plasma

<u>Interferon Gamma Gene Expression</u>
Result:-   858 copies/ml of plasma
Normal range:-   3,000 – 10, 000 copies/ml of plasma

Blood test results May '03

---

72   Therapy related Acute Myeloid Leukaemia is like oncology's dirty little secret. 10% of AML diagnoses are a direct result of prior therapy, either chemotherapy and/or radiotherapy. But it is this 10% minority that fare significantly worse, probably because of the accumulated toxicity from prior treatment resulting in an already depleted immune system.

'What does all this mean?' I asked. I was looking at normal ranges, and every test showed my results were wildly out of range. The tumour marker TM2PK seemed to be particularly alarming. I knew what it meant.

He handed me another sheet. 'These were results from the other blood test,' he said, his face giving little away.

'The deleted p53 protein, combined with the other blood results and your fatigue and night sweats, means you're really going to need to discuss all of this with your oncologist. She might suggest further chemotherapy.'

Further chemo! No way. I would do anything to avoid that.

I remembered that the p53 gene was a tumour suppressor. Shit! With this gene deleted it meant the brakes were now off for cancer to rampage through my blood and bone marrow. I looked at the results again and tried to remain calm. I didn't want to scare Andrew. But panic was gripping me.

'You have an abnormal immune response,' he added. 'Your Interleukin 5 reading, which measures your allergy or humoral response, is very high. Your Interleukin 12 and tumour necrosis factor beta results are both suppressed and these both control your natural killer cells. In other words when the allergy response is raised, the natural killer cells are suppressed.'

My Interleukin 5 (IL5) reading was 26,000. In a healthy person, it was meant to be between 3,000 and 4,000.[73] Did Dr Kenyon think I was in another slow-motion car crash, heading towards impact again? I felt a cold shiver down my spine. After everything I'd done to stay alive, perhaps I really was going to die after all.

---

73   Cimetidine helps to reverse the abnormal Th1:Th2 ratio but I did not make this discovery until 2007.

'I think we need to give you some more intravenous vitamin C for a few weeks,' he said.

'Can I start tomorrow?' I replied. He said he would make some arrangements. Thank God I'd been proactive about my health, and that I had a team on hand ready to help! This could easily have been missed by the usual 'standard of care'. Conventional treatments would be woefully inadequate, as I knew from the statistics.

I hugged Andrew in the car park outside and assured him this was a mere 'blip', that I'd sort it out with the intravenous vitamin C, that my SCC markers were still stable. I didn't dare mention it was almost certainly another cancer, so he just nodded and assumed everything was under control.

When I got home, I made the call to my oncologist and told her about the deleted anti p53 protein antibodies. I was shocked by her response. She was mad with rage. 'You can't just have a test done without proper counselling! Send me the result! Who has performed this test?' I was so upset by her reaction I clammed up and said nothing about the myelodysplasia. A blood cancer was not foremost in her mind, she was concerned about a recurrence of my cervical cancer. Those markers looked normal. If she discovered it was a possible blood cancer, she would want to give me chemotherapy and this might result in a row. I decided that it was best keep quiet. I was tiptoeing between my doctors, walking on eggshells. But I sent her the p53 test result and she had an immunologist review it.

I said nothing about the Live Blood Analysis as I thought she might be dismissive of this test too, but I did tentatively ask her about the TM2PK test. She had never heard of it.[74] The reason being that abnormal cancer metabolism is still not recognised as important, either for testing or for treatment. Conventional treatment is completely focused on the genes for which nice, expensive patented drugs are available or in development. There was apparently no drug available for the abnormal glycolysis, the breakdown of glucose, ergo it was deemed irrelevant.

I still had enormous respect for my oncologist, but I realised the failings of the conventional route and its denial of treating the abnormal cancer metabolism. I had no intention of travelling down the conventional path anymore if doing so meant further chemotherapy. I would have to work out how to deal with this without her help.

Lying awake that night my mind was racing. 'I might kill you with all of this' was the throwaway line she'd uttered as she had delivered the maximum doses of chemo and radiotherapy in the early days. Negative words had a way of getting stuck in my head. I was so sure I'd been doing everything right, keeping my SCC blood marker low. What more could I do?

I felt as though I'd been kicked in the stomach. I had been tootling along thinking the road ahead might be bumpy, but I hadn't been expecting this major side swipe out of nowhere. I had been proactive, ready to take on the monster if it returned. But I had been preparing for a return of the cervical cancer, not this! A blood cancer meant a whole new approach, as it obviously didn't respond to my diet or any of the supplements. It had

---

74 TM2-PK stands for Tumour Marker 2-Pyruvate Kinase (or PKM2), an enzyme that cancer cells use to produce their energy, which is not present to any great extent in normal cells. It tests for pyruvate kinase, a by-product of 'aerobic glycolysis', the abnormal metabolism or the 'Warburg Effect' present in cancer cells. Elevated levels are associated with the presence of cancer. Haiyan Zhu, Hui Luo, Xuejie Zhu, Xiaoli Hu, Lihong Zheng, Xueqiong Zhu: **Pyruvate kinase M2 (PKM2) expression correlates with prognosis in solid cancers: a meta-analysis. Oncotarget**. 2017 Jan 3; 8(1): 1628-1640.

been sneaking up on me despite my best efforts. With a sad and heavy heart, I felt I was back at square one. It was truly gutting.

I wanted to cry but I couldn't let myself crumple up in despair. It would hinder me in my efforts to work out what to do next. What nonsense that treatment for therapy-related myelodysplasia and acute myeloid leukaemia was yet more chemotherapy! Not only was it toxic and immune depleting, but chemo made the risk of a venous thromboembolism or a blood clot or even worse.[75] I was not going to take any more chemo, no matter what anyone said.

Many cancer patients are at risk of heart disease, strokes, DVTs (deep vein thromboses) or pulmonary emboli because of cancer's effects on the platelets and plasma fibrinogen. It can increase the risk of venous thrombosis from four to sevenfold. This is an unspoken side effect of the disease and I knew that this risk was under-appreciated, despite it being a leading cause of death among patients. Around 25% of cancer patients subsequently die of a cardiovascular event, which is never directly attributed to the cancer and so is not included in the statistics. The simple addition of a low dose aspirin prescription to every cancer patient would potentially save so many lives, or at the least extend many patients' survival.

Business was put on hold while I hunted for an answer. It had to be out there, I was sure of it, if only I had time to find it. I was desperate and terrified. But terror was not going to help. What had I missed? Focus, focus, focus, Jane!

I had subscribed to various journals, one of which was the Townsend Letter for Doctors and Patients. An earlier article on a drug for cardiovascular disease called dipyridamole had caught my eye. As I scoured the literature, I spotted a mention of dipyridamole again. A

---

75   Kirwan 2003.

small column in the 'Letters' section, written by a gentleman called Wayne Martin, made me sit up. His letter described dipyridamole, an antiplatelet drug for cardiovascular problems, and how its anti-cancer effects had been ignored. As I read the letter it became clear that here was a powerful anti-cancer drug that had direct effects on the blood. I felt a shiver of excitement as I read on. Was dipyridamole going to help rescue me? Somehow, I was sure of it.

I am reproducing Wayne Martin's letter here, because it contains so much valuable information.

'Anti-Cancer Effect of Dipyridamole:

'This is about the anti-cancer effect of dipyridamole. It is a harmless widely-used drug in treating patients who have survived an episode of thrombotic stroke or coronary thrombosis that has a vast potential of being a harmless anti-cancer drug.

'First let us look at the report in The Lancet in the March 23, 1985 issue, p. 693, by E.H. Rhodes *et al.* of St. Helier and Kingston Hospital in Surrey, England. These doctors for the past 11 years had been maintaining melanoma patients with Clark's level IV and III disease on dipyridamole, 300 mg a day. Thirty of these patients were maintained on this dose of dipyridamole. Of them, 26 had level IV disease and four had level III disease. At five years, the survival of the level IV patients was 74%. The five-year survival for the total thirty with level IV and III disease was 77%. None of the level III patients died. Reference was given that the expected five-year survival for level IV melanoma is 32%. In the case of melanoma, 100% of deaths are caused by distant metastases. Reference was given that when metastases in many forms of solid malignant tumors are formed from the vascular network, the tumor cells moving in the blood circulation, at the beginning of metastasis formation, are attached to the vascular endothelium. Reference is also given that dipyridamole tends to prevent this attachment of cancer cells flowing in the blood circulation to the endothelium and thus tends to prevent the formation of metastases.

'Dipyridamole, like aspirin, inhibits platelet adhesion, and thus tends to prevent the vascular thrombosis of heart attacks and strokes. In the Lancet in the December 12, 1987 issue (pp. 1,371-4) was the report of the European Stroke Prevention Study. The introduction to this report reviewed the indicated lack of benefit in treating with aspirin, patients who had survived a small stroke, a TIA, a temporary ischemic attack. In this trial, dipyridamole 300 mg a day was added to treatment with aspirin and the results were outstanding. Over a two-year period, stroke deaths were decreased by 50%, deaths from myocardial infarction decreased by 38% and deaths from cancer by 25%.

'The numbers of patients involved were small, however here is another indication of an anti-cancer effect of dipyridamole.

'I have had a long exchange with Dr Betty Rhodes who has been in retirement for about eight years. She treated melanoma with dipyridamole because she is a dermatologist and that is the kind of cancer that she treated. She has been disappointed that there has been no follow up on this most hopeful indication that she has demonstrated of dipyridamole in treating melanoma. She feels that dipyridamole may be just as effective in treating many other forms of solid malignant tumors.

'The above-indicated anti-cancer effect of dipyridamole may be due only to its prevention of metastases, however Eva Bestida *et al.* of the University of Barcelona had a report in Cancer Research in the September 1985 issue (pp. 4,048-4,062) on the inhibition of certain human cancer cell growths by dipyridamole. It caused an inhibition of greater than 80% of adenosine, thymidine and uridine. These are substances needed by cancer cells to prosper. This may indicate an anti-cancer effect of dipyridamole other than in the prevention of metastases.

'In 1958, Professor R.A.Q. O'Meara of Trinity College, Dublin Ireland, had a report on Coagulation and Cancer in the Irish Journal of Medical Science, vol. 394, pp. 474-9. I met with him briefly in 1965. At that time, he felt that with both the primary tumor or a metastasis, clotting factors are given off by cancer cells and then cancer cells tend to become coated with fibrin. He felt that our cancer cell-killing immunocytes can kill cancer cells more effectively if they can make contact with cancer cells. He felt that this fibrin coat on cancer cells acts as a protective barrier to prevent them from being killed by immune attack.

'I think that L. Michaels may have been one of O'Meara's students. In any event Michaels had a report in The Lancet in the October 17, 1964 issue (pp. 832-5) with the title 'Cancer Incidence and Mortality' in patients having Anticoagulant Therapy. In that time frame nearly every patient who had survived a heart attack or a thrombotic stroke was maintained for year after year on warfarin. The concept was that warfarin would prevent the formation of the red or fibrin thrombus. Michaels did a study of such patients to the extent of over 1,500 patient years. There only one death among them – that of a primary lung cancer patient, when eight cancer deaths had been expected in this group.

'Warfarin will tend to prevent the red or fibrin part of a blood clot. Dipyridamole, by preventing the formation of the white or platelet thrombus, will also be preventing the formation of a fibrin thrombus but without depleting vitamin K as warfarin does.

'The tendency of cancer cells to give off clotting factors puts cancer patients at a far greater risk of death from vascular thrombosis. They are greatly more at risk of death from a heart attack or stroke.

'At the time of the first O'Meara report in 1958, there was very little thought being given to the role of platelets in heart attacks and thrombotic strokes. Beginning in 1945, the standard treatment for survivors of heart attacks or thrombotic strokes was to anti-coagulate with warfarin or similar anticoagulating drugs. By 1970 the practice had almost completely come to an end. It was decided that anticoagulant treatment was not increasing survival. By then it was understood that in the vascular tree, there will never be the formation of a red or fibrin thrombus without there first being a white or platelet thrombus. The discovery of the factors in the arachidonic acid cascade and of the platelet aggregation substance thromboxane A2 was the basis for the Nobel Award for Medicine in 1982. It then followed that a platelet thrombus with no fibrin thrombus could be enough of an occlusion to cause a thrombotic stroke or a heart attack.

'With this understanding, along with the knowledge that aspirin will tend to reduce the aggregation of platelets, the entire medical establishment replaced warfarin with aspirin in treating heart attacks and thrombotic strokes.

'Since that time there have been three trials in England in using aspirin in the prevention of a heart attack and two in the USA. Of these five trials only one, the Physicians Health Study in the USA, showed any benefit at all. This one trial that did show some benefit in the prevention of a heart attack used Bufferin, and Bufferin contains aspirin and magnesium.

'There are many reasons to believe that dipyridamole at 300 mg a day will be far more effective in the prevention of heart attacks and strokes than aspirin. Moreover, dipyridamole has none of the harmful side effects of aspirin.

'As of March 1999, there is now a new light thrown on the harm of platelet aggregation, this time with respect to cancer. In Cancer Research March 1999, pp. 1295-3000, B. Nieswandt *et al.* of the University of Regensburg, Germany had a report on platelet aggregation and cancer. Using three different tumor cell lines in mice, it was demonstrated that tumor cells can activate platelet aggregation and that platelet aggregates deactivate cytotoxic NK cells, preventing NK cells from killing cancer cells.

'This is to suggest that dipyridamole is a harmless drug. The generic form of it costs less than one dollar a day for treatment. It has in one small trial been demonstrated that it is effective against melanoma. There is every reason to feel that it may be effective against a broad spectrum of cancers.

'If it were granted that all cancer patients are at a greater risk of heart attacks and strokes, it is hoped that many doctors will treat cancer patients with dipyridamole for this reason. However, if they do so, it will soon be found that dipyridamole will be having a marked anti-cancer effect.

Wayne Martin
25 OrchardDrive
Fairhope, Alabama 36532 USA
334-928-3975
Fax 334-928-0150'

I felt like Alice in Wonderland again, staring at another bottle with a 'Drink me' label. This drug might be the lifeline I needed.

From the letter I gathered dipyridamole would:

- Stop blood clots forming by breaking down fibrin.
- Stop platelet aggregation.
- Stop metastases forming.
- Work in synergy with aspirin and magnesium
- Allow the immune system to remain intact and not be deactivated.
- Allow natural killer cells access to circulating cancer cells.
- 'Starve cancer' of nucleosides for new cell DNA (e.g., adenosine and thymidine) and hold proteins in the circulation.

It was this or further chemotherapy. There was no question that I was going to take it, assuming I could get it prescribed. It was a no-brainer. But with all these anti-cancer effects, why was nobody using it? Surely it wasn't just because it was out of patent and cheap, and so ignored, forgotten and discarded? I knew enough about the workings of Big Pharma to know this was more than likely the reason.

Wayne Martin wrote in another letter that the Boehringer Ingelheim sales reps used to speak of dipyridamole's anti-cancer effects, but when their first patent ran out they didn't mention it again. Eli Lily re-patented it for proliferative disorders like rheumatoid arthritis, then

Boehringer Ingelheim got the patent back again in 1998. In my view, this all constitutes deeply suspicious behaviour. Medical patents are not meant to be renewed like this. Once a patent expired, it is open for other companies to produce cheaper generic versions. Why did Boehringer Ingelheim feel that they had to protect this cheap drug at all costs?

Who was Wayne Martin? I wondered whether he was a knowledgeable oncologist, or perhaps a complementary doctor. I discovered he was neither, and that he was ninety-one years old when he wrote this letter! He died four years later in 2006, sadly before I could shake his hand and thank him for saving my life. He was the most remarkable person, with an open, enquiring and scientific mind, and he was a prolific contributor to the Townsend Letter.

Martin's first interest in medicine was kindled in 1926, at the age of 15. His mother, aged forty at the time, was close to death, suffering from pernicious anaemia (for which there was no cure). A young Baptist Minister had been attending to her daily, ready to give her the last rites, and one day he arrived announcing that everything was going to be 'alright'. An article had appeared in his Baptist magazine citing research from Harvard where forty-six late-stage patients with anaemia had been cured by eating a pound of liver every day. The young Wayne Martin fed his mother liver three times a day and sure enough, after three weeks, she was cured. But his doctor had scoffed at the reasoning. 'Ridiculous,' he had said. 'Doctors do not learn medicine from the Baptist magazine.'

Ten thousand patients a year continued to die of pernicious anaemia until in 1938, twelve years later, the drugs firms launched a painful liver injection. It worked for some, but not all. It took until 1948 and the discovery of B12 to finally hail the cure for pernicious anaemia. Eating a pound of B12-rich liver would indeed have worked.

Early on, Martin realised that doctors in the US paid more attention if there was something they could sell, and only changed their practice when instructed to do so by the pharmaceutical industry. Doctors are encouraged to ignore studies, despite obvious truths staring them in the face. Randomised clinical trials paid for by Big Pharma companies were the only 'acceptable' data. Evidence from trials was the gold standard, anything less ran the risk of legal action.

After a motorbike accident in his teens in which he lost a leg, Martin's chosen career in biochemistry switched to metallurgy. He was an inventor of many important patents of aluminium alloys. But he never lost his thirst for medical knowledge and continued to be an avid reader of medical literature, searching for a cure for both cancer and heart disease, which were his top priorities. He would digest facts, gather all the research together and come up with theories, piecing the jigsaw together. He worked like a medical Sherlock Holmes, just as I was trying to all these years later.

Martin pulled together lots of studies on heart disease and cholesterol and in the 1970s, he was the first person to come up with the theory that HDL cholesterol was beneficial and protective for patients, not harmful as many have since been led to believe. This was decades before Dr Malcolm McKendrick and Kilmer McCully slammed the industry for using cholesterol as a biomarker for cardiovascular disease. Rather than testing for cholesterol levels, Martin suggested that platelet adhesiveness was a far more important indicator of heart disease as plasma fibrinogen has been definitively shown to be the biggest risk factor. The role of platelets has been continually ignored for both heart disease and cancer, yet these small forgotten structures have far more significance than most medics would have us believe.

Martin felt anticoagulants were not effective enough to prevent heart disease. He was a passionate promoter of dipyridamole for both prevention and treatment because of its effects on platelets.

By the 1970s, two opposing views on cancer had already been firmly established: orthodox versus alternative. Martin's dismay at how big companies ruthlessly abused data for their own ends and the ways in which they quashed medical innovation led him to author Medical Heroes and Heretics in 1977. It is long out of print, but I managed to get hold of an old, discarded copy from a library. It is now one of my most prized possessions.

It is a wonderful account of the history of medical giants. He discusses Max Gerson, John Beard, William Kelly, William Coley, Ernst Krebs Jr, and Otto Warburg, who first noticed the abnormal cancer metabolism. All these names will be familiar to anyone researching complementary cancer treatments. He relates the agony of new medical discoveries that came with an almost inevitable rejection by the establishment: we learn of Oliver Wendell Holmes Sr, who made physicians wash their hands; Louis Pasteur who postulated the connection between disease and bacteria; and of Jonas Salk, who solved the mystery of polio. He charted the paths of many scientists who have been ostracised, derided, vilified and had their lives ruined, only to be proved right in the end. All braved the wrath and scorn of the medical establishment. At first, they were viewed as heretics, but ultimately, they were all crowned heroes. It seems that little has changed since 1977.

Medical discoveries suffer in much the same way today. It has taken ninety years for Warburg's theories on cancer metabolism to begin to step out of the shadows. And it is only the use of social media and the Internet that is allowing growing numbers of patients to realise this glaring error, an error fuelled by the dogma taught in medical schools.

Martin identified four distinct groups of people involved in making up the medical establishment:

1. Sincere, honest, able investigators who can and have followed revolutionary lines of thought, to the everlasting benefit of mankind.
2. Men just as honest and sincere, but who are or have been enchanted with false concepts and who in a misguided manner would sponsor either worthless or harmful modalities.
3. Dishonest, incompetent or deceitful individuals who, in seeking self-advantage, would risk or actually cause harm to humanity.
4. Investigators who work for large profit-making corporations who often do not have the wherewithal to object to their work being distorted or shelved for reasons of profit.

From my own experience and knowledge of the workings of the pharmaceutical industry, this outlines precisely where we've gone wrong with advances in cancer treatment, where it has faltered and failed. Ultimately, it is all about profit over health. A healthy patient earns nothing for the pharmaceutical companies, whereas unhealthy individuals provide all sorts of lucrative possibilities.

Further research revealed that dipyridamole (DPM) had been used alongside AZT for patients with AIDS in the 1980s because of its antiviral properties. So perhaps it would help against HPV, Epstein Barr, CMV and other viruses now proven to be linked to cancer? In 2014 the University of Pittsburgh began recruiting for a trial to include dipyridamole once again for HIV immune activation, in combination with the antiretroviral drugs.

Dipyridamole beckoned to me like a siren to a sailor. But who could I get to prescribe it? I decided to ask Dr Callebout. Gripping my copy of the Townsend Letter in my hand I made an urgent appointment with him. Given that he is such a Guru, I felt sure he would know about it.

He rubbed his beard thoughtfully.

'I read about this in the 1980s,' he said. 'I wondered if there would ever be further developments for its use in cancer. I thought it had gone in the dustbin of history, never to be heard of again. Dipyridamole was thought of as relatively ineffectual for heart disease until it was used in conjunction with aspirin, at which point they realised it improved the effects of both significantly.'

It seemed as if the whole medical profession was neglecting the potential of dipyridamole. Even for heart disease and strokes it was only being used at later stages. Would it not be a good prophylactic drug to be used with aspirin and magnesium, instead of the widespread use of statins? Or should it in fact be used with statins? Later studies have suggested that this would indeed be a major improvement on the current guidelines; these drugs work in synergy, improving cerebrovascular circulation by 50% after a stroke.[76]

'Are there any side effects I should know about?' I asked.

'Well, your blood pressure may drop a bit, so we need to watch that, and you might get some headaches to begin with.'

He ran some checks on my blood pressure, along with some other standard tests and saw no reason why he shouldn't write out a prescription straightaway. I rushed, huffing and puffing to the nearest chemist to get it!

---

[76] A Cochrane Review has also suggested that dipyridamole should be used instead of statins for prevention. The European Stroke Prevention Study in 1985 in the Lancet showed adding dipyridamole to aspirin reduced the risk of stroke deaths by 50%, deaths from heart attacks were reduced by 38% and cancer deaths were reduced by 30%! And this without the addition of magnesium which would undoubtedly improve results even further.

From then on, I would take dipyridamole and aspirin, combining both with magnesium.

I hoped that dipyridamole might buy me some time. I couldn't risk more chemotherapy; it would see me off this planet. So, cautiously, I began by taking a 100mg dipyridamole pill daily for a week and then increased it to two doses per day, although the article had suggested 300mg a day.

I was nervous about what I was doing, but what had I got to lose?

Chapter Eleven:

An Arsenal of Big Guns

While my discovery of dipyridamole was like finding an angel in hell, I wasn't sure it would be enough to stop the impending disaster of leukaemia. I was still very uneasy about the state of my health and desperate to find more 'big guns'. Perhaps I could add other allies to my aspirin/ dipyridamole drug combination? What else might I have missed in the medical literature? I wondered whether there were any other drugs that had escaped the attention of the medical profession, having been ignored or forgotten.

I had put aside several journal reports over the years and I went through them all again, searching for anything I might have failed to spot. It was then that I came across a piece on lovastatin in the American Association of Cancer Research Journal from 2001. A study at the University of Toronto, Ontario had found that out of twenty patients who had either head and neck or cervical cancer, five had achieved stable disease after other conventional therapies had failed just by taking this simple statin drug. But would it also be useful for leukaemia?

I wanted to prevent any return of cervical cancer too, so naturally I investigated. For me, clinging onto life by my fingernails, anything that might offer stable disease was seriously exciting!

I wondered whether lovastatin was also helpful in treating other cancers, and whether it was the most useful statin. I found several pieces of research by the same team in Toronto, led by Linda Z. Penn, who had been exploring lovastatin and its use for cancers that responded to retinoid treatments.[77] Retinoids are vitamin A analogs, and Dr Callebout had already put me on a short-term dose of emulsified vitamin A by the name of A-Mulsin Hochkonzentrat.

Research suggested lovastatin was more effective and less toxic. The statin had caused pronounced apoptosis in acute myeloid leukaemias (hoorah!) and neuroblastomas and was also an effective treatment for various paediatric cancers, as well as head and neck and cervical cancers. Bingo. Another shiver of excitement went down my spine.[78]

But then I discovered something else. One of my regular reads was the monthly Life Extension Magazine, a great journal for health hackers like myself. It was in there I read a 'letter' structured by the editor for patients to take to their oncologists, proposing a combination of both a statin (they suggested lovastatin) and a non-steroidal anti-inflammatory drug. This combination was shown as being more effective for causing apoptosis (cell death) than using a NSAID (non-steroidal anti-inflammatory) on its own by triggering something called the 'caspase cascade'.

It was news to me that an NSAID such as ibuprofen, indomethacin or celecoxib (but not aspirin) caused apoptosis at all. How had I missed that? I thought the COX 2 enzyme inhibitors I'd investigated in 1999 would merely stop it growing. Perhaps aspirin, which had been the main focus of my research, was not a strong enough COX-2 inhibitor to perform this apoptotic function and it needed a more powerful NSAID to send cancer cells into a death spiral.

---

77 It was shown that retinoids exert their anti-cancer effect in part by targeting the same enzyme (HMGCoA reductase) as statins to produce their anti-cancer effects by stopping a growth substrate called mevalonate.

78 Differential Sensitivity of Various Pediatric Cancers and Squamous Cell Carcinomas to Lovastatin-induced Apoptosis: Therapeutic Implications. Jim Dimitroulakos, Lily Y. Ye, Mark Benzaquen, Malcolm J. Moore, Suzanne Kamel-Reid, Melvin. H. Freedman, Herman Yeger and Linda Z. Penn. Clin Cancer Res January 1 2001 (7) (1) 158-167

Life Extension Magazine suggested the combined use of Lovastatin and etodolac as a safer, more gut tolerated COX-2 inhibiting drug than many of the others. It was usually prescribed for arthritis. The journal had followed up a report in the *Wall Street Journal*[79] that COX-2 inhibitors were proving to be useful for the prevention and treatment of many cancers as COX was a fuel that drove them.

But the really interesting fact they shared was taken from the journal *Gastroenterology*,[80] which showed that taken together, the statin increased the cancer killing effect of a NSAID (in this case sulindac) by as much as five times! There was clearly huge synergy between NSAIDs and statins for triggering this normal process of cell death.[81]

This statin and etodolac drug combination were beckoning to me again; I couldn't believe that yet another elixir had been lost in the rabbit hole! I wondered if I could take both these drugs alongside the dipyridamole. Would there be a bad interaction, or would they be synergistic, further magnifying their anti-cancer effects?

Who could I get to prescribe the statin and etodolac combination? Dr Callebout wouldn't be happy about prescribing yet more drugs, so I decided to try my oncologist. She was forward-thinking and generally open-minded. I felt guilty that I was withholding so much from her – I didn't dare tell her about the dipyridamole, which might put her off prescribing the etodolac and statin. But this was my life in the balance, my decision, my choice, and discussing myelodysplasia would add confusion and delay. I was quite clear that I wanted no more chemotherapy, but if there were drugs that would help, I didn't want to have to wait until the cancer had progressed. I wanted them now.

---

79 Sept 7, 1999
80 1999, Vol.116, No. 4, Supp A369
81 http://clincancerres.aacrjournals.org/content/7/1/158.abstract

With huge trepidation I took the articles and the letter from *Life Extension* to my next appointment. I had expected a bit of a battle and debate after her reaction on the phone to the p53 protein test. In fact, I expected her to refuse. But she was far more receptive to the idea than I had expected. She had been investigating the use of statins herself, which was a real stroke of luck!

'You might have helped me shortcut some of my research!' she said.

She decided that prescribing the two drugs 'off label' (not for their intended use) was fine on balance, given my stage IV cervical diagnosis, but she was clearly still worried about my p53 status, or lack thereof. She also warned me of potential gut issues with the etodolac, and to look out for any muscle weakness with the lovastatin, which was a rare side effect. I promised her that I'd be careful.

When I got out of the consultation, I gave a jubilant yelp, hugged Andrew and told him I was going to be OK. I felt sure of it. He grinned, happy that whatever was happening was going in the right direction. He had every faith in his medical Sherlock Holmes.

I would check for interactions with Dr Callebout once I had the drugs in my possession. The statin would starve the cancer of mevalonate and cholesterol. The etodolac would quell the cancer's inflammatory COX component that fuelled its growth and tip it into a death spiral (apoptosis) when combined with the statin. The dipyridamole would starve the cancer of adenosine, thymidine and uridine, which are the proteins it needs for making new DNA. I would starve the cancer of glucose and other fats with my diet and supplements.

Both cervical cancer and leukaemia were driven by the Ras gene. I had deduced this from the research. And the Ras gene controlled the mevalonate pathway, which produced cholesterol. In other words, both cancers fuelled themselves in a similar way, so perhaps there was a common cancer stem cell that had started both.

But would blocking cholesterol be bad for the rest of my body? Many people were taking statins long-term, and the downsides seemed to be relatively few when you compared a statin to chemo. Besides, I was taking the statin for cancer, not heart disease. Chemo might shrink tumours, but when it came to survival it only helped advanced cancer by a pathetic 2.7%. The statin seemed to stabilise disease in leukaemia and advanced cervical cancer on its own. It was clearly a 'big gun'. I wondered what the effect of combining all the drugs together would be.

I decided that I would swap the aspirin for the stronger NSAID for three months, then go back to aspirin if my stomach was OK. I had already been on the dipyridamole/aspirin combo for a couple of months. I would withhold this for a month while I tried the etodolac/statin combination. The statin and NSAID seemed to be more important drugs for the leukaemia and the dipyridamole might or might not enhance the effect. I would take regular markers and find out.

I had nothing to lose and everything to gain by trying. The long-held 'magic bullet' theory was a dead duck. There was never going to be a cure-all drug. That much was obvious.

I was certain that what I needed was a combination of drugs, attacking from all sides, acting synergistically. It fitted my guerrilla warfare approach of hitting cancer with lots of bullets from different directions rather than employing one bigger, more toxic hit from a single source like chemo, which only allowed the cancer to reroute and become resistant.

Lovastatin was the first of the statin drugs on the market, extracted from the fungus Aspergillus terreus, and it opened the floodgates to a new pharmaceutical opportunity to lower blood cholesterol. A new drugs market had been created, whether it was necessary or not. No-one was entirely sure how statins worked back then; they just knew they did.[82]

I didn't care, either. Neither did I care about a lack of randomised clinical trials. All that interested me was that there were drugs already available and there was a strong chance that they would work. I didn't want to wait fifteen years for the results of a trial. I might not have fifteen weeks.

Taking the dipyridamole and aspirin for two months had already made my SCC markers drop. There had been no side effects, not even headaches. I switched to taking the combination of etodolac and the lovastatin for a month, and before I added the dipyridamole, I checked with Dr Callebout that combining was safe. He gave me the go-ahead. The research already suggested huge synergy and a multiplication of effects with the NSAID and the statin. Would the dipyridamole synergise too and multiply the effects even more?

I had worked out that each of the drugs would starve the cancer in a different way. Once starved of their major metabolic drivers, the statin and the etodolac combination would deliver a killer blow to the cancer cells, triggering apoptosis once they were weak and vulnerable. At least, that's what I hoped.

But would it work? I was about to find out.

---

82   The theory in 2003 was that it acted on the Ras gene, but it was only a theory. Cancer treatments back then were all about the genes, not the metabolism but Linda Penn had established it was also by inhibiting mevalonate, a substrate which is overproduced by Ras driven cancers.

Chapter Twelve:

Lab Rat

Taking this drug and supplement cocktail was a giant leap of faith. To my knowledge no-one had taken this combination of drugs to treat cancer before, and many would see it as too risky because of the lack of randomised clinical trials. I was confident from my research that combined with my cancer-starving diet, they would, at the very least, have powerful anti- cancer effects. I grabbed every ounce of courage I had and began taking them all together as a cocktail.

Self-experimenting was scary. It was like sailing across the Atlantic in thick fog with just a hand-held compass, with no chart and no radar. Would I make it across without sinking? I have sailed across busy shipping lanes in the English Channel in thick fog many times and I can tell you that even with GPS, radar and all the latest gizmos, it is still a frightening experience each and every time. In both situations, the worst-case scenario was unthinkable.

I had no idea whether my cocktail was going to put me into remission, or for how long. All I was hoping for was to buy myself some extra time.

My SCC blood markers had already dropped with dipyridamole alone, but I had no clue what the drug cocktail had done to my TM2PK blood result until I went to see Dr Kenyon seven months later for a repeat test.

He sat there with a big grin on his face as he handed me the result.

Blood test results Dec '03

Boom! My TM2PK markers had dropped from 397 to 21.5! Woohoo! I nearly danced with joy.

I was stunned, too. To begin with I didn't believe it. Had this little combination done what I thought? Had I stopped the progression of therapy-related leukaemia, known to be impossible to cure? A TM2PK result of less than 15 was 'normal,' but a reading of 21.5 was good enough for me! Had I stumbled on a magic metabolic combination, a way to starve and conquer my cancer?

Andrew and I celebrated quietly that evening – with advanced cancer there is never any certainty. I was also nervous about taking all these drugs for too long. I knew they were all relatively low toxicity (certainly compared to chemo) but I wasn't sure what effect they'd have long-term. I preferred a natural route wherever possible.

Did I need to continue with them? Would the cancer come roaring back if I stopped like it does with chemo? These were unchartered waters with no point of reference. I was making it up as I went along.

I decided to keep taking the dipyridamole for a little while longer, but I stopped the statin after about five months. I only took the etodolac (that strong NSAID) for three months as I was nervous about my stomach lining. I wasn't sure I was tolerating it that well.

All NSAIDs are associated with significant side effects and need to be approached with caution. Besides their gut effects, less commonly known is that they can also increase the risk for heart attacks and strokes over the longer term, especially if you already have cardiovascular disease.[83] Celecoxib, initially hailed as the answer because it was a selective COX-2 inhibitor with fewer gut effects (like etodolac), was nearly taken off the market when its significant cardiovascular risks came to light.[84]

But dipyridamole acts in the opposite way, relaxing blood vessels and lowering blood pressure, inhibiting platelet aggregation, undoing all the negative side effects of the NSAID. So, a NSAID combined with dipyridamole seemed an ideal marriage, and unbeknownst to me at the time, the statin improved the cardiovascular risk even further by acting in synergy with dipyridamole. Statins release endothelial nitric oxide, making the dipyridamole behave like a kind of mild Viagra (which is a PDE inhibitor) relaxing and improving blood-flow.

In 2011 and 2014 Linda Penn and Aleksandra Pandyra at the Ontario Institute for Cancer Research published more results on their work on statins. They noted the potency of the statin/dipyridamole combination for leukaemia, myeloma and breast cancer – causing apoptosis in multiple cell lines. I was right about their synergistic effects:

---

83   Except in the case of aspirin.

84   This cardiovascular risk is because along with inhibiting the bad prostaglandins that cause inflammation and pain, they also inhibit the good prostaglandins that dilate your blood vessels and increase blood flow, which you need to maintain oxygenation in the tissues. The result of this is higher blood pressure from narrower arteries and an increased risk of blood clotting.

A. Pandyra

Ontario Institute for Cancer Research, Toronto, Ontario, Canada

Statins are drugs that have been utilized for years to treat hyperlipidemia via inhibition of the rate-limiting enzyme of the mevalonate (MVA) pathway, 3-hydroxy-3-methylglutaryl coenzyme A reductase (HMGCR). Recent evidence has demonstrated statins to possess anti-cancer properties against a wide range of tumours without being toxic to normal cells. Multiple myeloma (MM) is largely incurable and in acute myelogenous leukemia (AML), less than 50% of patients with poor cytogenetic disease have a chance of long-term survival. Therefore, novel therapeutic strategies are urgently needed to treat these haematological malignancies, subsets of which are sensitive to statin-induced apoptosis. Through the use of a chemical library screen, we hypothesize that the identification of compounds which potentiate the anti-cancer effects of statins will uncover novel molecular pathways and/or targets that can be exploited in combination with the MVA pathway to maximize tumour cell death in MM and AML.

A pilot 100-compound library, composed of off-patent pharmacologically active drugs clinically used for a wide spectrum of diseases was screened in the MM KMS11 cell line. Dipyridamole (DP), a commonly prescribed anti-platelet agent potentiated the anti-cancer effects of atorvastatin. The DP-statin combination is synergistic and capable of inducing apoptosis in a variety of AML and MM cell lines as well as primary AML patient samples. DP is a wide-acting agent and known to elicit numerous effects at the molecular and global physiological level. Further investigations at the level of mechanism and evaluation of in vivo efficacy are currently underway. As both statins and DP are pre-approved for use in humans, off-patent, and readily available, they have the potential to directly impact patient care.[85]

Progress over the following months was good. After taking my etodolac-statin-dipyridamole combination, my blood markers remained within normal levels, but my immune system was still out of kilter. I was no longer resistant to colds and flu – in fact they would knock me down for weeks.

'At least your immune system is working,' said Dr Callebout. 'With advanced disease it usually switches off, and you're left with no reaction to bacteria and viruses.'

Was this why I'd been so 'resistant' before? Not because I was healthy, but because I still had advanced disease and no reaction? Had the immune-boosting nutrients helped at all, or had I been fighting fire with a water pistol?

---

85   A Pandyra, L. Penn et al; *Immediate Utility of Two Approved Agents to Target Both the Metabolic Mevalonate Pathway and Its Restorative Feedback Loop: Cancer Research* July 2014. 'The statin-dipyridamole combination was synergistic and induced apoptosis in multiple myeloma and AML cell lines and primary patient samples, whereas normal peripheral blood mononuclear cells were not affected. This novel combination also decreased tumor growth in vivo.' Lead researcher Alexandra Pandrya states 'there was a dramatic induction of apoptosis when atorvastatin was combined with dipyridamole with no effect of either drug alone.' It was the combination, the synergy that was important.

Chapter Thirteen:

Gifts and Dragons

Friends had no clue about my ongoing cancer concerns. Even Andrew didn't know just how close I'd been to another crisis. I wasn't going to make it a big issue. It was all under control.

I hadn't even felt ill or stressed on my drug cocktail. I hadn't felt nauseous. Nothing. The apparent ease made me sure that other patients could be cured of their cancers in a similar way. I was brimming with confidence that I'd 'cracked it,' or at least part of it. The answer seemed clear. Starving the cancer was the right path and my cocktail had been spectacularly effective. The question though was whether it would work for other cancers at different stages.

When I looked at the stress I'd been under, it was no wonder that I had developed the myelodysplasia. I had been desperate to launch the business, to produce this new range of toiletries, but it had been at great cost to my health.

These toiletries and spa rituals were my babies, plugging the hole in my life, and taking my attention away from the cancer. I was proud I'd managed to produce and sell them so widely – my first orders before I even launched came to £120,000. Not a bad start. But creating the brand was relatively easy compared to raising the money, producing the goods and then delivering them to the stores. As a woman starting a business on my own, I encountered many barriers. The banks wouldn't lend me a penny.

I ended up using a manufacturing outfit in the Midlands. I had nowhere else to go at the time, but orders were finally coming in and stock was expected in time for Christmas. I was very excited about the launch, finally seeing my baby being born and my product ending up on the shelves.

Then disaster struck. The manufacturers screwed up production. Removing parabens had proved too difficult for them and I discovered later it was something they had never done before. As a result, the toiletries had not been preserved correctly and to my dismay I discovered that every single product they had supplied contained the same bug, which smacked of poor manufacturing practices. All the stock had to be destroyed. I was gutted.

The autumn of 2001 was spent howling my eyes out as every penny of savings I had in the bank disappeared. I was distraught. All that effort had been wasted. I would have to find a new supplier and start again but with no money at all this time. Eventually, I cobbled together enough money, found a new supplier and started again. I was not a woman who accepted defeat in any area of my life! I was not a quitter.

The following year, in September 2002, I finally launched a range I was truly proud of. It was clean natural and smelled gorgeous. When my thirty-minute spa ritual with lovely thalassotherapy toiletries (listed as 'Bathrobics Beauty Spa') finally hit the shelves, the public response and press reaction was outstanding. I was delighted!

Not expecting anything, I entered my Beauty Spa pack into the coveted Gift of the Year competition. To my surprise I was shortlisted and invited to the Award Ceremony. When they announced I had won, I was truly stunned! It was a shock and a delight to be presented with the award by the lovely comedienne Ruby Wax at the Savoy Hotel in London. A proud moment!

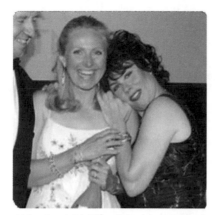

Winning UK Gift of the Year Award

Keeping the business afloat after its shaky start was getting more and more difficult. I could not afford to employ staff, so I was swimming in paperwork, juggling manufacturing, sales and PR.

I was trying to run before I could walk, performing the jobs of ten people. It was a crazily busy time.

I needed a business partner and I was desperate for investment. Andrew was too busy with his own projects to give me any assistance. Until my business made a healthy profit, he had to focus on keeping the log fires burning.

Chasing money now took up most of my time, when I should have been selling, marketing and fulfilling orders. I couldn't understand how anyone ever managed to make a business work in such a stifling financial environment. The advice I was given was to fold and start again, but that seemed too defeatist. Even if I did give up, I would still have no money.

One morning in June 2004, my bookkeeper came in and handed me the Evening Standard newspaper. She had spotted a small advert:

'Look! A new programme on BBC2 for business ideas that need investment.'

Well, it could be worth a try.

I applied for a strange new show called Dragon's Den.[86] In order to enter I needed to submit a business plan and cash flow forecasts for five years, which I duly sent. A week later, I received a call and an invitation for an interview. Yikes! What had I let myself in for?

Here I am, lamb to the slaughter, entering the 'Den'…

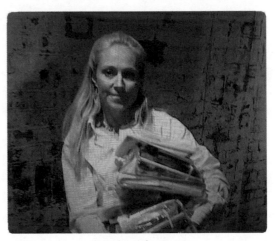

Entering 'The Den'

I never said a word about my cancer to the Dragons. Part of the entry process was signing a disclaimer to say I was fit and well. Had I had any major operations in the last three years? No, I hadn't. It was nearly five years. Had I suffered any heart attacks or heart conditions? No. Nowhere did they ask, 'have you been diagnosed with terminal cancer in the last five years?' So I decided to keep my cards close to my chest.

86　The US have an equivalent show called Shark Tank.

Had I known just how those Dragons were going to treat me, with a barrage of needlessly callous and cruel comments, I would never have gone in at all. Looking back at the subsequent series of *Dragon's Den*, they were particularly mean in the first, especially the lone female Dragon Rachel Elnaugh. I can't say I detected any hint of sisterhood from her!

Dragons Den was brand new. It was being filmed for BBC2, which in my mind was a bastion of old-fashioned English politeness and courtesy, known for their informative and educational shows. Surely they wouldn't be following the same armchair bullying technique, would they? This would be a proper business forum with proper business discussions, right?

Wrong. This was all about viewing figures. If you have a business idea, my advice is to avoid appearing on the show, no matter how tempting the extra PR may be.

As one of the first ever participants on *Dragons Den*, I had no idea how gruelling the experience might be. I was told very little about the show, other than that I would be presenting to five 'Dragons', who were all 'successful' businesspeople.

I arrived at the set with a mixture of unease and excitement. My worries were not helped by the attitude of the staff, who treated us like cattle. I was herded into a little room along with other participants with hardly anywhere to stand, let alone sit. I sat propped on the edge of a sofa for about an hour before being called.

I realised very quickly that the programme was being rigged and stacked in the producers' favour. I had to make a quick decision. Should I go in? I was still confident in the quality of my products, and there was nothing like them on the market. But I seriously considered backing out.

I decided to give it a go. It would give the range a bit of publicity, and I wasn't just after the money; I needed a business partner.

This is me on the show with a small selection of my products.

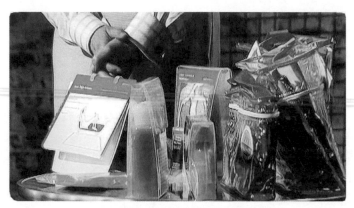

In The Den with some of my products

My three-minute pitch, which was never shown on TV, had been perfect. But I quickly realised that the blank faces in front of me were never going to invest in me. Anything that required the slightest effort on their part was of no interest to them. I made no mention of cancer, because the products were good enough to sell themselves without any of the emotional blackmail you saw on shows like The X Factor. I certainly didn't want to share my health struggles with these obnoxious individuals.

The tension in the Den escalated. I no longer wanted their money. They were so arrogant, and clearly had no intention of putting any effort into my venture. It was also evident that what they knew about toiletries you could tattoo on an ant's behind.

Telling this bunch of muppets that removing parabens, fake oestrogens, and other toxic chemicals was the future of this market fell on deaf ears. Since 2003, the rate of oestrogen-driven cancers has escalated beyond anyone's predictions. Ovarian, breast and non-small cell lung cancer are all oestrogen-driven. Rates of non-small cell lung cancer (NSCLC) have escalated from 12% to 40% of total cancer diagnoses in the last fifteen years and this is likely a result of the increasing presence of plastics and oestrogen mimickers in our environment. These diseases affect mostly young women in their thirties and forties. Most people are unaware that NSCLC is driven by oestrogen, not by cigarettes. Parabens in cosmetics and toiletries make up some of this oestrogen load, and microwaving food in plastic containers, which has become the norm for many busy families, is a practice that fills me with horror.

Of course, the BBC only showed a one-sided version of events. By the end of the session in the Den they had nearly managed to push me to tears, more through sheer frustration than anything else. I came out of the experience shaking with fury that I had been so badly abused by the BBC. But I came off lightly compared to many others. Two and a half hours of filming can give an editor a lot of material to work with. I was completely at his or her mercy. This was the first series, so of course the 'mighty' Dragons had to look invincible and the participants meek. It made for more interesting viewing that way.

As a strategy to get well, I may have got things just a teeny bit wrong! I wanted to do as much as I could in as short a timeframe as possible, to cram it all in. In the back of my mind, I was convinced I was going to die. The enormous stress of my health issues, financial hardship, business woes and – to top it all – the emotional and psychological battering I had taken in the Den really should have finished me off. Anyone feeling that cancer is just too much to fight and seemingly impossible to beat should take heart. Despite all this frenetic activity, I survived. Taking on so much was crazy, but at the time I just couldn't see it.

It demonstrates just how good my cocktail must have been. And it demonstrates just how resilient the human body can be; despite tension, stress and pressure, you can still get well in the direst of circumstances. There is **always** hope.

It was difficult enough just to stay sane knowing that cancer was still right behind me, snapping at my heels, watching my every move. I had carried on regardless. My dogged, bloody-minded refusal to accept defeat meant I had been oblivious to the damage that stress had caused. But I wasn't done yet.

Chapter Fourteen:

Danger Returns

Not surprisingly, after all of this, I was burnt out. I had never fully acknowledged just how much cancer had beaten me up. I had carried on as before, refusing to give in, believing I could cope, almost to the point where I was denying I had ever had the disease at all. I would hide the supplements and drugs I was taking, furtively swallowing them out of sight, trying to convince the world that I was fine.

If anyone learned about my diagnosis, I wanted them to think I'd made it out the other side unscathed. That cancer had not robbed me of 'me'. That what I'd been through hadn't been the most devastating experience of my life. When I look back now, I'm quite sure I had delayed post-traumatic stress disorder. I had powered on through, taking on more and more, rather than processing it all at the time. And business had delivered yet another blow.

It was a blow too far. I was aware of the link between stress and cancer, and I finally acknowledged that life mattered more. I made the gut-wrenching decision to let my business go.

But my company was my baby, with all those beloved creations I'd toiled night and day to produce. I would shelve them all. I told myself it would only be until I got myself on a better footing, regained my composure and felt more like me again.

I still had all the formulations, trademarks and copyright on the rituals and CDs, so perhaps holding off for now and relaunching in the future was for the best. With a heavy heart, I informed my buyers that the business was closing.

I was fast approaching my 40th birthday and I needed a break. My markers had remained steady, within normal levels, and it was time to rein back and have a breather.

I was still sailing regularly, and my birthday was going to coincide with Cork Week in Ireland, a great gathering of the sailing fraternity – brilliant sailing and even better après sail. It was time to let my hair down for the craic!

I had begun to truly believe that I could conquer cancer. It would not defeat me. But I was still being very careful with my diet. I could not relax completely about that. But I was no longer taking any of the drugs; they had been short term. Even the aspirin was only taken every now and then as I worried about the damage the etodolac (NSAID) might have done. I did not fully understand at the time how important it was to keep taking it.

Over that summer I did go off the rails somewhat. I was getting close to my five-year 'all-clear' date again (hah!) and I wanted to celebrate both that and my birthday. In Cork I found myself in the champagne bar on several occasions – on the eve of my birthday I was in there, diving into many willing hands, fuelled by Black Velvet cocktails, a mix of both Murphy's (a black stout like Guinness – full of iron, which is a disaster for cancer patients) and champagne. Yup, Jane was certainly letting her hair down!

But it was to be a mistake. After I returned home, my right leg swelled up with lymphoedema and a few weeks later, I began coughing and tasting blood. Night sweats returned with a vengeance. Had the leukaemia come back too? I panicked.

To my horror, my SCC markers had jumped to 200, above the level they had been at when I was diagnosed with the lung tumour. I couldn't afford to wait, because this was a clear danger signal. I immediately started taking my drug cocktail, the little stash I had in stock from the year before. I began to take more intravenous vitamin C alongside my cocktail of dipyridamole and the statin, and I tentatively took the occasional etodolac, scared about my stomach and how it might cope.

The cancer seemed to have come back hard and fast. I looked back through my research and found the piece from the 1999 *Journal of Herbal Medicine*. I realised I needed the **Mahonia aquifolium** with its potent berberine content. This big gun had been forgotten. I hastily added it to my cancer-starving cocktail again.

Two months later and to my enormous relief, my markers had plummeted back down to below normal again. By the time a CT scan was performed, there was nothing, if there had ever been anything there to see. Perhaps I had over-reacted, or perhaps I had averted another disaster. I would never know. But I realised that I could not afford to be reckless like that again. Cancer was a long-term problem that would need managing, much like diabetes or HIV.

Would cancer eventually completely disappear over time? Or would I always have it, lurking in the background, for the rest of my life? Perhaps I needed to take the drugs more regularly. If survival meant taking a few daily drugs, then that was hardly a problem. It was perfectly manageable.

Whatever had happened, I had got through another 'blip.' It confirmed the power of my cocktail. It demonstrated to me that it had worked against the cervical cancer as well as the leukaemia, but perhaps the addition of the berberine had helped boost the synergy further. I started to wonder whether cervical cancer was more reliant on glucose and fat than leukemia was.[87] (This is indeed the case. Leukaemia is more driven by amino acids.) [88]

My minor transgression had not been fatal. I was back in control, thank the Lord. This had been a valuable lesson. I would not let myself slip like that again. I decided to continue to take the statin and got another prescription from my oncologist. who agreed that it was worth taking longer term.

With my business closing I had a void in my life. I really wanted to focus on trying for a baby. I now felt confident I could beat cancer again if it came my way. I was no longer scared by it. I didn't care if others thought my actions reckless, that I might die and leave the child without a mum. With all the knowledge I had acquired over the past decade, I didn't feel like I was being selfish in wanting to bring another person into the world.

After lengthy discussions with Andrew, we decided that combining an egg donor and a host surrogate would be emotionally easier for all parties, even if = it was far more difficult logistically. We put out the word that we were looking and to my joy one of my gorgeous friends offered up her eggs. I was overwhelmed by her generosity; it was such a huge thing for her to do. We had lots of long chats, and she was totally happy about it. That she was prepared to endure hormone injections and go through this for us was the most amazing gift.

---

87   AKT Inhibitors Promote Cell Death in Cervical Cancer through Disruption of mTOR Signaling and Glucose Uptake. PLOS ONE 9(9): e107846

88   Inhibition of glutaminase selectively suppresses the growth of primary acute myeloid leukaemia cells with IDH mutations *Emadi, Ashkan et al.* *Experimental Hematology, Volume 42, Issue 4, 247-251*

We had also found a surrogate in an old school friend but getting both women to synchronise cycles was easier said than done! With huge hopes, we started treatment at a well-known fertility clinic in Harley Street.

There was no reason why it should fail. Both parties had already had children of their own, and both had a track record of success. My donor was still under 35, which is a good age for donating.

But the first cycle gave us a very disappointing number of eggs and in the end, we only managed to produce eight viable embryos. Of those, only two were of reasonable quality. I remember looking at them through the microscope, thinking how amazing it was that these bundles of cells could eventually transform our lives.

The implantation of our two little embryos took place. We had to wait an excruciating few weeks to see if one – or both (gulp!) had implanted.

I will never forget the crushing blow of discovering that neither had taken. I couldn't understand why not. Both women had managed to have children of their own. Why was this fertility business so difficult? Had the clinic done something incorrectly? Should the transfer have been done in the dark, as I later learned was standard in another clinic?

I had scaled so many mountains to get to this point, so I told myself this was a mere bump in our journey to parenthood. Hey, this was only our first attempt!

Our surrogate was extremely disappointed and took the failure personally. I had not been expecting that. I tried to reassure her that it often failed, particularly on the first go, but she felt too emotionally drained to carry on. It was indeed asking a lot of her. Without meaning to, I must have shown my dashed hopes and disappointment. It was an intense situation. I was sorry she wanted to stop but understood.

Would my friend consider donating eggs again? Thankfully, yes. But now we had to find another surrogate. Fortunately, the agency (COTS) came up trumps with a surrogate, but she lived near the Scottish border and we were in London! Still, distance didn't matter. Once visits and all the vetting procedures had been completed, which all took several months, we were anxious to get started again. But just as we were about to proceed, the surrogate discovered that she was pregnant by her husband for another baby. We were hugely disappointed.

She had already been a surrogate for two for other women and this was baby number seven for her. After another wait, COTS found us another angel, a lovely lady called Rebecca, who lived much closer to us in London. Perfect.

Once again, we went through the same implantation process. We crossed our fingers and waited to see if it worked this time.

I tried not to pick up the phone every day to find out how she was, because I didn't want to sound too desperate. Somehow, I was totally convinced it was going to happen this time. Then, one morning, my mobile rang. I picked up the phone, nervous with excitement.

'My period has started,' she said quietly. 'I've taken a pregnancy test just to be sure. I am so, so sorry, but it hasn't worked.'

She told us she'd started a relationship with a new man and that he wasn't keen for her to do it again. I was floored. I pulled myself together, thanked her and told her we should meet up for a drink anyway, but I wasn't sure what we would do next.

A few months later the lady up near the Scottish Borders became available again. She had given birth to baby number seven! She was so fertile, how could it fail? Her doctor wasn't happy about her becoming a surrogate again, but she was perfectly happy to go ahead with it after taking a break for a few months. I would not give up hope! We waited until she was ready, then the two remaining embryos were defrosted and the transplantation took place.

I remember taking her call standing in a changing cubicle in a shop, half-dressed. I took a deep breath as I answered. Were we finally going to be parents?

But it was not to be.

My friend who had donated her eggs had now been through two cycles for us. I hated subjecting her to all these unnecessary hormones. I just couldn't ask her to do it again, it was unfair. I went over to her house, we had a long chat and I told her that I was going to find someone who could do 'straight' surrogacy instead, without the involvement of a clinic. Besides, we just couldn't afford to do it through a clinic again.

We both shed a few tears that it hadn't worked and hugged each other. It was sisterhood at its very best. I will never forget her generosity. I was simply overwhelmed by all the women who up to this point had been on this journey with me. What incredible angels there are in the world.

But now Andrew and I were back at square one. We had no more embryos, and no more money in the pot to fund more attempts through a clinic. Even though I was gutted, I held onto the belief that somewhere out there was someone special who could help us. One day I would be holding my own little baby, looking into his or her eyes, feeling the love and bond between us. Please, God.

Chapter Fifteen:

Devising My 'Metro Map'

My immune system had been wiped out by chemotherapy and several years later it seemed I still had not fully recovered from the onslaught. In 2002, I had swapped the immune-boosting and glucose-lowering berberine for gymnema, as I had forgotten the long list of reasons why I had chosen berberine in the first place. In fact, berberine is so effective as an antimicrobial, the army are investigating it as an anti-anthrax supplement.

I reintroduced it into my regime in 2004 when my markers had shot up again, but there was still no other research I could find about it, so with hindsight I still failed to take it as regularly as I needed to. Instead, I began to look for other ways to boost my immune system.

It was in 2007, during an outbreak of avian flu in the UK which caused mass panic and hysteria, that I discovered cimetidine as an immune booster as well as a potent anti-cancer drug. I was concerned that if I did pick up a potentially deadly bug such as avian or 'bird' flu, I might fare worse than others because I was struggling so badly to fight off any infection I contracted. I was picking up one bug after another, and they would lay me flat for weeks. Despite defeating cancer, I was not thriving. I was merely surviving.

I wondered whether I had to reboot my innate immune system from scratch. Maybe it needed to relearn how to react to colds and flu. Perhaps the trick was to build it back up again slowly, allowing it to relearn how to recognise pathogens. But this approach wasn't working. Every cold was as bad as the last. I was not building up my immunity at all.

I discovered that my Th2 immune response, the humoral response to allergens, was permanently raised (this was what Dr Kenyon had tested – my IL5 result). It was this that was preventing me from raising my Th1 (pathogen) response to opportunistic infections. When one goes up, the other drops. Antihistamine drugs helped reverse this problem: by dampening the Th2 response it allows the Th1 response to come back up. Research showed that cimetidine would do just that.[89] It was an old drug, no longer available over the counter in the UK, despite being liberally prescribed in the 1980s for gastric ulcers.

It was still available in other countries like Germany and the US. I should have asked one of my friends in America to buy it and send it over to me, but instead I used an online pharmacy in Canada. As it was an antacid, I only used it for just three months as I was concerned it might mess up my digestive system long-term. Having an acidic stomach was important for proper digestion. It was all such a juggling act trying to get my body back in balance! But it worked. After being continually blitzed by bugs, I was suddenly back to my old self. Hurrah! I felt especially spritely when I added berberine back into my regime.

It was also in 2007, digging around for drugs for other cancer patients, that I concluded that metformin (a common drug in diabetes treament) would help starve cancer of glucose. And I have since discovered that it has many other cancer-combating effects too, like blocking IGF-1 and mTOR (a key enzyme for cell division), boosting good bacteria in the gut so also improving immunity, while blocking hexokinase 2, one of the steps in the oxidative phosphorylation pathway, reducing the

---

89   Pantziarka, Pan *et al.* "Repurposing drugs in oncology (ReDO)-cimetidine as an anti-cancer agent." *Ecancermedicalscience* vol. 8 485. 26 Nov. 2014, doi:10.3332/ecancer.2014.485

conversion of lactate back to glucose, and increasing insulin sensitivity.[90] Metformin, I decided, was a 'big gun'; it would help boost any cancer-starving diet, but rather than taking it after a meal as many diabetics do, I wondered whether it might be best for cancer patients with 'normal' blood sugar levels to starve the cancer by taking it **before** meals, before the rise in glucose occurred at all.[91] Timing, just like when to exercise (which I decided was best utilised fifteen minutes **after** meals to reduce insulin and glucose), must be of critical importance. A large part of metformin's effects take place in the gut in a similar way to berberine, modulating the 'microbiome', which can be unfavourably altered by both high saturated fat as well as too many simple sugars. Both metformin and berberine improve the number of health-promoting short-chain fatty acids in the gut, helping to reduce inflammation and keep the intestinal barrier intact.[92]

Both berberine and metformin were added into my daily regime. I alternated between the two, but occasionally I added them together. Perhaps I should not have done this without a glucometer to check my glucose levels, but I suffered no ill effects. I was not a diabetic and metformin is 'normo-glycaemic', in other words it doesn't drop glucose levels below normal readings. It is safer than many doctors believe; for years it had been tarred by its more dangerous sister phenformin.

By now, word was spreading that I was a stage IV survivor and that I might know something about achieving remission in impossible

---

90   Madiraju AK, Erion DM, Rahimi Y, Zhang XM, Braddock DT, Albright RA, Prigaro BJ, Wood JL, Bhanot S, MacDonald MJ, Jurczak MJ, Camporez JP, Lee HY, Cline GW, Samuel VT, Kibbey RG, Shulman GI Metformin suppresses gluconeogenesis by inhibiting mitochondrial glycerophosphate dehydrogenase. Nature. 2014 Jun 26; 510(7506): 542-6.

91   Naguib A. et al, 'Mitochondrial complex I inhibitors expose a vulnerability for selective killing of Pten-null cells' Cell Reports, April 3, 2018.

92   Xu Zhang, Yufeng Zhao, Jia Xu, Zhengsheng Xue, Menghui Zhang *et al.* Modulation of gut microbiota by berberine and metformin during the treatment of high-fat diet-induced obesity in rats. Scientific Reports Sept 23 2015

circumstances. I was finding myself taking more and more referrals from friends and friends of friends. I really wanted to put cancer behind me, but I also knew I now possessed valuable information that could help others. Reluctantly, I took on a few cases – kidney, bladder, pancreatic, colorectal and breast.

I tried to stay at arm's length, as researching for them brought back all the bad experiences I was trying so hard to forget. I needed to stay detached, so I rarely met the patient and only communicated through emails.

Alongside natural and alternative therapies, I found many off label drugs that might offer benefits to these patients. Propranolol was a beta blocker that would help reduce VEGF, the growth factor that stimulated the growth of new blood vessels to feed cancer. Propranolol also blocked matrix metalloproteinases 2 and 9 (MMP-2 and MMP-9), so it prevented the tissue scaffold around tumour cells breaking down to allow it to metastasise, changing it from being cancer-promoting to becoming cancer-hostile. But it would interact with dipyridamole as both can potentially lower blood pressure. However, dipyridamole, I discovered, also blocked MMP-9 and blocked WNT signalling, with the latter often being altered in cancer. Sulindac was a NSAID that seemed very useful for colorectal cancer, but it was very difficult to obtain.

I encouraged people to make their own Spot of Bother Charts. But it was clear that after a couple of years, this arm's length approach wasn't working, and the list of supplements seemed too long and confusing. What were the 'big guns', which were the most effective drugs and supplements, and why? People continued to die, and no-one was able to get any of these off-label drugs prescribed from their oncologists. I had some spectacular successes though: two stage IV patients are still alive and very much kicking as I write, both at least fourteen years after their terminal diagnoses, having used natural therapies alone.

These successes were the patients I had met in person. Only then had they fully grasped the importance of the low glycaemic diet, the need for a fully integrated approach and regular supplements. Without this extra level of support, I realised that patients could drift from their diets too easily and simply revert to their oncologist to get them better (a doomed approach with stage IV disease).

The more I discovered, the more I deduced that every patient would need to stop all three dietary 'macros': the bad fats, simple carbohydrates (especially glucose) and the protein (e.g. glutamine) together to achieve the best results.

Despite lengthy explanations on the phone and sending my patients articles from PubMed and Medline, I felt I was mostly wasting my time. Most failed to understand just how important it was to modulate their diets or the importance of adding more to their armoury to boost the woefully inadequate 'standard of care.' Combinations were key. Professor Jane Plant's book *Your Life in their Hands* was all well and good when it came to reducing IGF-1 by cutting out meat and dairy, but I felt it just didn't go far enough. I had been ruthless about sugar. No honey, no bananas, no grapes, no alcohol – you had to really starve that cancer. No half measures.

Jane Plant still thought pizzas and honey were okay, whereas they were definitely on the banned list to me. It was important to reduce the 'glycaemic load' and that dangerous post-meal insulin spike. Cutting out IGF-1 was only one angle, but cutting out glucose and lowering insulin, reducing saturated fat and protein alongside reducing the IGF-1 was surely better.

From observing the behaviours of other patients, I could see that most were still eating white potatoes, white rice, bananas, bread, honey, grapes and fruit juices. I knew they would not fare well without the drugs to help them and a better understanding of how cancer was feeding itself.

With a sigh of resignation, I knew I had to take a more active role. I found myself helping patients design their own Spot of Bother Charts, sitting down with them face to face, discussing what changes they needed to make and who to see. I became a 'facilitator', steering them in the right direction to find the drugs, doctors and supplements they needed.

To explain what had worked for me in simple terms, I put together a basic triangle diagram which showed how each of the drugs I'd taken had worked to starve each 'macro' of the diet that cancer needed. My theory was that you had to starve all three sides of the triangle – the fat, protein and simple carbs – *together* for maximum effect. As cancer became more resistant, it switched from glucose to using glutamine. If you only blocked one route it would simply use another. In fact, it does this through a great many fuel lines. Cancer can utilise not just glucose and glutamine, but also fatty acids, acetate and hydroxybutyrate (ketones) and lactate.[93] Determining what fuel was being used by the cancer was important, but the research regarding this in those days was hard to find. The metabolism wasn't seen as important, and the focus was all on the genetic changes.

93 Butyrate inhibits growth in some cells but accelerates it in others. Rodrigues, L.M., Uribe-Lewis, S., Madhu, B. *et al.* The action of β-hydroxybutyrate on the growth, metabolism and global histone H3 acetylation of spontaneous mouse mammary tumours: evidence of a β-hydroxybutyrate paradox. *Cancer Metab* **5**, 4 (2017). https://doi.org/10.1186/s40170-017-0166-z

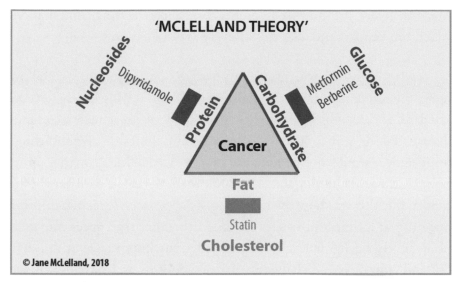

Figure 15.1. *My Triangle Theory to starve all three macros.*

This 'Triangle Theory' to starve cancer was a very simplistic diagram, but it explained my theory visually and easily, based on my sparse knowledge ten years ago.

- Dipyridamole starved cancer of the nucleotides and other proteins.
- Metformin and berberine had starved the glucose.
- Lovastatin had starved the fat (cholesterol).

Once the cancer had been starved, I had delivered the killer blow with the intravenous vitamin C, ozone, the etodolac (NSAID) and lovastatin combination; all had triggered apoptosis. In fact, what I had done to 'starve' my cancer was much more detailed than I have drawn above, and it has only been in recent years that I have been able to piece together exactly how good my combination really was. This simple triangle diagram became a template for me to include other fat, glucose and glutamine pathways that I had blocked, and as my knowledge about the fuel pipelines increased, this triangle eventually evolved into my Metro

Map (see later). It is now a comprehensive cancer-starving combination, which can be used and adapted for every type of cancer.

To newly diagnosed patients, I emphasised the importance of taking more than one treatment at a time, and not relying solely on the standard of care, which is currently inadequate to treat such a complex disease. Taking just a little bit of metformin alongside chemotherapy, for instance, would not be enough. Nor would taking any drug on its own. Nor would ignoring the many abnormal metabolic pathways of the cancer. But this was how their oncologists approached treatment, using one drug at a time and when that failed (because the cancer mutates), using another drug, failing to acknowledge the importance of the stem cell and how it is the change to its metabolism, as I have concluded after much research, that is the real reason why cancer becomes resistant. When under pressure, it shifts its fuel source to continue to feed itself in a new way. The constant search for new 'genetic' drugs only serves the pharmaceutical industry, not the patient. The genetic drugs, while useful for temporarily suppressing growth, all eventually failed. I had to remind my friends that they were not in a trial. This was the real world and combinations were the key, especially when the medications I suggested they should investigate and ask for had little or no toxicity, as shown by years of safety data. Treatment absolutely had to be an integrative approach. My theory was that the major fuel sources needed to be blocked at the same time to starve it. You cannot give cancer any quarter.

Despite all of this, it was frustrating to watch patients make the same mistakes time and time again. Most would not realise the level of effort required to get well. Some felt they would rather die than change their diets or take lots of supplements and pills (and there are a lot!). Patients are naturally resistant to the idea of taking many drugs. And some were reluctant to offend their oncologist, the majority of whom remain resolutely against anything complementary and dismiss diets as useless.

Patients would rather meekly do as they were told, because all their faith entrusted to the white coat and the 'system'.

I was wasting my breath on patients like that. I could only help those who were ready and willing to take on the disease, patients who recognised the failings in the current medical system and were able to take those extra necessary steps. The more advanced the disease, the more they had to do. I could only offer my suggestions and support.

Chapter Sixteen:

Two Slow Car Crashes

One day in 2012 my friend Louise phoned me.

'Rachel has just called me from Dubai,' she said, her voice breaking. 'She told me her triple negative breast cancer has spread. Can you help her?'

Rachel was a mutual friend from Guernsey. She had two children under five and she'd moved out to Dubai with her husband. I winced. Triple negative has the worst prognosis of all the breast cancers – it does not respond to hormonal or herceptin treatment. Treatment usually involves a gruelling combination of surgery, radiotherapy and chemotherapy. If you don't get rid of it first time, it progresses rapidly. Survival with a recurrence is measured in months.

I spoke to Rachel directly later that week. She was in tears.

'The oncologist told me bluntly that everyone has to die as if it were normal,' she sobbed. 'But I'm only forty. I have young kids. Cancer **isn't** normal. I don't want to die. I want to see my children grow up and have families of their own. This just isn't fair.'

I was horrified by her doctor's heartless comment. Not for the first time I wondered whether some oncologists get a perverse kick out of telling patients they're going to die. So much power is handed to them – they wield the axe by either palliative under-treatment or conversely by over-treatment with large amounts of chemotherapy and immunotherapy drugs.

Rachel had been diagnosed with a secondary in her mediastinum (the section between her lungs) months earlier, but she had only just been told her prognosis. Many oncologists feel they're protecting the patient and the family by saying nothing early on, and I can understand why they shy away from revealing the true facts. But this is backhanded cruelty, albeit unintentional. If patients are kept in the dark until they're almost on their deathbed, it leaves them no time to accept the diagnosis, make plans, or find other treatments. The desperate search for alternatives at this stage is heart-breaking. I see it time and time again.

Oncologists view the slow car crash as inevitable, unstoppable and messy. Their job is to merely cushion the blow with palliative treatments and leave the family to pick up the pieces. That's their job as they see it. It is no wonder that oncology attracts only the hardiest personalities.

Often, a patient is given a piece of paper with a cryptic code like T3N2M1 on it, in the hope that they will go away and discover for themselves exactly what this means from Dr Google. The code can easily fool patients into thinking they're only a stage III when in fact the M1 means a distant metastasis, or stage IV. Patients are lulled into a false sense of security, only to be confronted with the harsh reality of their situation when time has passed and the chance for any effective use of other treatment modalities has already become harder.

'I think you should come back to the UK for a second opinion,' I said to Rachel.

So, she made an appointment with one of the UK's top oncologists, Professor Justin Stebbing in London. When she arrived, Rachel, Louise and I sat around my kitchen table and spent the whole afternoon going through some research I'd found her. I drew up her Spot of Bother Chart. On it I had included metformin, the lovastatin and etodolac. I talked her through the reasoning.

I suggested she take her chart to her appointment with Professor Stebbing, but she was reluctant. She was too overwhelmed with her diagnosis to know what to do.

So off she went to the appointment with Louise with a list of questions instead, to ask about being prescribed metformin and lovastatin, to ask about whether her tumour was inflammatory and to ask for a NSAID. I'd tried explaining how inflammation drives cancer.

At the time, I couldn't find enough data to support the inclusion of dipyridamole for triple negative cancer,[94] but I hoped Professor Stebbing might think the other three drugs were worth prescribing, given she was stage IV, 'terminal'. It was surely only reasonable that patients should be allowed to seek treatments that might help save their lives. Was this not humane?

Rachel forgot to ask anything about the off-label drugs during her consultation. Louise reported back to me that she'd only spoken to Professor Stebbing while hidden behind her scarf, probably to hide her tears. I insisted that I come with her on her next visit. She agreed.

A month later, I walked into Professor Stebbing's consulting room with Louise and Rachel. It must have been an odd sight, all three of us trooping in together. After our introductions, I explained that I was there to help Rachel make some decisions. With Rachel's permission I stood up and spread out the A3 Spot of Bother Chart on his desk. His eyes widened in surprise! I could tell the professor had never seen anything of the sort before! Who was this audacious woman?

The chart had many different suggestions, from intravenous vitamin C, stereotactic radiotherapy, sono and photodynamic therapy and high

---

94 I have since uncovered an article published in Clinical Experimental Metastasis published in Jan 2013. Researchers in Naples, Italy have discovered that dipyridamole stops triple negative cancer progression in mice.

intensity focused ultrasound, to the more conventional PARP inhibitors (he was already investigating these). It listed her supplements, diet and detox suggestions too. And (of course) it also included the metformin, lovastatin and an NSAID like etodolac.

Completely ignoring his stunned reaction, I stood there rattling off the possible merits of metformin and a statin. Had he ever prescribed those? And did her tumour express COX2? What did he think of using a nonsteroidal anti-inflammatory?

After he recovered from his initial shock, we had a lengthy discussion about the use of complementary treatments.

He was unsure about the intravenous vitamin C but agreed she could try it, and the photodynamic therapy. After much deliberation, but not outright dismissal, he said he couldn't prescribe the drugs.

'They are not regarded as standard treatments for cancer, and I do not want to prescribe these without randomised clinical trials,' he said.

No matter, I had anticipated this outcome and had already booked another appointment for her around the corner with Dr Kenyon, who I hoped might be able to prescribe some of the drugs.

By now Rachel had quite a large tumour in her mediastinum. Both Professor Stebbing and I knew the standard medical treatments on their own were never going to control her disease for long. They would only buy her a few months, not that we said so in her presence.

An hour later, Dr Kenyon ran some tests. Rachel still appeared to have good liver function and she hadn't been wrecked by chemotherapy at this stage. All was looking good if she wanted to start photodynamic therapy. But Rachel had other ideas. She just didn't feel comfortable with alternative treatments. She wanted to stick with convention, although she did agree to the metformin, so Dr Kenyon, with a bit of encouragement from me, wrote out a prescription for her.

I met Professor Stebbing several times with Rachel and he gave me his email address. Together we discussed various treatments she eventually decided to pursue, such as stereotactic radiotherapy. And despite the huge tumour resting between her lungs, Rachel stayed alive for a further twenty-two months. Precious time with her young family.

When she died, her passing felt like a personal failure to me, despite my efforts. I wished I had managed to get her all the drugs I felt she had needed. A proper cocktail that targeted several fuel lines. Triple negative breast cancer was tricky. What fuel did TNBC use that others didn't? It was one of the hardest cancers to cure. In her honour, I would make it my mission to find out how. If I could find out what it was and how to block it, perhaps it would help reverse this dreadful disease that afflicted too many young mums.

A few months later, I was asked for help again by a lady who'd been diagnosed with malignant melanoma. I met with Beth and her two sons, both in their twenties. We all sat in my kitchen and made a treatment plan together. I sketched out a Spot of Bother Chart and showed them the rudimentary cancer-starving triangle. We investigated lots of different natural approaches that Beth might want to try as well as old drugs. Everyone was happy with Beth's chosen path. It was important that the decisions were made by her. She felt it would be useful if I accompanied her to see her consultant at the Royal Marsden Hospital in London, the best-known cancer hospital in the UK.

From the research done by Dr Betty Rhodes at St. Helier Hospital on melanoma patients in the 1980s, I knew that dipyridamole would be helpful for her. I even managed to acquire the original paper from the Lancet. But convincing oncologists to prescribe anything off label would be particularly hard at this bastion of traditional treatments. Still, we agreed that it was worth a try.

We added a statin and an NSAID to her list as I'd found good articles on both that related to melanoma. I couldn't find much evidence for metformin at the time so stuck to just three drugs: dipyridamole, a statin and an NSAID. The following week I met Beth at the hospital.

She greeted me as I entered the waiting room of the Royal Marsden, which was rammed full of gloomy, silent patients and families. It was standing room only. Her sons could not attend that day and Beth introduced me to her brother and sister who had come instead. They both eyed me with suspicion; clearly they did not approve of my presence.

When we entered the consultant's room, I realised with some dismay that he was 'old school.' He peered at us over his reading glasses as we sat down.

Beth, buoyed up by her new treatment plan and feeling more in control of her disease, launched into quick speech about how much better she felt to have cut out sugar from her diet. Unfortunately, this set the tone for the whole meeting. Diet was the last thing that the oncologist wanted to discuss.

'I have already explained that changing your diet is a waste of time,' he said, as if scolding a disobedient child. 'It has never been shown to help cancer patients and all you are doing is depriving yourself at a critical stage when you should be relaxing and eating what you like best,' he added.

So she might as well be gorging on chocolates because she was going to die anyway? No wonder patients call it The Royal Mars Bar.

'I wondered what you thought about her trying some photodynamic therapy?' I asked, regretting the words as they fell out of my mouth.

I could see his calm demeanour changing from one of tolerance to one of irritation.

He looked me straight in the eye with an icy glare.

'There is no evidence that will help either,' he answered curtly. 'She will just be wasting her money.'[95]

If this was a difficult subject to tackle, then broaching the subject of off label drugs was going to be really hard. For Beth's sake I had to try and get her something. Sticking to the standard of care alone would fail.

'Okay. We'll park that idea,' I said, just to humour him. 'I've also been looking at some off label drugs that might help,' I added nervously. 'This is an article in The Lancet showing that dipyridamole, an antiplatelet drug, might help stop metastases. It stopped progression in several patients with stage IV disease.'

I handed over the article. He took the piece of paper from me, said nothing and stared at it. I carried on,

'Dipyridamole also has antiviral properties, and the article suggests there might be a viral component to melanoma.'

'This is not evidence! This isn't a randomised clinical trial! It is a study on a few patients in 1985!' He made a snorting sound and the article was thrust back at me. Beth stole a look at me, winked and rolled her eyes to say, 'Exactly the reaction we expected.'

'I know it's old, but what if it's been overlooked?' I added, cross that he was dismissing a potentially life changing drug just because it wasn't new. It was like saying The Beatles were rubbish because they split up in 1970.

---

[95] I had read a report that clearly showed photodynamic therapy might benefit stage 3 and 4 melanomas: *https://www.ncbi.nlm.nih.gov/pubmed/22653896*

'How about looking at a statin?' I asked, bringing out the next article and aware that I was rapidly losing ground.

'And what date is that research?' he asked.

'Um… 2005, published in Melanoma Research,' I said.

'This is 2013! If these were in any way useful, wouldn't we already be using them?'

'So you don't think they might be of some help? Do you want to read the article?' I said in a small voice. Obviously not. The oncologist turned to Beth.

'I want a word with you. Alone.'

Crikey. That hadn't gone well. I knew I was going to meet with some resistance, but it had been far worse than Beth or I had expected.

He stood up, opened the door and beckoned for her brother, sister and me to leave the room. We filed out and once again, he threw me a huge scowl. I turned to see that Beth was okay and he slammed the door shut in my face.

I could hear him talking in heated tones to Beth. I felt bad. I'd been trying to help, and it wasn't fair that she'd been caught in the crossfire between us. I was also upset he had been so dismissive without even examining all the evidence. Where was patient choice?

But what happened to me next was truly shocking. As soon as I was in the corridor her brother and sister turned on me. Dave towered over me and pinned me against the wall.

They both began yelling in my face, Dave jabbing me in the chest with his finger.

'Who the hell do you think you are? Are you a doctor? How dare you make suggestions to the oncologist! You have no right interfering with her treatment!'

I stood there trying to breathe calmly, 'I…I'm just trying to help her,' I stammered.

Nothing like this had ever happened to me before. I was desperate to escape. There was little point in entering into a discussion with them, because they were in no mood to listen. I wriggled my way out of their grip and quickly headed for the door.

'Don't you dare contact her again!' shouted her sister at my back as I sped to the exit.

Cancer is a confusing and frightening experience for the whole family, and I knew they were only acting in what they thought were her best interests. As much as I told myself that they were only being over-protective, I was very shaken by this physical and verbal abuse.

Once safely outside the hospital, I sent Beth a text with an excuse about having to go home urgently. She probably guessed they had been rude to me, but I never told her what they'd done. Beth and her sons would have been mortified if they had ever found out. She had enough on her plate already.

Helping a desperate patient was one thing, but dealing with protective, angry relatives was quite another! I vowed to never accompany anyone on a visit ever again. It was not good for my own health! But how would patients ever get hold of these drugs? It seemed an impossible task. Oncologists were bound by rigid protocols.

Later I sent Beth off to see Dr Callebout, but she never asked for dipyridamole or any of the other drugs. I believe her oncologist at the Royal Marsden put her off. Why had he been so antagonistic and angry? And why shouldn't she try and save herself by any means possible? Had the oncologist felt threatened by me questioning his authority? This was not patient-centred care!

To my dismay I learned that she died six months later.

I felt that I had failed again. I couldn't help but wonder how she would have fared if only she'd taken a drug cocktail. When would the oncology profession wake up? Could they not see how rigid and inflexible they were? They seemed closed to every suggestion, apparently for no good reason at all. How had this arrogance got so bad? I couldn't understand what could have gone wrong with the profession to make them behave like trained killers, refusing to allow patients to save themselves. 'My way or the highway! I decide how you are going to die.' Oncology was so messed up, and the losers were the patients.

Once you're diagnosed with stage IV, you're given few options but to go on a treadmill of approved drugs, none of which have ever cured anyone with advanced disease. New drugs and trials are so overhyped in the press that people have too much faith in them. The pharmaceutical industry has hoodwinked the medical profession and especially the vulnerable patient into believing that modern medicine and their patented drugs hold all the answers. It is only natural to believe the latest drug is going to be better than the last. But if you examine the statistics, this, sadly, is not the case.

The NHS budget is so tight, it relies on most patients with stage IV dying with the first treatment option, which is invariably high dose chemotherapy, the cheapest but least effective treatment for cancer. A dead patient is a massive saving! It is far cheaper for the NHS if you die as soon as possible than if you hang on, clinging onto life and requiring lots of nursing care and costly medications. And just to kick you when you're down, the side effect of high dose chemotherapy is that it will markedly reduce your chances of recovery by crushing your immune system, an essential ingredient to your long-term survival.

If, against the odds, you have proven yourself a 'worthy' candidate by surviving the high dose chemotherapy, the NHS reserve the newer and often staggeringly expensive immunotherapies for the people who make it this far. By then the immunotherapies are, of course, less effective after the chemo. And we wonder why the UK has the worst cancer survival rates in Europe.

As a stage IV patient in the NHS, you're playing a deadly game of snakes and ladders by using conventional therapies alone. If you survive the chemotherapy, when the cancer comes back (as it will – chemotherapy alone fails to kill the cancer stem cells) you may then be offered a lifeline, a ladder in the form of a targeted drug to climb back up. If it's available you grab it gratefully, while still utterly exhausted from the previous treatment. If you're lucky, this new drug will work for a while, but the effects are only short term – average life extension with targeted drugs at this stage is around two or three months. Boom! You land on another snake and slide back down again. If you're still lucky they 'rescue you' once more with another line of treatment, perhaps a newer immunotherapy drug. How grateful you are to the wonders of modern medicine! Your hopes are raised yet again, only to be dashed when the hype fails to live up to expectation. There are no more ladders – only snakes.

The whole paradigm of cancer treatment is wrong.

Cancer has two types of cells: stem cells and fast dividing cells. The ones targeted by oncologists are the fast-dividing cells; the treatments they provide do nothing to address the cancer stem cell itself. And cancer stem cells are the ones that cause the cancer to spread. These are located at the heart of every tumour and are untouched by conventional treatments. Chemotherapy, radiotherapy and the newer targeted drugs are all short-term solutions, because they leave the stem cells behind to regrow and become more resistant.

It is a medieval, cruel and heartless game. And it could so easily be different if the medical profession would look at using cocktails of drugs, not just ones to target the genes and fast dividing cells, but substances that actually attack the stem cells too.

As patients, we need to be aware of this despicable game that the pharmaceutical companies play with us while we desperately cling to life, our bodies mercilessly used like laboratory mice. When would oncologists prescribe off label drugs alongside conventional care? Surely it had to happen soon. As the doctor at the Royal Marsden had pointed out, this was 2013. When would the profession wake up?

Chapter Seventeen:

Finding My Tribe

In February 2015, I was quietly reading the newspaper with my morning cup of tea (green, of course), when I noticed an article in The Telegraph.[96] I sat up when I realised it was all about cancer and the use of old off label drugs! At last!

A Professor in psychology, Ben Williams, had been diagnosed with an incurable brain tumour twenty years earlier. He had followed traditional conventional medicine having surgery, chemotherapy and radiotherapy, but he had healed himself completely using a few drugs that he'd researched and added into his cancer regime. Finally, here was someone else who had been cured using a cocktail of old drugs! Hoorah!

He had used verapamil, a calcium channel blocker (something which is also a property of berberine), during his chemotherapy, an antibiotic called Accutane normally used for acne. It is a vitamin A analogue (which weakly blocks mevalonate – I had used a statin -and it also promotes a cell death process called autophagy), and to obtain it he had travelled across the border to Mexico. He had also used tamoxifen which, besides its oestrogen-blocking effect, is an IGF-1 inhibitor (I was now taking metformin daily as an IGF-1 blocker, both for its anti-cancer and anti-ageing benefits).

---

96   http://www.telegraph.co.uk/lifestyle/wellbeing/healthadvice/11424747/The-professor-who-cured-his-cancer-with-a-cocktail-of-everyday-pills-and-20-years-on-remains- disease-free.html.

As I read more, I nearly fell off my chair. There was a new clinic in Harley Street, right here in London, investigating an almost identical drug combination to my own: metformin, a statin and two other drugs. My God. This new clinic, called the Care Oncology Clinic, were studying the use of these drugs as adjuncts to conventional treatment, just as I had always suggested. Two of the drugs I had not seen or heard of in oncology before, doxycycline (an antibiotic) and mebendazole (an anti-parasitic drug). There was no sign of dipyridamole anywhere, though. But they were looking at adding a NSAID to some of the treatment programmes in the future. Perhaps they could add dipyridamole into their programme too!

What was more incredible was the chief oncologist at the Care Oncology Clinic was none other than Professor Justin Stebbing! According to the article, he was overseeing this new clinic in Harley Street, prescribing the very same off label drugs I had begged him to prescribe to Rachel!

I can only describe what came over me as a metaphysical rush. Goosebumps, shivers, call it what you will; the sensation was incredible. My feet and legs began to tingle, and a hot prickling sensation swept all over me, up my back and down my arms.

They say you have two great moments in life, the first when you're born, the second when you realise why you were born. This was that moment.

As soon as I'd finished reading the article, I was convinced that someone had finally cracked the cancer code, that the answer had indeed, as I had always believed, been in using combinations to starve the cancer. I had to meet these people. I wanted to find out more about the drugs they had chosen and why they might work.

Doxycycline was an antibiotic, mebendazole was an anti-helminth or worming pill, commonly used for children with pinworms. I had always wondered if cancer might be caused not by 'random genetic mutations', but maybe it could be triggered by something as simple as a co-infection of various microbes? There was no doubt that these drugs had other effects beyond their antimicrobial ones. I wondered whether microbes affected the mitochondria, or whether doxycycline worked because it acted on mitochondria, on the metabolism, as they were both once ancient bacteria. If viruses were known to cause cancer, was it such a stretch to think that other microbes, like bacteria, yeasts and parasites, could affect cancer too? Perhaps an altered microbiome (the environment or terrain around the cancer) also affected it.

The article listed several drugs being investigated by the ReDo (Repurposing Drugs for Cancer) campaign for their anti-cancer potential. It listed cimetidine, which I had also taken for a few months a few years earlier because of its immune-stimulating and anti-cancer effects, but dipyridamole was nowhere to be seen. No matter, the Care Oncology Clinic were on the case with the other drugs. I cannot begin to tell you how delighted and excited I was!

I stood up, danced around the kitchen like a lunatic, and then promptly burst into tears. Emotion poured out of me. I realised that this would change everything. I was elated to think that finally there might be a serious step change in cancer treatment. Two fingers up to all those arrogant oncologists who had ignored me! This trial would prove me right, I knew it! I was so excited to finally have somewhere I could send the many patients who approached me for help. This clinic meant I no longer had to fight the medical profession on my own, having doors shut in my face, being sneered at, laughed at, belittled, with fingers jabbed in my chest. Here was validation of everything I had said and thought about cancer – even the parts which had been dismissed as ridiculous.

How could a lowly physiotherapist, albeit a stage IV survivor, have lived when so many eminent cancer scientists died? In the eyes of the medics,

I was a spontaneous remission, an anecdote, a medical anomaly. Now I had found my army, fighting back against these entrenched doctrines, not on the other side of the world, but right here in London! I could hardly believe it!

I realised with dismay that this meant I would finally have to write my book and writing it would stir up many painful memories. But without my help I was worried this clinic would struggle. I knew about the Cancer Act 1939, which meant they were not allowed to advertise. They would need a patient to champion their cause. And I was patient zero.

I didn't want cancer to start playing a central role in my life again. I desperately wanted to bury it, for my struggles to be forgotten, for people to never know what I had been through. But my story would have to be told. Patients would need to know that I had walked in their shoes, that I too had felt the sorrow, the sadness, the despair. I needed them to know there was hope for them, and that there was so much more they could do. But it would mean revealing intimate details of my illness, my relationships and my struggles. I would be unmasked. Damn.

But this time I would not just be fighting for better treatments for myself, I would be fighting for all the mothers, fathers, daughters and sons affected by this dreadful disease, each one of them badly let down by the current inadequate standard of care. Patients deserved better, but they were too ill to fight for themselves or realise just how badly they were being treated by the pharmaceutical companies. I was convinced that with the right cocktail, we had all the drugs we needed to cure cancer already.

I needed to find out who had started the clinic and what they expected to gain. Who was funding it? It couldn't be a big pharmaceutical company, as these were all cheap off-patent drugs and would be of no financial interest to the powers that be. I was confused, but equally thrilled. This clinic could shake up the entire medical profession! One thing was certain: it was not going to be popular with Big Pharma.

If it became as successful as I believed it should, this clinic would rock the pharmaceutical giants to their core. I knew they'd need all the help they could get to overcome resistance and attempts to shut them down. I immediately phoned my friend Louise. We agreed to meet at a café for lunch.

'That is incredible!' she said when I showed her the article. 'What a turnaround by Stebbing! He's prescribing the very drugs he didn't want Rachel to have only a few years ago!'

'To be fair, I don't think he could have prescribed the metformin as she wasn't diabetic, and the statin is for lowering cholesterol and not normally used for cancer, so he was in a very difficult position. Oncologists have their hands tied by strict protocols. It is difficult for them to prescribe these drugs – in many ways it seems harder now than it was seventeen years ago when I got hold of them, even though there is more research to support their usage now.'

The waiter handed me my cup of green tea, which I would have gladly swapped for a celebratory glass of red. 'It's not easy for doctors to step outside the narrow options laid down by NICE. They have to be very brave and know that the patient or their relatives aren't going to come back and sue them. People are so litigious nowadays.'

'Yes, but he knows that the patient is dying. If something might work, surely the doctors should try it?'

'I agree with you, Lou. The red tape is crazy.'

'You're going to do that embarrassing thing with the tea bag now, aren't you?'

She watched me squeeze the last few drops from the bag into my hands and smear it over my face. 'That's better! Young and beautiful!'

She laughed. 'I admit you don't look too ancient given your advancing years.'

I had done a lot of research into moisturisers and anti-ageing ingredients for my toiletries range and found a lot of overlap with nutraceuticals. Green tea was a consistent winner both internally and externally – I couldn't give a rat's arse what people in a café thought. The benefit of being the wrong side of forty is that you aren't particularly bothered what people think of you.

'I distinctly remember Stebbing telling you to sit down when you spread out Rachel's Spot of Bother Chart,' she said, re-emerging from behind the menu. 'I think you terrified him.'

I laughed. 'Scary Jane!'

Perhaps I had. Most patients and relatives are so terrified and compliant they're ready to do anything the oncologist suggests. They would jump out of a window if he or she said it would make them better. This gives some oncologists an unhealthy sense of power and an air of arrogance and superiority. Professor Stebbing was not like that; he gave patients his phone number and was ready to help at any time of day or night. He was their hero. To have me striding into his consulting room, determined and demanding, must have been an unusual sight, nonetheless.

I hadn't meant to come across as confrontational. I was merely trying to add to Rachel's list of medications and enhance the standard treatments.[97]

---

[97]   N.B. Confrontation is not the best way to approach your doctor! The best way? Evidence, evidence, and yes, more evidence. Know as much about the treatment as you can.

As I sat there with Louise, there was no doubt in my mind what I needed to do. 'I am going to write to Professor Stebbing today,' I said. 'This clinic is up against it. These treatments are going to meet with a lot of resistance from Big Pharma and probably a great many oncologists. Stebbing is really sticking his neck on the line. Behind the scenes, I sent him many emails and we discussed lots of things I never told you about during Rachel's care, not just about these drugs. Perhaps I ground him down in the end!'

'Perhaps you did! You are persistent, that's for sure! Write to him and I will back you all the way,' she laughed.

Later that day, I fired off an email:

Dear Professor Stebbing,

I am sure you remember when I first met you a few years ago with Rachel T-C, demanding she should have metformin and a combination of lovastatin and etodolac! Apologies for that. A mixture of frustration and um... more frustration, I think. I can't tell you how delighted I am to see some joined up thinking treating cancer as a systemic disease and not just a local problem. There is too much emphasis on micro-targeted therapies nowadays and scant regard to the macro. I am so pleased to see a cancer clinic offering to use these cheap 'dirty' drugs as I used many of them myself to overcome cancer back in 1999, alongside dietary changes and detox. You may have forgotten, or I may not have told you, but I had stage IV cervical which had spread to my lungs sixteen years ago. I persuaded two integrative doctors to prescribe dipyridamole (Persantin) and later metformin. I am still taking the latter and I also later took cimetidine for a short while, which I am ashamed to admit I bought direct from a Canadian online pharmacy. Lovastatin and etodolac were a combination my oncologist (now retired) decided had enough research behind it to prescribe to me in a high dose for three months. She was in fact delighted when I gave her my research as she was investigating statins at the time! I know you are chair of the World Vaccine

Congress and I wondered if you have you read the following article in The Scientist about probiotics and vaccines?

http://www.the-scientist.com/?articles.view%2FarticleNo%2F40973%2Ftitle%2FBacteria-Boost-Viral-Vaccine-Response%2F

I am sure this is old news, and this article relates to flu, but I firmly believe the gut and the immune system are inextricably linked and that to get the best effect from a vaccine the patient should be on a good probiotic for a few weeks prior to being injected with the vaccine. Intravenous vitamin C would also prime the immune system for cancer vaccines. Are you also looking into 2-methoxyoestradiol? And I am sure you know all about the exciting vitamin D research. Sulindac/lovastatin for colon cancer, gemcitabine/ curcumin and low dose naltrexone and alpha lipoic acid for pancreatic cancer, I could go on... I would love to come and do some voluntary work for you. Would there be anything I could usefully do? Anyway, DELIGHTED to see this clinic up and running! I will be sending patients your way! And I am serious about a job as I want to do something meaningful whilst I write my memoirs!

Best regards,

Jane McLelland

I hit the send button and wondered how Professor Stebbing and the clinic would respond.

Chapter Eighteen:

Mobilising the Troops

Whichever way I looked at it, the Care Oncology Clinic were trying to achieve something monumental, and I knew I had to help. If they proved successful, they would threaten not just pharmaceutical giants but also major cancer charities like Cancer Research UK (CRUK). The latter survive both on cancer being incurable and through keeping the pharmaceutical industry supplied with a steady stream of guinea pigs for their trials and new patents. CRUK's mission was to get more patients onto clinical trials, to 'stop more patients dying' (whilst taking lots of expensive medicines), not to find a cure.

Drug companies base new drug launches on a thirty-year profit return, with drugs developed to encourage repeat prescriptions over many years rather than one-off cures. Old off-patent drugs make them very little money.

So who were the brave people behind this clinic who were daring to challenge the status quo? With a bit of background digging, I discovered that the Clinic is owned by Seek, a private Biotech company with some seriously clever scientists. They are redeveloping metformin and other old drugs as well as ibuprofen, so that they can be delivered more efficiently to the areas needed with fewer side effects. Genius.

They don't hope to make much money from the Clinic – it's there to study the drug combinations, put into practice a metabolic approach and allow doctors to do the job they signed up for as medical students: to improve lives and get patients better. Not to poison them with ever more toxic drugs and make their last few months on Earth a misery.

The very next day, a return email arrived in my mailbox from Gregory Stoloff at the Care Oncology Clinic. It appeared that they were equally excited to have discovered me too! Gregory and Dr Robin Bannister wanted to meet me as soon as possible to share ideas. Holy moly. I can't tell you what a shock this was. For years I had been challenging the way oncologists prescribe treatments, quietly waging a little war on my own, championing the old drugs, and losing. To be asked what I think? And to share my ideas? To me, it felt like these concepts were alien to most of the medical profession. Trying to get through to most oncologists was like trying to get through to a brick wall.

When I met Gregory and Robin, I was blown away by their enthusiasm and commitment. We were so much on the same page I felt like crying. We had travelled completely different roads to arrive at the same junction, and we were now driving off in the same direction! Even though their cocktail is currently dismissed by the medical profession at large, I found nothing controversial in their approach. It totally matched mine. Combine the old drugs and attack the different metabolic drivers. Stress the cancer, starve it, weaken it and then trigger apoptosis.

Gregory had worked on mergers between pharmaceutical giants. He saw first-hand how old drugs were left on the shelf collecting dust. It's hard to get Gregory to speak about himself but I've gathered that he initially studied medicine before switching to finance, and his eyes remained open to the broader view and the big problems which are still rife in medicine. But despite setting up his own pharmaceutical company to explore his ideas, he has always been an outsider in that world. His fresh and lateral approach to problems is what the industry needs, but that kind of thinking is unwelcome in a world dominated by large corporates with vested interests in maintaining high prices and profits ahead of patient wellbeing. He doesn't fit the profile.

It was an incredibly emotional meeting for me. I don't think they understood just how much it meant to be finally acknowledged for all the time and effort I had put in to researching cancer, not just for myself but for friends and family too. They couldn't know the obstacles I'd faced. To keep going despite the rejection and scorn. The realisation of just how close I might have been to saving some of my friends if only I'd got them on more of the repurposed drugs. Used appropriately, at the right time, in the right combination, at the right dosages, I knew they held so much potential to save lives. There will always be patients for whom treatment comes too late. Nothing, no matter how amazing, is going to work if organ damage is too severe from other treatments or from the cancer itself. Long-term remissions, even with late-stage patients, will be the aim of the Clinic, and I have every confidence they can do it.

It's hard to talk about cures. I haven't had a cancer 'episode' for years, but I can never say I'm cured. I am confident that my disease is controlled, but 'cured' is a big, uncomfortable word. Certainly, the longer I remain disease free the more confident I am.

When I said I felt I'd been over-treated with chemotherapy, they completely agreed. What? I had to keep pinching myself that I was hearing correctly. Indeed, they plan to get patients back to normal using low dose chemotherapy where possible, by getting their oncologists to agree.

When I came out of that meeting I had never felt so totally, passionately driven. I knew I would do whatever it took to get this therapy accepted by mainstream doctors. Patients had suffered long enough.

How was I to spread the word? When I mentioned how I had cured my cancer with a handful of old drugs and how there was a new clinic offering a similar cocktail in a few Facebook groups I did not get the enthusiastic response I'd expected. Patients were unsure of using any drugs, no matter how low the toxicity. Most wanted natural cures, if anything. Patients would need to be educated. It was time to 'come out' and admit publicly that I had been terminally ill, with a closed Facebook group dedicated to off label drugs with anti-cancer effects.

Directly promoting the Care Oncology Clinic was not allowed by law. The Cancer Act 1939 is an antiquated ruling that prevents advertising for cancer treatments. While I understand it helps prevent corrupt salespeople selling fake cures, it also stops people discovering effective help too. Ultimately, it keeps Big Pharma in control. I had to be cautious, only mentioning the Clinic by name when asked.

The Clinic needed patients through its doors. Without the statistical data to show that combination therapy works, it risked being shut down. It still does. Over the next few years, they hope to recruit about 5,000 patients on the study, and so it's become my mission to spread the word to the masses. With the Cancer Act dangling over my head, this is proving more difficult than I thought. I have also run into quite unexpected resistance from friends and doctors.

A few weeks ago, I was telling a friend about the Clinic over dinner when she mentioned her father had advanced cancer. 'You must send him over to the Clinic!' I said, expecting her to be as enthusiastic as I was. I'd explained the treatments and how they'd help starve his cancer. But her response took me by surprise.

'I don't believe it. If it's so good, then how come my dad's oncologist isn't giving it to him already?' She said looking completely unconvinced.

I should have known that this might be the reaction. It's an instinctive question and one that comes up regularly. As a layperson you only realise the failings of the medical system when you've been in the thick of it and it has let you down. Even then most people still have unerring faith that everything possible was done to save their loved one. But was it?

It is not unusual or even unexpected for a well-meaning relative of a patient to remain closed to suggestions of treatments outside the conventional path. Relatives can unwittingly be the largest obstacle to a patient's survival. Taking a less orthodox approach is too risky in their eyes – they may think that complementary treatments will only hasten their demise. New immunotherapy drugs or exciting vaccines are very enticing, but you shouldn't put all your eggs in one basket. Adding metabolic drugs that starve the cancer will weaken the enemy and stop drug resistance. By adding extra weapons to your anti-cancer armoury, you can raise the cancer-busting power of traditional drugs. Combinations are the answer to this 'emperor of all maladies.' It is not immortal.

Fear of the unknown and an unquestioning faith in the system is a driving force behind pharmaceutically-fueled oncology. Treading an alternative path can cause terrible arguments, depression, anxiety and family break-ups at a time when everyone should be pulling together. Often, the patient is being pulled in so many directions, it's easier just to keep the peace and stick to doing as they're told.

Even my own GP is resistant to the idea of using a combination of old drugs. When I mentioned I was going to be volunteering in a cancer clinic he said, 'That's the last place you need to be.' I had taken a press cutting with me from The Independent newspaper, about Dr Bannister, the Clinic and how his wife's tumours were shrinking with the treatment, hoping my local doctor's surgery wouldn't mind me putting it up on their noticeboard. I'd shown the receptionist who thought the story was amazing, particularly in light of my own experience. 'Of course you can put it up,' she said. Before I did, I decided I ought to run it past my doctor first.

He took one look at the article, speed reading, and dismissed it. 'This is all very well but there's no science behind it. Where's the evidence?'

What! There was a ton of science. I couldn't believe my ears. Apart from the ample science cited in the article, the proof was sitting right next to him, living and breathing, despite a terminal diagnosis. I think he'd been looking after me for so long he'd forgotten I had been stage IV.

'Results will eventually be published in a peer reviewed journal like the BMJ, but you know I took statins, etodolac and other drugs. You even prescribed the statin after my oncologist suggested I keep taking it. You can see it worked for me. My markers plummeted during that time.'

'If it's that good then add it to the water.' This was a typical knee-jerk reaction I might have expected from a doctor. Yes, that thought had been mooted years ago when statins first appeared on the market amidst much hype about their miracle effects. Lovastatin, the first statin and the one I took, was far weaker than more recent statins and had far fewer side effects. Since then, statins have become stronger and side effects have become more likely. The conflicting research about whether we really need to reduce cholesterol for heart disease continues to mount while other benefits of statins, like their anti-inflammatory effects, are suppressed. Dipyridamole had been the first drug routinely prescribed for heart disease. When statins were discovered, they stopped prescribing dipyridamole. No-one thought to combine the two together, yet the two drugs work synergistically, enhancing the effects of each other.[98] For cancer, though, the beneficial effects of statins are quite clear. There is a growing heap of research on simvastatin, atorvastatin and lovastatin (the lipophilic statins) for nearly every cancer, showing their clear benefits.

---

98   Kim, Hyung-Hwan *et al.* 'Additive Effects of Statin and Dipyridamole on Cerebral Blood Flow and Stroke Protection.' *Journal of cerebral blood flow and metabolism: official journal of the International Society of Cerebral Blood Flow and Metabolism* 28.7 (2008): 1285-1293. PMC. Web. 25 Jan. 2018.

'Yes, you could argue a good case for everyone being on metformin,' I countered. 'Our diets are far too high in carbs. We were not designed to eat the way we do. Our Western diet is a disaster for the metabolism. Taking metformin regularly would stop a lot of health problems developing and decrease your workload significantly!'

If he wanted science, I would blind him with it. I started to talk about metformin and its impact on the mTOR pathway, and the impact of statins on the Glut receptor and the mevalonate pathway. I could tell he wasn't really listening. He was still staring at the article, glazing over. After feigning interest in what I was saying for a minute he piped up with a smile, 'There's the problem!'

What had he spotted? 'They are just after people's money!' he exclaimed.

'What?' At the clinic, the total cost of treatment including four consultations and medications for an entire year came to a mere £1250, roughly £100 a month, which included the cost of the drugs! In what way could that be seen as costly for a Harley Street clinic, when the total average cost of cancer care was estimated to be roughly £100,000 a year? How did he expect the Clinic to pay their staff and overheads? On fresh air? And how exactly were the patients going to get hold of these drugs? They couldn't get them on the NHS.

'Well, good luck with it, but I bet it won't work,' he added.

Oh really? I thought to myself. 'How much do you bet? A million?'

We bet on a measly pound, which I'm going to hold him to. And he still wouldn't let me put the press cutting up on the surgery noticeboard. When I came out of his consulting room, I told the receptionist his reaction. She read it again. 'Can I photocopy it and take it anyway?' she asked. 'Of course,' I said, 'take it!'

My doctor may have had a point. Being involved with an oncology clinic is potentially a psychologically disastrous choice for any cancer patient to make, even a healthy one. The loss, grief and trauma gave me deep physical and emotional scars I continue to bear. But over the years I've found the strength and courage to shelve my personal feelings and help many friends and relatives through their diagnoses. I've been able to help many survive long after their predicted expiry dates.

Most cancer clinics are deeply depressing places that fill me with dread. I cannot stand the ritual of cutting, burning and poisoning the cancer, while you are fed pizza, chips and ice cream, served with a muffin on the side and a bottle of Coke to wash it all down. With the Care Oncology Clinic, I no longer have to battle an antiquated system. If a cancer patient asks me for advice, I draw up a Spot of Bother Chart, work out the dominant metabolic drivers of their cancer, use my Metro Map (see later) to give the patient some treatment options and point them in the direction of the Clinic to see a doctor. Then I sit back and sigh with relief, no more tense meetings with blinkered and arrogant oncologists! Phew.

In a few short months, I helped get two major articles published in the Sunday Times and the Daily Mail, spoke at a key Metabolic Conference on cancer, visited Adam Afriye MP in Westminster several times,[99] met with the former Deputy Prime Minister and helped push through some small changes in legislation with off patent drugs. At last, I started to feel like I might be getting somewhere, albeit slowly.

What I achieved with Professor Stebbing was an unusual working relationship in oncology. In other areas of medicine, say in neurology, doctors work with multidisciplinary teams that may include a physiotherapist, occupational therapists and an extended nursing team. Integrative teams in oncology are woefully inadequate. To me they

---

99   Mostly to talk about the Off-Patent Bill and Saatchi Bill, which have now merged together into the Medical Innovations Bill.

should include a complementary or functional medicine practitioner, a nutritionist, lifestyle coach, a dentist and a physical therapist. Not just an oncologist, surgeon, radiologist and oncology nurses.

With Professor Stebbing we collaborated to work out an integrative strategy, and guided Rachel's treatment choices by working together as a task force. As a result, she had taken metformin, received photodynamic therapy, intravenous vitamin C and stereotactic radiotherapy (Cyberknife), as well as traditional treatments, several supplements and diet modifications. It was so refreshing to receive encouragement and a blessing for suggesting these treatments, rather than derision and scorn. And there was absolutely no doubt that our joint efforts had helped her survive much longer than anyone had ever thought possible.

Professor Stebbing is a genuinely caring man, and it was no surprise to me that he had teamed up with the Care Oncology Clinic. As one of his colleagues says on his charity web page: 'Professor Stebbing is a tireless and creative protagonist in the battle against cancer. Always open-minded and receptive to new ideas, he has the intellectual courage and stamina to bring the fight to the enemy. He is a risk-taker, and we desperately need more like him.'

Indeed. We certainly do.

What makes this clinic really stand out for me though is that they collate information not just on these drugs, which would be awesome enough on its own, but on the patient's other supplements and treatments. During the consultation it's noted whether the patient is having intravenous vitamin C, hyperbaric oxygen, vitamin D, laetrile, cannabis oil or any other off label drugs, and the best bit is they don't bat an eyelid at any of it. No more lying or deceit. The data becomes a melting pot, where the truth about what really works for each cancer type will eventually float to the top.

The savings from these cheap drug cocktails, alongside appropriate conventional treatments and proper nutritional advice, could be so vast I can't begin to imagine it. Could this on its own save the NHS? The price for treating most cancer patients is roughly £5,000 a week, while metformin costs just five pence a day! Even metformin on its own is a wonder drug that reverses many diseases of ageing. It could potentially change the health of an increasingly obese nation at risk of metabolic syndrome, diabetes, cancer, heart disease and Alzheimer's.

My hope is that one day soon, prescribing medicines off label for cancer will become the new normal and that powerful natural supplements will rightfully be given their place in our medicine cabinets. The time has come for radical changes in medical thinking, and it can't happen soon enough. But the impetus for change must come from the patient. Doctors are too constrained by their protocols and too governed by fear and bullying from NHS bureaucrats. Persuading doctors to break rank must come from a groundswell of public and patient pressure.

Someone called me an activist this week! Who, me? Golly, I suppose I am. Who would have thought? Yes, I am now on some kind of a mission. I feel destined to do this, whatever 'this' is. It certainly involves informing as many people as possible about this cocktail and getting the message out there. Doing nothing has no longer become an option for me. But what should I do next?

Maybe I should lead a march against the corruption of Big Pharma? But perhaps I should just treat them with the disdain they deserve. The best punishment may be to 'starve' them too by killing off their obscene profits and letting them die quietly, as tempting as it is to give them a good kicking while they're down. Perhaps we patients should start a class action and sue the biggest companies for unnecessary suffering. Boehringer Ingelheim are withdrawing dipyridamole from the market, despite knowing its anti-cancer effects.

Or maybe the best way is just to continue spreading the word about these cheap old drugs and getting patients on board. My Facebook page arms the patient with knowledge, strength, hope and solidarity. If it encourages them to stand up to their oncologist like the man in front of the advancing tanks in Tiananmen Square. Once there are enough of us, I believe that, with strength in numbers, there will be a gradual shift in attitudes. We absolutely must do something. The health of the nation, both literally and financially, demands it.

What is important to me now is to ensure that other patients don't have to suffer the woefully inadequate cancer treatments we have today. People are dying and suffering needlessly, families are torn apart, and the medical profession is painfully slow to change. But all of this can and will change with the introduction of low-cost medications and supplements. Barbaric, outdated cancer treatments will eventually move aside. Social media is now too strong for Big Pharma to have it all their way in the future. The knowledge once learned cannot be unlearned. My Facebook group is growing every day.

I put enormous effort into educating and empowering my patients with daily updates on the latest research. But this means I find myself in an awkward place. I stand somewhere in the middle, between conventional medicine and the complementary approach, not approved by either. The divide between the two approaches is still a yawning chasm, so much so that it often seems there's outright war between the two. The clamour of the alternative camp is now so loud that many patients are no longer sure whether they should try any conventional medicine at all. Some patients who would benefit from chemotherapy are now too frightened to accept it. The patient is left floundering in the middle, utterly confused, not knowing which way to turn. Conventional doctors can be hostile at the mere mention of complementary advice, while on the other side there are die-hard advocates of all things natural who will not let a single drug cross their lips. 'No drug comes without side effects,' is their standard retort.

As I stand here in the middle, I can hear the war of words flying over my head. Any attempt at drawing attention to these old drugs is drowned out by the din of the conventional doctors yelling 'Quacks!' at the integrative doctors, and the integrative doctors yelling 'Poisoners!' in return. I wondered how I could change these entrenched, dogmatic and polarised views.

Instead of targeting the medical profession or integrative doctors, I decided that the solution would be to reach out to patients. Given that both sides are still failing to provide a cure, more and more patients are investigating my middle path and joining my online revolution. This cocktail therapy has global implications ethically, socially and financially, and this patient-led revolt is happening right now. We patients have far more power than we're led to believe and we must learn to wield it. One by one, my lone voice is being joined by more and more patients. Most are not interested in the arguments. All they want is to get better.

Gregory Stoloff, Robin Bannister and their team of doctors, scientists and researchers are staking their reputations on these cheap old drugs and so am I. They are brave pioneers. They are nothing short of amazing.

Chapter Nineteen:

Parenthood at Last

It's March 2015, and I am sitting in a studio just off Carnaby Street, an area of London full of cool media types wearing hipster clothes, with their barely decipherable marketing speak. I glance around the room and survey the dozen other hopeful parents with their array of talented offspring. I wonder how many of them had struggled with infertility too, or how many were divorced or separated, caring for stepchildren or half-brothers and sisters? Families are so complex these days. Against all odds, Andrew and I had finally made it to parenthood. It had taken us ten years of heart-breaking failure, but finally we had become the proud parents of two gorgeous boys. Hardly anyone thought surrogacy bizarre or unusual anymore. Not that I had told many people. At Jamie's school, only a couple of the other mums in his class knew.

At that moment, Jamie emerged from the audition room, his face beaming.

'How did you get on?' I ask. I'm never allowed into auditions with him, so I had no clue what they had asked him to do.

'I told them I had a KCF Big Value Bucket last night and it was the best meal I've ever had!'

The other mums laugh at his muddle-up of the name but inwardly I groan. I had bought him said meal as 'research' for the KFC audition. I was curious about his reaction as not one morsel of fast food had ever passed his lips, which hadn't been easy to achieve with an eight-year-old. In 2006, KFC had been in the dock because of their use of hydrogenated fats. And after all my time educating him about healthy food, just one taste of the chemical flavour enhancers and tasteless poultry pumped full of hormones and antibiotics, and Jamie was hooked. Damn it!

Visions of Jamie in the future float through my head. I see him lounging around in a shared bedsit with out-of-work actors, a pile of greasy cardboard in the bin and unwashed dishes in the sink.

'Well done! Let's see if you get a recall, darling,' I say as I usher him out of the building. If he did get a recall, I'd have to turn it down on principle and that would annoy his agent. He was only there for audition practice – the last thing I wanted was for him to land the job. Hopefully KFC would be put off by his name muddling. How on earth could any eight-year-old not know their brand in this day and age?

Jamie had started acting the year before, and I know what you're thinking. No, I promise you, I'm not a pushy mum. Honest. He is a natural and it seemed only fair to boost his confidence by encouraging something he was obviously destined for. Friday nights have always been either a magic show with his younger brother Sam as his trusty assistant, or the pair of them performing a dynamic dancing display, or a funny play. He'd already appeared in several TV commercials, some short films and was about to film a speaking part in *Call the Midwife* for the BBC. We were also waiting on word for a feature film.

Jamie can stand in front of a crowd of people and just talk, about anything at all, with no apparent stage fright. I am in total awe of the ease in which he learns his lines, then mucks about without a care in the world until the word 'Action!' is uttered. Then he switches to delivering with total conviction, even in a cockney accent if required. Not easy for a boy brought up in plummy Southwest London.

I've always been fearful of making a fool of myself in public and had crushing shyness as a teenager. Nowadays, I have a more devil-may-care approach. Defeating terminal cancer makes you feel you can take on most things. But I'm still a bag of nerves if asked to speak about my cancer experience, something that seems to be happening more and more. I'm hoping it gets easier, although it can't possibly be as bad as my gruelling experience on Dragon's Den. Perhaps it was good training for the position I find myself in now. I may have to talk at events with a hostile reception. The idea of taking any drugs, no matter how safe, is still abhorrent to many.

As we leave the audition, I check my watch. We should make it home for Sam's bedtime cuddle. Jamie's younger brother arrived three-and-a-half years after he did, by the same wonderful surrogate. Sam was another bundle of total gorgeousness. He is super sporty and not at all interested in drama. I don't think I could cope with two actors in the family – the sibling rivalry is intense as it is!

We take the bus back home and Jamie tackles his homework on the top deck. We never take the tube unless it's late, as I can't stand the over-crowding and smell of B.O. As usual, Jamie is not the slightest bit interested in his book. It's during these moments alone with him that he often asks about his birth, particularly when we take the number 14 bus past Chelsea and Westminster Hospital, where he had first entered our lives like a tidal wave of joy.

His questioning has progressed from 'How are babies made?' to slightly more in-depth questions, but they always make for interesting and entertaining eavesdropping.

'When Tabatha gave birth to me did you take me home straightaway?' I can see the man in front pretending to read, his head turned slightly towards us. I have no issue telling Jamie about how we created him and how amazing his 'tummy mummy' Tabatha is.

A pretty young blonde girl opposite catches Jamie's eye and he grins cheekily at her. He's such a flirt! Fortunately, he has grown out of sticking his tongue out at anyone smiling at him. When he was two years old, he once went around the entire carriage pointing to each person in turn saying, 'He's got a willy. She hasn't got a willy. He's got a willy…' while I blushed furiously and tried to stop him. Mortifying! But very funny. Shyness is a word that doesn't feature in his dictionary.

'Is having a baby painful?' he asks. He has obviously seen something recently on TV. I'm trying to prepare him for his role in *Call the Midwife* so I'm quite relaxed about it. As part of our chat, I discuss how childbirth is different for every woman. I describe how a TENs machine works to make the whole birthing experience easier. The man in front of us has been reading the same page for quite some time.

Surrogacy is something I have always been open about with both Jamie and Sam. Jamie loves to hear the story of how he was born, the rush to hospital, how he nearly arrived in this world on the back seat of our car, how we had driven through red lights to get to the hospital from Kent, and what complete and utter joy it was for us when I first got to hold him. Andrew and I had waited so long for that moment. 'Hello Jamie,' I'd said as I cradled him in my arms, looking down into his bright blue eyes, uncannily like my own. He blinked back at me from his scrunched up little face with a knowing look as if to say, 'ah, I'm in hospital and you must be my mum. Hi Mum.' If I had known then how much he would love drama, I would have realised what he was really saying was 'Tada!' I will never ever forget it.

What I haven't told Jamie was the finer detail of how the nurses sadly failed to understand our surrogacy. I attended several antenatal classes at the hospital but was eyed with some suspicion as I had no bump. With hindsight it would have been best to attend with Tabatha rather than on my own, but she lived quite some distance away. Logistically, it was difficult.

When we had arrived at the hospital, Tabatha was already ten centimetres dilated and her contractions were coming in quick succession, so I was more than a bit panicked. We had phoned ahead to tell them it was a surrogacy arrangement and that we were on our way. It turned out the hospital had only seen one surrogacy birth before, and it had been a gay couple. On the assumption we were also gay males with a female surrogate they had assigned a gay midwife to come to greet us. He was all smiles to begin with, but his attitude immediately changed when he discovered it was a heterosexual arrangement. His disapproval was obvious. Was a gay arrangement perfectly acceptable, but not a woman asking another woman to carry her child for her? He was so dismissive of our concerns that we asked for another midwife. I am convinced that he then tainted the entire staffroom with tales of how dreadful we all were.

Tabatha was moved to the delivery suite. They told us that the delivery room was too small for us all and that Andrew would have to wait outside. He looked gutted. 'Too crowded,' they had said, but neither of us were going to miss the birth of our son. Tabatha and I told them quite clearly that we wanted Andrew to attend, so in we all went, disobeying orders. And there was more than enough room.

Jamie then steadfastly refused to come out. But after a bit of persuasion from the obstetrician, there he was! My world changed in an instant. A baby boy. Our boy. My Jamie. I was instantly in love.

Tabatha lay there smiling, relieved it was over. The last stage had been exhausting for her.

'He is just perfect,' I said, taking him over to her. 'How can we ever thank you?' I was filled with happiness.

'Well, he's all yours now!' she grinned. 'I've done the easy bit, over to you!'

'You have truly been an Angel.' I kissed her and passed Jamie to Andrew. He had his first proud dad moment. He too was overwhelmed.

There was no show of joy or jubilation from the staff. It wasn't how I'd imagined it at all. They had no idea how to react in this situation. Was I stealing a child? Should they be happy for me? Sad for Tabatha? In the end, all I got was a stony silence and frosty stares. I ignored it all. I was in heaven with my little man.

The hostile attitude didn't end there. To my dismay, it continued when we got back to the ward. The atmosphere was thick with disapproval and judgement. The staff either glared at me or acted as if I didn't exist. I was snubbed, ignored, talked over, and they were downright rude. Everything I did was criticised. Without the surge of female hormones at birth, how could I possibly know what to do? The hormones taught you everything you needed to know about childcare, right? Of course not.

Tabatha was a neonatal maternity nurse. She too was shocked at their attitude. The nurses came over to us both, but instead of speaking to me, they addressed all aspects of the mothering, breastfeeding, nappy changing and bathing to Tabatha, completely ignoring me. She politely told them that she was not the mother and please could they talk to me. It was so unnecessary.

They certainly didn't like the fact I refused to wash Jamie straightaway, neither did they approve of me taking off my top and giving him skin to skin contact. How dare I?!

Seeing the bonding I was establishing, one midwife told me curtly, 'That child is too cold. He needs to be dressed.' Rubbish. The ward was so hot a mother had just fainted with the heat, and everyone was complaining. When I finally dressed him, reluctantly, in a light romper suit, another midwife remarked, 'That child is too warm.' Sigh.

Because Jamie had taken a while to emerge, he needed to be kept in hospital overnight, to check his lungs.

'You will have to go home and leave the birth mother with the baby,' the staff nurse told me brusquely. What? And leave Tabatha to bond with him? How could that be the best decision? Tabatha was equally confounded.

'There is no way I'm going home without my son! I am going to stay right here,' I said. 'If there are any decisions that need to be made about him, I am going to be here to make them.'

This did not go down well. The staff refused to let me stay on the ward. There were apparently no beds available for me, although I counted at least eight free on the ward and another five empty side rooms. How many did they need? I legged it down to the private ward to see if I could take a room for the night, but no, there were none available there either. I dashed back to the ward and begged them to let me stay. Tabatha said she would go home, and I could have her bed, but apparently this was not acceptable. 'Not hospital policy.' There seemed to be no good reason as to why.

I argued, but they failed to see just how important it was for me to remain with Jamie. I explained it would be unfair on Tabatha to have that time with Jamie; it was crucial bonding time between him and me. Unbelievably, they summoned the hospital bed manager to come and have a word with me. This large, overbearing woman told me curtly that there wasn't room for me, and I would have to go home. Wow.

I couldn't see the hospital filling up with a wave of expectant mothers. So I waited until the nurses changed shift at 7 o'clock that evening and the bed manager had gone home. Cheekily, I just moved myself into a side room, moved Jamie in and said nothing. I wasn't going home and that was final. They would have to call the police.

No-one questioned me, so I sat on the bed with my beautiful baby in my arms. 'Hello Jamie,' I said again to the little blue eyes looking up at me. 'Hello Mum,' said his scrunched up, wrinkled little face. Oh joy! It was the best feeling in the world. To hell with the rude staff. My world was right here in my arms. No one was going to ruin the best day of my life!

Later, with Jamie asleep on my lap, an older night nurse visited me and explained why they were being so mean. She confided that they all thought I'd coerced Tabatha into giving him up. They assumed she would be distraught and upset by giving up a baby. In fact, she was absolutely delighted with her 'job' and was handling it very well. She was over the moon to have achieved a healthy baby boy for us after all we'd been through.

'I hear them talking in the staff room. They just don't understand. None of them have ever seen a surrogacy arrangement before. I think it's an amazing story, so just try and ignore them. Don't let them upset you.'

I tried, but they had already tainted what should have been a completely wonderful experience. It was only one night, I told myself. I had a lifetime of joyous evenings ahead of me!

That night I didn't get a wink of sleep. I was savouring every moment staring at my little man, so calm and peaceful in my arms. I was full of awe for this tiny little thing, which was so totally dependent on me. I WAS A MUM! Wow.

The next morning the bed manager stormed into my room, furious. She shouted angry words at me, but I really wasn't in the slightest bit bothered. She could be as cross as she liked. Frankly I couldn't give a flying fruitcake. Her words just washed off me.

'Surely it isn't policy to split up a mother from her child?' I said. 'I will be writing to the hospital manager about your despicable treatment of me. And you can have your bed back right now. We are not staying a moment longer.'

I phoned Andrew to bring the car round with the new baby seat. I needed to be at home. We packed our bags and left. Tabatha came with us, all four of us leaving the tense atmosphere behind. As we left, we roared with laughter at the attitude of the staff and the furious bed manager! You had to see the funny side. I was elated to finally be home with our baby boy. A baby boy! MY baby boy!

When it came to Sam's birth, again by the same amazing angel Tabatha three years later, we had no intention of repeating the same sorry birth experience. We chose Kingston Hospital instead. We'd learnt a lot and realised that the staff needed coaching, so they were given a full list of 'What To Dos' if anything went wrong during the birth and a brief on how we expected to be treated. We made it clear that if Sam needed to stay in hospital and Tabatha was fine to go home, that I was to stay instead of her.

The staff present at Sam's birth could not have been more different. Sam's arrival was greeted with the kind of joy and happiness from the midwives I had expected with Jamie, not with stares of disdain.

Sam's birth was far easier, and the staff even allowed me to deliver him, which was an amazing experience. Another perfect little boy. Our family was complete! The family I had always yearned for and thought I would never have. I felt so blessed and so lucky! I was overcome with love, and totally smitten by them both.

The struggle for a family had been long, painful, difficult and expensive. After giving up on egg donation, we had contacted COTS again and asked if they had any surrogates prepared to offer 'straight' surrogacy, where the surrogate self-inseminates. We were introduced to Tabatha a few months later and I knew instantly that she was right for us. She was warm, open-hearted and was doing it for all the right reasons. Tabatha, herself a midwife with a child of her own, made it abundantly clear that she wanted to do it for us because she had lost friends to cancer. As I got to know her better, we developed an amazing sense of sisterhood. She really is an incredible, selfless person.

From then on, I had organic deliveries sent to Tabatha's house every week, provided her with multi-vitamins, folate, probiotics, massage and reflexology. I wanted her to feel as special as she was. Even then we had three failed pregnancies and two years of trying before we finally achieved a healthy pregnancy. On each failed occasion, I expected Tabatha to turn around and say she'd had enough but every time she told us resolutely that she would carry on and try again. Like me, she was not a quitter. I love that woman.

When we got home from the audition, Sam had been dozing off in bed, but as soon as he heard the front door he leapt out and ran down the stairs to hug his older brother. He really does adore Jamie. As good and healthy as this brotherly love is, I secretly felt a bit miffed not to have had first dibs on the hugs.

I got to have my cuddles with Sam later, snuggled up in his bed while I sang him a lullaby and massaged his back. Jamie stopped me singing him lullabies when he turned five. Frankly I can't blame him – it was always the same song and my skills in that department are woefully lacking. Jamie told me he was no longer a baby and please could I stop. Sad face. I'm dreading Sam saying the same thing. I'll feel ever more redundant in the motherhood department as their independence grows.

As I kissed each of them goodnight, I said my daily silent prayer of thanks to Tabatha, without whom the crazy life we lead would be so different. She has transformed our universe beyond measure. The joy I see on their faces when we play in the park, at home or muck about on the boat, and the easy cuddles they have for me, makes me burst with happiness. They have the biggest hearts and beautiful loving natures. They are truly special. They did not arrive without the usual challenges, but our boys are the most wonderful gift anyone could ever give us.

Chapter Twenty:

The Future?

'At this date, we are not limited by the science; we are limited by our ability to make good use of the information and treatments we already have. Too often, lives are tragically ended not by cancer but by the bureaucracy that came with the nation's investment in the war on cancer, by review boards, by the FDA, and by doctors who won't stand by their patients or who are afraid to take a chance.'

Dr Vincent DeVita, former director of the NCI (National Cancer Institute), editor-in-chief of *The Cancer Journal*, and author of *The Death of Cancer*

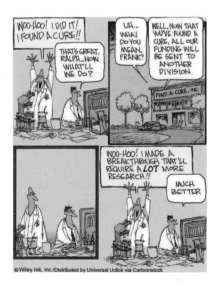

It has become increasingly obvious that genetics only make up one part of the cancer equation. Even James Watson, DNA pioneer (with Francis Crick and Rosalind Franklin), is deeply frustrated by the slow progress being made in the field of cancer. Although initially hopeful about the Cancer Genome Atlas project that mapped out our entire genomic code, he recognised that sequencing DNA did not reveal the answer in the way that everyone hoped. Recently, Watson was heartened by the discovery that Stat3, a transcription code for the genes to tell them what to do, is involved in most if not all cancers. Importantly, Stat3 is now being recognised as a crucial key modulator of mitochondrial 'respiration', the way cells generate energy, which firmly supports the metabolic theory, rather than the genetic or 'somatic' theory of oncogenesis (how cancer begins).

Stat3, a transcription factor, has been shown to be altered first, a process which is triggered by inflammation. This then results in mutagenic changes that increase cancer's appetite for more nutrients, driving ever more rapid cell proliferation. There is now emerging evidence that metformin, the diabetes medication, blocks this malfunctioning pathway, enough for James Watson to take metformin daily as prevention. But he is frustrated by the slow uptake of this simple intervention for every cancer patient. He has recently stated that:

'The depressing thing about the cancer 'moonshot' is that it's the same people getting together, forming committees, and the same old ideas and it's all crap…'

Quite.

Despite this, he is still positive that in five years' time he will see 80% of cancers becoming treatable. I am similarly optimistic, if my revolution takes off.

I believe that almost all stage IV cancers can be reversed from being incurable to becoming treatable, unless organ damage is too severe, with the right combination of drugs, given at the right time and in the right order. All too often, death is a result of excessively aggressive chemotherapy or a side effect of the toxic therapies currently on offer, as nearly happened to me. My brush with fatal therapy-related leukaemia was a little too close for comfort.

We need to embrace a more comprehensive approach, combining lower toxicity drugs and natural therapies, to achieve a 'gentle' remission, one that gets the patient better without killing them in the process.

Currently, patients receive aggressive and cruel treatments, using too much chemotherapy, too much radiotherapy and indeed excessively aggressive surgery. I firmly believe that we can cure cancer if we take a better approach to which pre-existing drugs we should use, and how we should use them.

I am convinced that the answer to cancer has been out there all along, with many of the solutions buried and lost in piles of old scientific journals just waiting to be uncovered. And discovering them was a matter of piecing the old information and newer data together like a jigsaw, fitting the metabolic parts together, both natural and pharmaceutical, into cancer-starving combinations. Had I stumbled across a cure?

The 'McLelland Moonshot'

Instead of the current deeply flawed approach of treating genetic changes alone, surely the answer is to treat the genetic, metabolic and altered cell signalling **together**.

This is **my** 'moonshot':

1. STARVE YOUR CANCER (my 'Metro Map')
2. STOP ABNORMAL CELL SIGNALLING (Hedgehog, Wnt, Notch, PPAR gamma, inflammation)
3. STOP IT SPREADING (block growth factors and MMPs)
4. SNUFF IT OUT (trigger apoptosis in a more gentle and natural way through the caspase cascade and oxygenation, use lower doses of chemotherapy, radiotherapy and the new approach of ferroptosis)

5. RECOVER! Which includes detox, recovering the immune system and mitochondrial loss.

Those steps, employed in that order, can yield exceptional results – particularly when paired with 'pulsing' the apoptosis so that any dead cells can be safely cleared without too much toxic build up.

Dr Chi Van Dang, director of the Abramson Cancer Center in Pennsylvania, also believes the answer is to deprive the cancer of its fuel, recognising the insatiable appetite of the cancer cell. He acknowledges that they are 'addicted' to nutrients and that without enough fuel, they just 'wither and die'. Without a constant supply of food cancer cannot survive.

So, is it possible that managing cancer or even a cure could be as simple as taking a handful of cheap old drugs, with few side effects, alongside a modified lifestyle and cancer-starving diet? Imagine that if in the future you are unluckily diagnosed with cancer, but only a stage 1 or stage 2, how simple and convenient it would be if all you had to do was wander down to the chemist to pick up a prescription for a few drugs and then receive some dietary and lifestyle advice.

Advanced cancers might need more than just this approach, with longer term management of diet and lifestyle and with the patient continuing to take a few of the drugs. Could this be the answer to maintaining a lasting remission, much like the way in which HIV is controlled today?

In my vision of the future, I see oncologists and patients working together with many other health professionals. But they will need to be specialists. Each cancer patient will need a tailored diet and exercise regime. Every cancer is driven by different metabolic and genetic changes, which is why there can never be one specific recommendation. If your disease is more glutamine-driven (e.g. cancers with an over-expressed MYC gene), it may be important to follow a more vegan diet, cutting out protein. Melanomas, androgen -driven prostate and 'Braf-driven' cancers that rely more on fat and glutamine should avoid ketogenic diets.

I have long since given up trying to change attitudes in the medical profession. Instead, it is the patients who are joining my revolution, individuals who have tried everything else, both conventional and complementary, who still have cancer continuing to rampage through their bodies. They are the ones who are joining me in using these old drugs and other natural cancer-starving therapies. Slowly and surely, as more patients get results and more incredible remissions occur, the word is spreading. Egged on by success with other patients, more and more patients are turning to this multi-drug approach. Yet despite seeing results before their eyes, many oncologists continue to ignore the metabolic approach, concerned that prescribing anything different will lead to disciplinary action.

Even when you are first diagnosed, there remains a lack of understanding about the need to control the tumour's abnormal cell signalling, its demand for nutrients, the influence of stress, and the urgent need to quell inflammation. After a cancer diagnosis, you are normally sent home with nothing. No pill, no immediate treatment, just a head churning over all sorts of frightening scenarios.

Understandably, you can't help but imagine the parasitic lump inside continuing to grow whilst nothing is being done. Why haven't the doctors prescribed anything? Is the problem so enormous that taking anything is worthless? Yet at this point, right at diagnosis, is the prime opportunity to begin to control its growth. The prescription of something as simple as an anti-inflammatory, other cancer-starving drugs and an immediate visit to a skilled functional medicine practitioner and nutritionist could have an enormous impact on our dire survival statistics.

Years from now, when oncology practices finally change, as they must, I feel sure we'll look back with sadness at how many patients died and suffered needlessly. We'll be amazed that the medical profession persisted for so long with cruel and destructive treatments, duped by the hype and false promises of the newer pharmaceutical drugs.

Ever since 2003, when my eyes were opened to new and exciting possibilities, I have been looking on, helpless, while disastrous toxic approaches were used on friends and loved ones, knowing that they would almost certainly die as a result. I felt so alone championing old drug cocktails, despairing as the new 'game changing' targeted treatments inevitably failed. These were the bad old days, with the 'whack-a-mole' drug approach, constantly chasing after genetic mutations in a losing race. All I could do was wait patiently for science to back me up. Now the articles are mounting up about old metabolic drugs. There is undeniable proof of their efficacy. But there are few 'Randomised Clinical Trials' and because of this, medics remain dismissive of these drugs.

Despite the incredible potential of the cheap, off-patent, low toxic drug cocktail I describe in this book, you must take a rounded approach. If you take them without addressing your immune system, your diet, your gut health, your lifestyle and your levels of stress, you will not achieve the best results. A fully integrated approach, preferably with an oncologist who helps guide you through your choices (both orthodox and complementary), who understands the metabolic nature of the cancer, will be key to the future of the profession. High dose chemotherapy will eventually disappear, and a raft of new drug cocktails will be used, amongst them much lower doses of chemotherapy.

Research on 'repurposing' drugs is still very much in its infancy and continues to be viewed as experimental. But it works. Should the patient have to wait until Randomised Clinical Trials are completed, in another ten or fifteen years? Should the medics continue to do as they're told and ignore the very patients they are supposed to help?

Even the British Medical Journal in October 2015 reported that a retrospective analysis of recently approved immunotherapies revealed that only five out of thirty-six new drugs had any significant effect on overall survival.[100] The fact that they got approval in the first place is very worrying indeed. But with the stakes so high for every new drug launch, is it any wonder that desperate pharmaceutical companies are giving out misleading data for approval?

Getting these old off-patent drugs accepted by doctors and the public as cancer 'game changers' may be hard, purely because they are so very mundane, familiar and cheap. There's no schmaltzy, shiny new packaging. There's no fanfare or media party unveiling the next generation breakthrough. There are no exotic destinations for the oncologists' annual conference paid for by the pharmaceutical company. No one can afford that kind of marketing budget when the drugs cost less than five pence a day.

Both doctors and patients have a natural tendency to believe the newer the treatment, the more expensive a drug is, the better it is going to work. But this is not the case. New is not always better, and age and experience often trump youth and beauty. These drugs are indeed game changers, to use the parlance of Big Pharma.

Stories from other patients using off label drugs and other metabolic approaches are pouring in.[101] Slowly and surely, as more patients achieve disease stabilisation and incredible remissions occur using old drug cocktails and other cancer-starving therapies, the word is spreading. I

---

100 Doshi Peter, Jefferson Tom. The evidence base for new drugs BMJ 2015; 350: h952
101 I will be posting patient survival stories on my website *www.howtostarvecancer.com*

know I have already made a big difference to many, but so much more needs to be done.[102]

It is early days, and the metabolic approach is still viewed as highly experimental, but the success rate looks very promising. When more results are eventually published from the Care Oncology Clinic, the efficacy of these drugs will be available for all to see. Yet despite seeing the results before their eyes, many oncologists continue to ignore them. Worse, this approach continues to be treated with derision and scorn and much resistance, which makes life tricky not just for the patients who struggle to get hold of the drugs they need, but for the doctors working in this field. It is hard to raise awareness of the importance of these metabolic drugs in the face of such opposition.

So out with the new and in with the old!

Most patients that join my Facebook group are diagnosed with terminal cancer. Many have been told that there was nothing more conventional medicine could offer them. So, with nothing to lose and everything to gain, a brave few started using the old drugs in 2015, and despite grim prognoses, many of them are still alive today. One by one, others have followed. My page is now growing fast, purely through word of mouth, and I am witnessing my crew (they're like family to me) achieve some incredible remissions before my very eyes! Patients with incurable brain tumours given only weeks to live, home-schooling their kids because they want to spend every second with them, passing over all their worldly belongings to relatives and preparing for their imminent funerals. Then, suddenly finding that they have their lives handed back to them! Brain tumours, liver and lung metastases are disappearing... wow, wow, wow!

---

[102] Search #positiveprogress posts in my Facebook Group to see hundreds of patient stories and watch the video testimonials in my online course.

Social media is creating a rumbling militant spirit of rebellion amongst patients, upset about their unnecessary suffering. You don't need to be a vocal revolutionary: changing your oncologist or simply getting yourself enrolled in the Care Oncology study, demonstrating the value of these medicines, is perhaps all that is required. And although change will happen more slowly, it will happen. Hurrah!

For me, it has been a long hard road back to 'normality' and getting my life plan back on track. At times the obstacles looked too high to climb. When it all seemed too much, I concentrated on placing one foot in front of the other, taking it one step at a time. And very slowly, with every step I took, I inched closer and closer to the top.

I stand here looking down at every difficult path I forged to get here. The sun has broken through the clouds. The view is simply breath-taking.

Facebook entry: April 2016

Today is a very special day. Many years ago, I was told I would never have children but thanks to an incredible angel, 10 years ago that gloomy prediction was turned on its head. Fighting traffic jams to pick up our amazing surrogate from her home we raced from Kent up the A2 to the Chelsea and Westminster Hospital, the anxious parents-to-be leaning out of windows shouting at slow moving pedestrians to get out of the way while we put pedal to the metal, breaking speed limits, running red lights and darting down bus lanes to get to the hospital in time! Jamie was so nearly delivered on the back seat! We made it, and out came the most amazing bundle who continues to delight, surprise, amuse and fill me with absolute joy. And we got lucky again three years later with my wonderful Sam! They are both so adorable. They are both funny, witty and so super-talented.

So, to celebrate J's birthday, I took him on a special weekend, just me and him on a cultural tour of Paris. What culture did we see? The Louvre? Musee D'Orsay? No! We went on an evening Ghost tour, we ran in and out of fountains and rolled down grassy banks by the Eiffel Tower, jumped up and down over big ventilation grilles near the Arc de Triomphe, watched street performers, had both our caricatures sketched (: -o!), went on a great cycling tour of the city and chased bubbles outside the Pompidou Centre! The Lego display in Les Halles was the closest we got to art…

Happy 10th Birthday to my gorgeous boy!! What a wonderful, wonderful weekend! I can't wait to do it all again with Sam.

I love you both so much.
Mummy xxxx
Mummy. The word still sends a rush of joy through me.
I may have survived cancer, but you Tabatha,
you gave me back my life. I am forever in your debt.

Part Two

The Metabolic Protocol

Chapter Twenty-One:

Your Cancer-Starving Cocktail

In this section I describe what I believe are currently the best, least toxic drugs to starve and snuff out cancer. As with all science this is a fast-moving area, so updates and important new information is regularly sent out through my blogs on my website. I appreciate that some of you are not familiar with the terminology, or the drugs and supplements mentioned and taking in all this information in one go is a lot. Do not despair! I have also created an online course with lots of diagrams to help you understand how cancer works, its key pathways and which drugs and supplements may help your particular cancer. You will find details on my website (*www.howtostarvecancer.com*). Also, you will find it easier to understand Part Two if you haven't skipped Part One.

Jane's 'Piccadilly Circus' Analogy

Fifteen years ago, few cancer researchers understood the stem cell, at the heart of every cancer, the cell responsible for drug resistance and metastasis. Neither was it understood how 'metabolically flexible' the cancer stem cell was, able to shift from using one fuel supply to another, re-routing itself to maintain its constant supply. Without a comprehensive cocktail blocking off each fuel pipeline, cancer becomes 'resistant'. But don't imagine the resistance as merely a 'genetic adaptation', it also requires 'metabolic adaptation'. This is where the approach to treatment has being going wrong for decades. Instead of just treating the genes, we should be treating the altered metabolism that goes with them.

To make this easier to understand I now explain this to cancer patients as my 'Piccadilly Circus Analogy'.

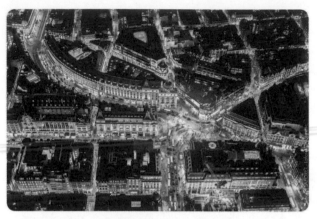

Piccadilly Circus at night

This is an aerial view of Piccadilly Circus at night. The place is buzzing, with lots of pedestrians, buses, taxis and cars. It is an exciting and vibrant place to be! Even after living in London for nearly twenty years, I still find it thrilling. Bars, restaurants, theatres, cinemas, clubs, galleries – the list is endless – all packed together so tightly.

Looking down from above, you can see the pedestrians heading in different directions and the vehicles moving up and down Regent Street, Shaftesbury Avenue, St James' and Piccadilly.

This is similar in some respects to the behaviour of a cancer cell. It is accepted that cancer cells possess distinct bioelectrical properties because they utilise different ion channel transport (e.g. calcium channel transporters). And there are common genetic changes in many cancers, such as p53, the tumour suppressor gene. The different directions of the traffic and the shifting routes of pedestrians represent the genetic changes. They can move in many different directions, altering their direction of flow. In the same way, a tumour can contain up to 2000 different mutations, allowing a tumour to evade genetically targeted treatments.

What is less visible is what happens below the surface, or at the heart of the cancer. Below the surface is the underground system, a kind of 'Tube' or 'Metro' network. And this has a finite number of routes. These are like the fuel pipelines of the cancer stem cell. To get to Piccadilly Circus if one tube line is out of action, you can travel around the underground and still reach your destination by another line. Similarly, the wily cancer cell is able to re-route and still feed itself with a different fuel source when one of its lines is blocked.

Unlike the genetic changes where cancer can endlessly mutate, below ground there are fewer options for rerouting and better opportunities for blocking its growth. It is the stem cell that is cancer's real Achille's heel and yet this is currently ignored by the mainstream, which treats only the fast dividing cells.

Explaining the complexity of cancer to a patient with no medical knowledge is not easy, many want an easy option with just one or two supplements. I wish it were that simple. My Spot of Bother Chart and my first Cancer- Starving Triangle, while useful, did not really explain the more numerous metabolic routes and the need to use a bigger cocktail. I had worked out how to starve my own cancer, reversing the altered metabolism by blocking each side of my Cancer-Starving Triangle diagram. The same combination would also help others in the same way. I believe that the combination of my drug cocktail together with the Care Oncology Clinic cocktail would work very effectively on a great many cancers by blocking off a larger number of pathways at the same time. There are synergies with combinations and much greater responses when the correct cocktail is used.

I decided to research more fuel lines used by other cancers in an attempt to understand how each behaves differently and seek off label drugs that should be added to my triangle to starve more aggressive cancers such as triple negative breast cancer, GBM and pancreatic cancers.

With much scratching of head, rubbing of chin, contemplative baths and further digging through hundreds of research articles, I have pulled together one comprehensive and (I believe) thorough cocktail of drugs, based on the findings of top researchers working in the field of cancer metabolism (e.g., Professor Thomas Seyfried, the Care Oncology Clinic, Dr Laurent Schwartz, Professor Gregory Riggins, Professor Michael Lisanti, Dr George Yu, Dr Michael Retsky, Dr Pan Pantziarka, Dr Ahmed Alsekka, Dr Abdul Slocum and many others). The more drugs you add, the less of each you should need, as long as they target different pathways. In theory, at least, this means chemotherapy and toxic immunotherapy drugs could be drastically lowered.

My Hallmarks of Cancer

I have narrowed down and identified five key steps that happen as a cell becomes cancerous. It starts with inflammation and finishes with the fast-dividing cells.

These steps or my 'hallmarks' of cancer are:

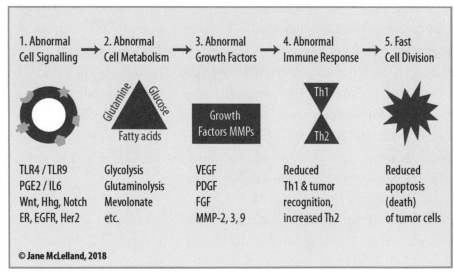

Figure 20.1. My Five Hallmarks of Cancer

I think that this is a little less confusing than the Hanahan and Weinberg Hallmarks of cancer (identified in 2000),which are 'sustaining proliferative signalling, evading growth suppressors, resisting cell death, enabling replicative immortality, inducing angiogenesis, and activating invasion and metastasis'.[87] All of these were linked to genomic instability and tissue inflammation and it wasn't until 2011[88] that they realised they had forgotten the reprogramming of energy metabolism (which Otto Warburg had discovered in 1924) and the evasion from the immune system. Doh! Embarrassing.

Many of the steps will need to be treated, whereas the standard of care focuses on the fast dividing cells with chemo and radiotherapy. It is clear to me from the published research that tackling the altered metabolism and starving the tumour is key to achieving lasting remission. Cancer cells need nutrients. The faster they are growing, the more they need. So let's go through each step and let me show you how to treat each one.

Abnormal Cell Signalling

 Some of these signals are 'cause' and some of these are 'effect'. The symbols are only representations of the cell membrane receptors that receive these signals and are for illustrative purposes only.

Emerging evidence suggests that the cause of cancer is either prolonged exposure to inflammation known as inflammatory cytokines (e.g. the cytokine IL6 released from deep visceral fat, chronic infection or prolonged exposure to a carcinogen), or prolonged stimulation of 'Toll Like Receptors', or stimulation of growth factors and hormones like IGF-1 and insulin. The Toll Like Receptors are ancient pathogen pattern

87 D. Hanahan, R.A. Weinberg; The hallmarks of cancer *Cell*, 100 (2000), pp. 57-70
88 Hanahan D, Weinberg RA. Hallmarks of cancer: the next generation. *Cell* 144(5), 646-674 (2011).

detectors – TLR1 to 9, but mostly 4 and 9 are activated in cancer.[89] Because IGF-1 and insulin signalling drive growth by increasing nutrient availability, they are included in the next section, the abnormal metabolism. Cancer may be a result of all these factors combined. Research has yet to establish this definitively.

How to treat Abnormal Cell Signalling

This differs in individual cancers. You will need to do your own research online and quiz your doctor to find out if your cancer 'expresses' any of the following to determine which of these you need:

Hedgehog Signalling – this is present in the vast majority of cancers. Berberine, Metformin and particularly the anti-helminth (de-worming) Mebendazole are effective treatments against this.[90] Arsenic trioxide – a chemotherapy, targets this and despite its hugely toxic sounding name, could be very useful for TNBC.

Wnt/beta-catenin – Wnt signaling is controlled by miR-34a, an epigenetically-controlled micro RNA strand with antiviral activity, so it may be linked to many viral-driven tumours.[91] Deregulation of Wnt signalling is responsible for the invasion and progression of herpes viruses (e.g. CMV, Epstein Barr, HPV). These viruses have evolved to manipulate and control this vital pathway to promote viral propagation, evade host immune recognition and maintain latency. Wnt also appears to play a part in encouraging bone metastases by interfering with the

89   Sato, Y., Goto, Y., Narita, N. *et al.* Cancer Microenvironment (2009) 2(Suppl 1): 205. https://doi.org/10.1007/s12307-009-0022-y

90   Larsen AR, Bai R-Y, Chung JH, *et al.* Repurposing the antihelmintic mebendazole as a hedgehog inhibitor. *Molecular cancer therapeutics*. 2015;14(1): 3-13. doi: 10.1158/1535-7163.MCT-14-0755-T.

91   Smith JL, Jeng S, McWeeney SK, Hirsch AJ. A MicroRNA Screen Identifies the Wnt Signaling Pathway as a Regulator of the Interferon Response during Flavivirus Infection. Diamond MS, ed. *Journal of Virology*. 2017;91(8): e02388-16. doi: 10.1128/JVI.02388-16.

normal activity of osteoblasts and osteoclasts. And it affects the c-Myc gene and cyclin D1. The cyclin D1 gene is amplified and the protein overexpressed in many cancers and about one-third of breast cancers. Wnt/ß-catenin signaling is activated in most colorectal cancers (CRC) through mutation of the tumor suppressor APC.

Other Wnt-driven cancers include ovarian, renal, cervical, hepatocellular and sarcomas.

Treatment: Aspirin and dipyridamole help stymie this abnormal cell signalling. Both also have beneficial effects on bone remodelling[92,93] and antiviral effects. Niclosamide, NSAIDs and Vitamin D3 also improve this abnormal signalling pathway. Itraconazole inhibits Wnt in combination with chemotherapy targeting both stem cells by and fast dividing cells in colorectal cancer.[94] Ivermectin may be a safer choice as it targets many pathways in cancer, including Wnt. It has less interactions with other drugs as well as helping reverse multi drug resistance, the reason many treatments fail.[95] Flavonoids such as Genistein, kaempferol, and baicalein inhibit Wnt/ß-catenin signaling by decreasing the expression of ß-catenin.

Notch – I never had any of these abnormal cell signals tested in my day, but Notch is now known to be associated with cervical cancer. To combat this, the natural flavonoid luteolin is what you need.[96] Unknowingly, I

---

92 Kok-Yong Chin, 'A Review on the Relationship between Aspirin and Bone Health', Journal of Osteoporosis, vol. 2017, Article ID 3710959, 8 pages, 2017. doi: 10.1155/2017/3710959

93 Mediero A, Wilder T, Perez-Aso M, Cronstein BN. Direct or indirect stimulation of adenosine A2A receptors enhances bone regeneration as well as bone morphogenetic protein-2. *The FASEB Journal*. 2015;29(4): 1577-1590. doi: 10.1096/fj.14-265066.

94 Semiramis A. Popova & Simon J. A. Buczacki (2018) Itraconazole perturbs colorectal cancer dormancy through SUFU-mediated WNT inhibition, *Molecular & Cellular Oncology*, 5:4, DOI: 10.1080/23723556.2018.1494950

95 Tang M, Hu X, Wang Y, *et al*. Ivermectin, a potential anticancer drug derived from an antiparasitic drug. *Pharmacol Res*. 2021;163:105207.

96 Zang M, Hu L, Fan Z, *et al*. Luteolin suppresses gastric cancer progression by reversing epithelial-mesenchymal transition via suppression of the Notch signaling pathway. *Journal of Translational Medicine*. 2017;15: 52. doi: 10.1186/s12967-017-1151-6.

had obtained a dose of this naturally in my daily celery-rich vegetable juice (although it is more potent in celery seed) but for better suppression it may be best taken as a supplement. Luteolin is also a SREBP-2 inhibitor (see later) so getting a proper dose is important. The supplements sulforaphane, delta tocotrienol, orodonin and quercetin also target this abnormal cell signalling. Notch is associated with an alteration in the surrounding fibroblasts and the gene c-MYC. Both may make cancer especially aggressive. This pathway affects thyroid cancer (through Braf activation) and can be helped by iodine[97] and is Notch-driven cancers (e.g. gastric cancer, head and neck, cervical squamous cancer, some breast cancers, colon, leukaemia, glioma, medulloblastoma) might benefit from the drug niclosamide, an old parasitic drug. Evidence shows niclosamide targets multiple signalling pathways – Notch, OxPhos, NF-κB, Wnt/ß-catenin, ROS, mTOR, and Stat3.[98] Arsenic trioxide inhibits both Notch and Hedgehog and when it was combined with the natural anticancer agent Gossypol it led to complete elimination of some deadly glioblastomas.[99] Wnt signaling promotes the switch from normal mitochondrial respiration (OXPHOS) to aerobic glycolysis and glutaminolysis (via ASCT2). We will discuss these later with the Metro Map.

Treatments: Luteolin, sulforaphane, quercetin, niclosamide, arsenic trioxide. All have multiple targets in cancer but if you take sulforaphane and luteolin, they will need to be stopped temporarily when you want to trigger a ferroptosis 'kill phase' of treatment (see later).

---

97   Fuziwara CS, Kimura ET. High iodine blocks a Notch/miR-19 loop activated by the BRAF(V600E) oncoprotein and restores the response to TGFβ in thyroid follicular cells. Thyroid. 2014;24(3):453-462. doi:10.1089/thy.2013.0398

98   Pan J-X, Ding K, Wang C-Y. Niclosamide, an old antihelminthic agent, demonstrates antitumor activity by blocking multiple signaling pathways of cancer stem cells. *Chinese Journal of Cancer*. 2012;31(4): 178-184. doi: 10.5732/cjc.011.10290.

99   Linder, B.; Wehle, A.; Hehlgans, S.; Bonn, F.; Dikic, I.; Rödel, F.; Seifert, V.; Kögel, D. Arsenic Trioxide and (−)-Gossypol Synergistically Target Glioma Stem-Like Cells via Inhibition of Hedgehog and Notch Signaling. *Cancers* **2019**, 11, 350. https://doi.org/10.3390/cancers11030350

Toll Like Receptors

TLR4   Low Dose Naltrexone, NF-kB inhibitors, Berberine, CBD

TLR9-
LDN	Many advanced tumours
Imiquimod –	BCC, malignant melanoma
BCG –	Bladder, m. melanoma, colon, urothelial, breast, AML
MPL –	NSCLC, breast, ovarian
Poly-L-Lysine –	advanced cancer, esp. melanoma, Glioma (synthetic amino acid)

These are present in every cancer.

TLR-4 – The role of this 'Toll Like Receptor' in cancer has only recently been studied but it is present in head and neck, oesophageal, gastric, colorectal, liver, pancreatic, skin, breast, ovarian, cervical and breast cancer.

Treatment: Berberine.[100] Low Dose Naltrexone (LDN), Berberine, CBD

TLR-9 – This is linked to oncogenic viruses.[101]

Treatment: Low Dose Naltrexone. Professor Angus Dalgleish, oncologist at St George's hospital in London was so impressed after witnessing the disappearance of some advanced tumours that expressed TLR-9 using Low Dose Naltrexone (LDN) he investigated it further and applied for a patent to repurpose the drug for cancer treatment as its effects on both oncogenic

---

100 Chu *et al.* Role of berberine in anti-bacterial as a high-affinity LPS antagonist binding to TLR4/MD-2 receptor BMC Complementary and Alternative Medicine 2014, 14: 89

101 Martínez-Campos C, Burguete-García AI, Madrid-Marina V (February 2017). 'Role of TLR9 in Oncogenic Virus-Produced Cancer'. Viral Immunology. doi: 10.1089/vim.2016.0103. PMID 28151089.

bacteria and viruses make it a good immune modulator.[102] Despite learning about it in 2001, it was only recently that I began taking LDN every night before bed. Since taking it, I have had an improvement in my lymphoedema.

Other treatments Chloroquine, imiquimod, BCG, MPL, Poly-L-Lysine (hydroxychloroquine or chloroquine sulphate) an antimalarial drug, is also a possible treatment for TLR-9 that also prevents macropinocytosis (see later in the abnormal metabolism section).

Integrins – Integrin protein molecules are located on the surface of cells, spanning the phospholipid (fat) cell membrane, and they normally 'grip' healthy cells in place like Velcro to form tissues and organs. Faulty p53 signalling causes integrins to retreat inside the cell and be sent to the wrong part of the cell surface, allowing the cancer cell to break away and travel in the blood stream.[103] Evidence is in short supply for treatments, but I hypothesise that dipyridamole may have some effect as it has an affinity for protein, so it may help prevent the integrin retreating into the cell, keeping it on the surface of the cell to perform its Velcro-like function.

Oestrogen Receptor (ER) – these receptors are found inside cells. They are upregulated in breast, ovarian and endometrial cancers but other less obvious cancers may also be oestrogen positive, such as gastric, NSCLC, gliomas, and even colon and liver cancers. Indole-3-carbinol (I3C or DIM)[104] and melatonin[105] help block oestrogen receptors, as

---

102 https://www.cancerdefeated.com/cheap-off-patent-drugfound-to-be-a-cancer-game- changer/3963/

103 Vousden, K. et al Mutant p53 regulates invasion via integrins and EGFR NCRI Cancer Conference5 October 2009

104 Aggarwal BB1, Ichikawa H. Molecular targets and anticancer potential of indole-3-carbinol and its derivatives. Cell Cycle. 2005 Sep;4(9): 1201-15. Epub 2005 Sep 6.

105 del Río B1, García Pedrero JM, Martínez-Campa C, Zuazua P, Lazo PS, Ramos S Melatonin, an Endogenous-specific Inhibitor of Estrogen Receptor α via Calmodulin J Biol Chem. 2004 Sep 10;279(37): 38294-302. Epub 2004 Jun 30

does metformin.[106] Stimulating the ER-beta receptor (rather than the ER alpha) can inhibit ERα and androgen receptor function, suppressing cell growth, and improving the response to hormonal therapies.[107] Siberian Rhubarb has a strong affinity to ER- beta and only a very weak affinity to ER-alpha. This supplement can have positive effects on mood as well as the bones, brain, skin and temperature control, so helps to alleviate those hot flashes in both oestrogen deprivation and androgen deprivation. Research in Adelaide, Australia has shown that double positive, i.e., oestrogen and progesterone positive cancers, fare better than oestrogen (ER) positive cancers alone. When progesterone was given to these ER positive patients, it slowed tumour growth.[108] The reason for this may be because progesterone is an autophagy inhibitor – also why megestrol acetate, a synthetic progestin, is prescribed for cachexia. White button mushrooms are natural aromatase inhibitors and have been shown to slow both breast and prostate cancer. Eat them daily if you can! Resistance to oestrogen therapy (Tamoxifen, Flaslodex, aromatase inhibitors) is common and driven by glutamine pathways (glutaminase) and the mTOR pathway, so adding these is essential for any oestrogen-driven cancer.[109]

Androgen Receptor – hugely relevant for prostate cancer patients but also important for triple negative cancer as some subtypes express this receptor. Ivermectin makes another appearance here as it helps blocks one of the ways that cancer cells exposed to ADT treatment become

106 KIM J, LEE J, JANG SY, KIM C, CHOI Y, KIM A. Anticancer effect of metformin on estrogen receptor-positive and tamoxifen-resistant breast cancer cell lines. *Oncology Reports*. 2016;35(5): 2553-2560. doi: 10.3892/or.2016.4675.

107 Omoto Y, Iwase H. Clinical significance of estrogen receptor β in breast and prostate cancer from biological aspects. Cancer Sci. 2015;106(4):337-343. doi:10.1111/cas.12613

108 Wayne D. Tilley Jason S. Carroll et al Progesterone receptor modulates ERα action in breast cancer Nature volume 523, pages 313-317 (16 July 2015) DOI: 10.1038/nature14583

109 Demas Diane M., Demo Susan, Fallah Yassi, Clarke Robert, Nephew Kenneth P., Althouse Sandra, Sandusky George, He Wei, Shajahan-Haq Ayesha N. *Glutamine Metabolism Drives Growth in Advanced Hormone Receptor Positive Breast Cancer* Frontiers in Oncology vol 9 2019 DOI=10.3389/fonc.2019.00686

resistant (through succinate and the heat shock protein Hsp27).[110] Androgen deprivation therapy works because it stops a glutaminase enzyme (kidney type) which makes the cancer unable to use glutamine. When it becomes resistant it is then using another glutaminase enzyme (C type). In the future I predict the cruel use of ADT will be swapped for glutaminase inhibitors and anti-inflammatory drugs.[111] Another approach is to block glutamine through ASCT2 transporters and the many other glutamine pathways I describe in the next section. Direct suppression of androgen receptors can be achieved by including a couple of the following into your protocol: xanthohumol, chrysin, danshen, permixon and pao pereira.

EGFR (epidermal growth factor receptor) – Present in about 30% of epithelial cancers (about 90% of all cancers) especially lung, brain, anal, head and neck cancers. I do not know whether my cancer expressed an active EGFR, but if it did, berberine, EGCG (green tea) and curcumin are natural antagonists, so I already had it partly covered. Unlike gefitinib, erlotinib and lapatinib, these natural alternatives come without severe side effects. Chloroquine and hydroxychloroquine, normally used to treat malaria, may hold the key to preventing resistance to EGFR and HER2 targeted treatments (see macropinocytosis and autophagy inhibition).[112] An opposite approach is to stimulate more autophagy, which is how ivermectin works. So in some cases, taking Chloroquine and Ivermectin together may reduce the efficacy of each, so to be safe, avoid combining the two unless you find research to the contrary for your specific cancer. However using metformin (stimulates autophagy)

110 Lucia Nappi, … , Gary D. Brayer, Martin Gleave *Ivermectin inhibits HSP27 and potentiates efficacy of oncogene targeting in tumour models* December 17, 2019 *Clin Invest.* 2020;130(2):699-714. https://doi.org/10.1172/JCI130819.

111 https//scienceblog.com/521886/new-therapy-approach-to-cut-off-prostate-cancers-fuel-source/

112 Autophagy can work to kill cancer or it can help progression, so has been thought to be controversial, we will discuss this further and my online course may be useful for clarification about when and how to use it in different contexts.

with an autophagy inhibitor (chloroquine) is synergistic, they enhance each other's effects death, the exception is when triggering ferroptosis, a special form of programmed cell death. EGFR sends signalling cascades down the RAS pathway which is partly blocked by statins and down the mTOR pathway, partly blocked by metformin. EGFR also sends signals down the MAPK pathway, a key pathway in many cancers and this can be blocked by indomethacin.[113] Aprepitant, an antiemetic drug used to treat nausea during chemotherapy, has shown it has considerable potential. It helps block both EGFR, HER2, glycolysis and other pathways. Natural treatments include reserpine, melittin and bromelain.

HER2 – (human epidermal growth factor receptor 2)- Not just present in 10-20% of breast cancer, it can also affect gastric and gastroesophageal junction adenocarcinoma, salivary duct carcinomas, and this gene can be amplified in non-small cell lung, ovarian, colon and pancreatic cancer. Use of Herceptin with cancers displaying this gene expression can show a good response, so it is worth finding out if you have it. Again ivermectin and aprepitant may be a good choice to add to your mix. Good supplements are cyclocreatine, (cautious use of creatinine), moringa oleifera leaves, GLA, danshen, resperine.

Interleukin 1 beta – this inflammatory cytokine releases COX (cyclo-oxygenase), an enzyme that fuels cancer growth but it can be neutralised by a non-steroidal anti-inflammatory (NSAID). Everyone needs to reduce this interleukin as it drives progression and metastasis through NF-κB as well as stimulating 'bad' immune cells that work for the cancer rather than against it.

113 Chi-Chuan Lin, Kin Man Suen, John E. Ladbury,Targeting the Shc-EGFR interaction with indomethacin inhibits MAP kinase pathway signalling, Cancer Letters, Volume 457, 2019, Pages 86-97, ISSN 0304-3835, https://doi.org/10.1016/j.canlet.2019.05.008.

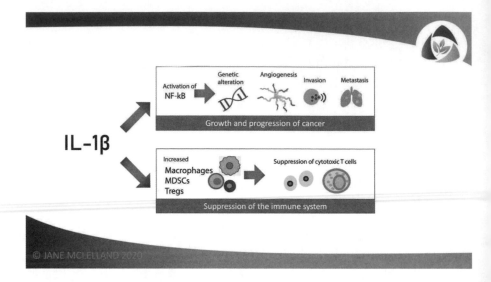

Treatment: Either aspirin, a stronger type of NSAID or Boswellia. Initially, I used aspirin and then switched to etodolac for three months. I never took the two together as the stronger non-steroidal would cancel out the anti-platelet effects of the aspirin and raise the risk of stomach bleeds significantly. Today, I continue to take a daily 75mg of aspirin as part of my prevention strategy and only use the stronger NSAID occasionally and even then only with a meal. I have added Boswellia as a regular part of my prevention programme to reduce inflammation, I believe it should be on everyone's protocol especially if you have a sensitive stomach to NSAIDS.

IL-6 stimulates the JAK-STAT pathway which we will discuss in the next section.

PPAR gamma (peroxisome proliferator-activated receptor gamma) – This is a receptor in the nucleus that is a master controller of fatty acid storage and glucose metabolism. When Wnt signalling is upregulated, PPAR gamma is downregulated. This occurs in many cancers. The PPAR gamma also controls inflammation and insulin, which makes it important to regulate in all metabolic disorders including cancer. It is the target for several diabetic drugs, the glitazones, which reduce insulin resistance and increase insulin sensitivity, but they have significant side effects. Statins,[114] Berberine[115] and another natural extract called Honokiol activate PPAR gamma. It is also partly activated by ibuprofen. Whilst they work, these are a bit like sticky plasters for activating this receptor. The root problem is linked to low gut flora (bifidobacteria in particular), and not enough fish oils (omega-3), vitamins A and D and omega-7.

Once you have worked out which of these abnormal cell signals are applicable to your cancer, you can get to the core of your treatment: how to starve it.

114 Grip, O., Janciauskiene, S. & Lindgren, S. Atorvastatin activates PPAR-y and attenuates the inflammatory response in human monocytes Inflamm Res (2002) 51: 58. https://doi.org/10.1007/BF02684000

115 Chen, F.L., Yang, Z.H., Liu, Y. *et al.* Berberine inhibits the expression of TNFα, MCP-1, and IL-6 in AcLDL-stimulated macrophages through PPARγ pathway. Endocr (2008) 33: 331. https://doi.org/10.1007/s12020-008-9089-3

Chapter Twenty-Two:

How to Starve Cancer

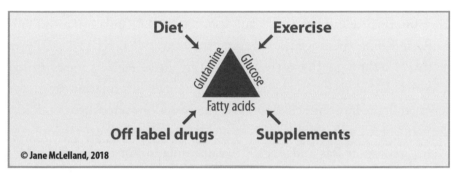

Figure 21.1. *My Four Pillars of Starving Cancer*

Treatments for the Abnormal Cell Metabolism

It would be nice to think that you could stop the abnormal metabolism in the tumour with just a handful of drugs and supplements and not bother with the exercise and diet side of things, but from what I have witnessed, this is just not possible, or wise. Those that make the effort to cut out the appropriate fuel source (mostly glucose) from their diet are the ones who do the best. Starving cancer, I believe, is **the** most important step to treat cancer. Once starved, it is weak and vulnerable. Then kill it. Boom.

Although this is a radical new approach to defeating cancer, evidence is mounting fast to support this idea. It is not about starving the body, although fasting intermittently helps. It is about targeting the tumour with drugs such as metformin to reduce glucose and statins to reduce its ability to make cholesterol. I often hear 'I have normal cholesterol levels,

I don't need a statin', but this is missing the point. Patients reject statins for the wrong reasons. Statins work, they starve cancer, there is a ton of evidence to support their usage. If you doubt this, type in your cancer, e.g. 'melanoma + statin + PubMed' into a Google search.

So how does the abnormal metabolism happen? (More science alert – Skip this section if this is not your thing!)

The abnormal cell signals, especially prolonged IL6 (inflammation) and TLR signalling (pathogens) trigger something called STAT3 pathway in the cell through the activation of tiny little RNA strands called microRNA that take epigenetic (environmental) information from the cell membrane into the cell. Stat3 is a 'transcription factor'. Stat3 talks to the genes of the cell and this leads to an alteration in their expression (e.g. overexpression of Ras and AKT). An upregulation of these genes (they do not have to be mutated, they just become 'overexpressed') triggers an excess production of Acetyl-CoA. Acetyl-CoA is a central node both for generating new 'daughter' cells and for its role in regulating gene expression. It is the principal building block for the generation of fatty acids, sterols, amino acids, and nucleotides needed for manufacture of the 'daughter' cells. The cancer cell will use whatever fuel is available in the primary tumour site to maintain its growth and specialise its metabolism towards growth.

Excess production of Acetyl-CoA leads to 'acetylation' of the DNA histones (the scaffold surrounding the DNA), which alters the polarity of the DNA. Acetylation has the effect of neutralising the electrical potential from positive to neutral, so that histones are no longer attracted to their polar opposite, allowing the DNA strands to part or 'loosen', thereby allowing carcinogens and viruses to enter the DNA or to become reactivated. Genetic mutations then result. (In other words, carcinogens pour fuel on the fire).

Before we get to the Metro Map, let's discuss the pathways that link interleukins, the inflammation signals to the Metro Map .

IL-1 stimulates the NF-kB pathway.

IL-6 stimulates the Jak and STAT3 pathways.

These routes are really important as they are 'upstream', i.e. they occur before the metabolic changes. TLRs and IL-1 and IL-6 inhibitors are upstream of these which is why 70% of bladder cancer patients can be put into remission purely with the BCG vaccine which targets TLR9. Adding drugs and supplements that block all these major routes above will make blocking the 'downstream' routes easier. See them as a priority.

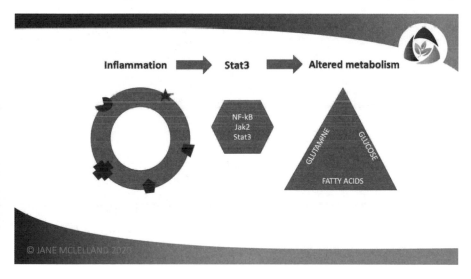

As NF-kB is linked to inflammation, it has a great many effects 'downstream' leading to metastasis and progression which makes it a really important target for every cancer. Anti-inflammatory drugs such as sulfasalazine, celecoxib, sulindac and my choice etodolac are the most potent. Interestingly tamoxifen makes it onto this list too. AKBA, a component of the Ayurvedic plant Boswellia serrata, a good anti-inflammatory supplement that does not have gastric effects like some of the drugs, can be safely included in the majority of protocols.[116]

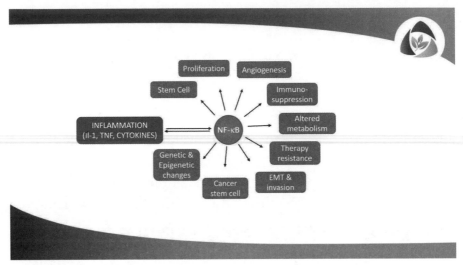

NF-kB has many effects on cancer

Jak2 can be inhibited by berbermine (often found with berberine) and ellagic acid.

Stat3 is another central node, it is a critical metabolic check point for the proper functioning of the immune system (see kynurenine pathway in the immune chapter). It is inhibited by metformin, nifuroxazide (an old, virtually non toxic anti-infective) and flubendazole. Natural supplements to suppress Stat3 are berberine, baicalein and nimbolide.[117]

116 Takada Y, Ichikawa H, Badmaev V, Aggarwal BB. Acetyl-11-keto-beta-boswellic acid potentiates apoptosis, inhibits invasion, and abolishes osteoclastogenesis by suppressing NF-kappa B and NF-kappa B-regulated gene expression. J Immunol. 2006 Mar 1;176(5):3127-40. doi: 10.4049/jimmunol.176.5.3127. PMID: 16493072.

117 Susmitha GD, Miyazato K, Ogura K, Yokoyama S, Hayakawa Y. Anti-metastatic Effects of Baicalein by Targeting STAT3 Activity in Breast Cancer Cells. Biol Pharm Bull. 2020;43(12):1899-1905. doi: 10.1248/bpb.b20-00571. PMID: 33268707.

The Metro Map

It has taken me a lot of time to research which treatments and pipelines are the best to target, but here it is, your route map to guide you to the drugs, supplements and therapies you need to starve your own cancer, no matter the type or stage of disease. My Metro Map represents the metabolically flexible cancer stem cell, present in every cancer, able to shift its different nutrient supply routes, with some routes proving easier to block off than others.

Like the underground and the over ground at Piccadilly Circus, there are two separate systems in a tumour, each behaving very differently and representing two different types of cancer cells; fast dividing cells and cancer stem cells. The two varieties are distinct from each other and require two completely different approaches to treatment.

My 'Metro Map' has not only helped me work out how the cancer cell is feeding itself, but it also makes it much easier for the patient to visualise what is going on in their own body. Bit by bit, as I have researched and added more fuel lines, I have gradually worked out how cancer rewires its metabolism. I have been able to see beyond the complexity of the disease and unravel much of its mystery. I no longer think of cancer as being impossible to cure. I believe all that is required is to attack the stem cells with the right cocktail of drugs alongside the fast-dividing cells. This differs slightly in each cancer type, depending on how it has 'specialised' its metabolism. Cancer will adapt how it feeds itself to the fuel available in the location of the primary tumour as it develops.[118] So the clues to starving and defeating cancer lie in determining what fuel it is using; you

---

[118] Matt Vander Heiden, Associate Professor of Koch Institute for Integrative Cancer Research, Massachusetts Institute of Technology is researching this theory and although it is hard to prove, he agrees that lots of data supports this hypothesis. (Confirmed by personal email). But different breast cancers metabolise nutrients differently so other factors must be at play, such as any pathogenic influence.

will need to work out your cancer's 'metabolic phenotype'. This you can do with the aid of PubMed articles and a helpful oncologist.

Fortunately increasing numbers of articles tracking cancer's 'metabolomics', the metabolites that each type of cancer prefers, are being discovered and written up. Metabolomics will reveal exactly how a specific type of cancer rewires its pathways during chemotherapy, targeted drugs and immunotherapy treatments. All these treatments cause metabolic effects on particular pathways in the cancer cell, often making the cancer cell addicted to particular metabolites, for example some become addicted to glutamine, others to serine, some to arginine. These discoveries will allow us to outsmart the cancer cell, to predict its moves and block off its ability to use these key metabolites. Cancer is merely a game of chess; we only need to know what it is likely to do next to win. Those answers are coming in folks!

As you search, type in words from each Metro fuel line, (e.g., HER2 breast cancer + chloroquine or macropinocytosis), working through each fuel line in turn. It might take you half an hour or so. For example, a search reveals that adding chloroquine works for HER2 breast cancer patients, so we can deduce that this type of cancer uses macropinocytosis to scavenge extracellular protein and fat.[119]

However, there are two problems with this.

1. Researchers are only just working out each cancer's metabolic phenotype, so not all of the information may be available yet. However, you can still get a good idea of the major fuel pipelines and whether it is driven by glucose, glutamine or fat.

2. Once you have worked out the fuel lines that need blocking, how to get hold of the drugs you need?

119 Cufí S, Vazquez-Martin A, Oliveras-Ferraros C, *et al.* The anti-malarial chloroquine overcomes Primary resistance and restores sensitivity to Trastuzumab in HER2-positive breast cancer. *Scientific Reports*. 2013;3: 2469. doi: 10.1038/srep02469.

Unable to obtain the drugs from either their oncologist or their GP, I have little doubt that patients will start up 'Buyer's Clubs' much like HIV patients had to do in the 1980s. Although this will be frowned upon by the establishment, why shouldn't a patient try to save their own life? If they have been told there is nothing more that can be done, why should they have to meekly go home to die?

So here it is, my Metro Map of how you too can starve your cancer. Each side of the triangle represents either a glucose pathway, glutamine or fatty acid pathway.

Note that some of the drugs target several pathways across both sides.

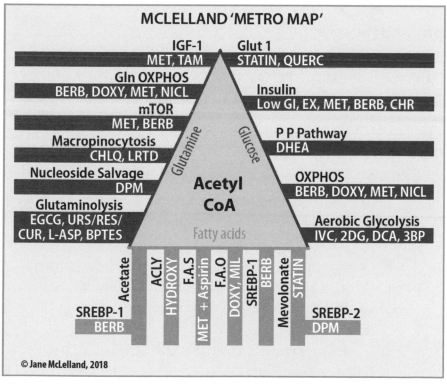

Figure 21.2. *My Stem Cell 'Metro Map'*

METABOLIC PATHWAYS

Glucose Pathways

Glut 1 = Glucose Transporter 1, Insulin, PP Pathway = Pentose Phosphate Pathway, OXPHOS = Oxidative Phosphorylation, Aerobic Glycolysis

Glutamine/Amino Acid Pathways

IGF-1 = Insulin like growth factor-1, Gln OXPHOS = Glutamine oxidative phosphorylation, mTOR = mammalian target of rapamycin, Macropinocyctosis (Autophagy) Nucleoside Salvage (Autophagy), Glutaminolysis, Acetate Pathway

Fatty Acid Pathways

SREBP-1 = Sterol Regulating End Binding Protein-1, SREBP-2 = Sterol Regulating End Binding Protein-2, ACLY = ATP Citrate Lyase, F.A.S. = Fatty Acid Synthesis, F.A.O. = Fatty Acid Oxidation, Mevalonate Pathway

TREATMENTS (written in colour)

MET = Metformin, TAM = Tamoxifen, BERB = Berberine, DOXY = Doxycycline, NICL = Niclosamide, CHLQ = Chloroquine, LRTD = Loratadine, DPM = Dipyridamole, EGCG = Epigallocatechin Gallate, URS = Ursolic Acid, CUR = Curcumin, RES = Resveratrol, L-ASP = Asparaginase, BPTES = bis-2-(5-phenylacetamido- 1,2,4-thiadiazol-2-yl)ethyl sulphide, MIL = Mildronate, IVC = intravenous vitamin C, 2DG = 2-Deoxyglucose, DCA = Dichloroacetate, 3BP = 3-Bromopyruvate, Low GI = Low Glycaemic Diet, CHR = chromium picolinate, QUERC = Quercetin

These words may seem like medical mumbo jumbo to you, but it really doesn't matter if you don't fully understand each pathway or how they work. The sad truth is that oncologists don't know about them either. Yet. But what you do need to understand is that to starve your cancer and obliterate the cancer stem cell it is critical that these pipelines are blocked off. And this can be achieved mostly by using low toxicity drugs and supplements that won't kill you in the process. Hurrah!

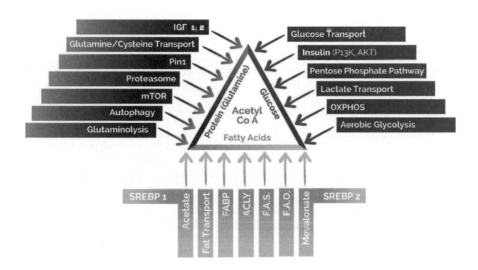

My 2021 Metro Map above includes a few more important nutrient pathways including lactate, fat and glutamine transport and the xCT antiporter, a really important fuel line for chemo-resistant cancers and for the process of ferroptosis.

Both maps show the major routes a cancer stem cell takes to feed itself. The altered metabolism in cancer is far more complex than just aerobic glycolysis! Otto Warburg was only partly right with his discovery in 1924, as these pathways demonstrate. Although I show these pathways as separate, there is crosstalk between them and not every route is exclusively blocking one nutrient macro, for example Mevalonate not only stops the production of cholesterol, but it also stops protein prenylation too. But for simplicity's sake, it is a handy reference guide to working out which drugs and supplements you need for your cancer's metabolic phenotype.

Almost all the drugs and natural supplements that I have chosen have 'pleiotropic' effects. In other words, they work on several targets at the same time, so you will find that the drug and supplement list is less extensive than you might expect.

With the current standard of care, only around 50% to 60% of all cancer patients will survive longer than five years (far fewer will make it to ten years), and these statistics have remained the same for decades. And, for many patients, the thought of a long 'battle' or 'war' armed with the barbaric weaponry currently on offer is just too great. Many fly the white flag and accede defeat with little resistance almost from the start.

Using the word 'war' or 'battle' is tantamount to literary suicide for a cancer book nowadays. Counsellors are told never to use these words or other bellicose phrases when talking to cancer patients. These terms are, quite rightly, being shunned by cancer patients as they try to grasp the enormity of what faces them. Many books now focus on 'making peace' and 'learning' from your cancer. Sure, do that if you think it is going to help, but that alone is not going to get you well. So, I am going to buck the trend. Yes, you need to wage a war, but of a different kind. Be smart. Be sneaky. Outwit your cancer. I don't believe you have to suffer to slay it.

Looking back at history, we have much to learn from the ancient Greeks and how they played out a great many of their wars. It was a very simple, very effective technique and casualties were few. If we were to employ a similar approach, our bodies would be spared the hugely toxic high doses of chemotherapy and this dreadfully damaging treatment would be consigned to the dustbin of history where it belongs. 'Making peace' with your cancer (whilst you slay it) would be an easier thing to achieve as a result. Did I ever 'make peace' with my cancer? Did I learn 'lessons' or feel it was a 'gift'? I guess I am not afraid of it, if that is making peace. I learnt to live with it. I have learnt a lot about the human body, especially mine, and the various aspects of the disease. But making friends with it, being thankful for it? No. Never. Cancer was always the enemy. But how you choose to approach your disease is entirely up to you.

Leaving the psychologically terrifying aspect of the disease aside for a moment, on a cellular level it is indeed a battle, however you choose to think about it in your head. Whilst you 'make peace' with it, understand there is a very real power struggle taking place, a turf war between your healthy cells and cancer cells, not just for territory, but for nutrients. Cancer behaves like a parasite, taking up your body's supplies, your immunity and gradually growing until it encroaches on your own life systems. As frightening as this sounds, there is, I believe, an easy and far less damaging approach to defeating it.

To illustrate my approach, let me take you back to a city called Plataea, located South of the city of Thebes in a Spartan controlled region called Boeotia, located in Ancient Greece in 431 BC…

Plataea was a well defended small city which somehow managed to survive being overthrown by Spartan led forces and was one of the last strongholds in Southern Boeotia that still swore allegiance to Athens. Unfortunately, its location made it incredibly vulnerable. Knowing that they would be attacked, the Plataeans had built up incredibly strong defenses. Despite being vulnerable, the citizens of Plataea felt sure that in times of trouble they could rely on their old ally Athens to come to their rescue.

The citizens of the nearby city of Thebes were under the control of Sparta. They were getting fed up with this neighbourly Athenian-controlled nuisance and decided that they had had enough. Knowing that Plataea was fiercely defended with strong, high walls, lots of weaponry and many fit young soldiers, they hatched a plan to take it in a different way. The idea was to use stealth and cunning and by doing so hopefully use less force and cause less bloodshed.

The Thebans had heard that there were some Plataean citizens in the city who, knowing their vulnerable position, felt very unsafe. They knew an attack would come from Thebes sooner or later. A few of the inhabitants of Plataea decided they would rather surrender and live to fight another day without the risk of a war.

The Thebans persuaded one of these nervous citizens to become a traitor and help them carry out their dastardly plan.

One night at about 3 o'clock in the morning, the traitor opened one of the gates of Plataea to an advance party of about three hundred soldiers from the Theban army. They met no resistance and they marched straight into the market square of Plataea, taking the city by surprise. The plan was that this smaller troop would occupy the city until the larger attacking force arrived later during that morning. This nearly worked, like the Trojan Horse.

The Plataeans were so shocked by this unexpected invasion, that they immediately surrendered. During the night however it became clear to the Plataeans that the Theban army was only small, so the men, women and even the slaves gathered together and mounted a full fight back in the middle of the night. Some Thebans escaped, some were killed, but the Plataeans took 180 of the invading army hostage and regained control of their city.

When the large attacking force of Thebans arrived as per the original plan, they were upset that their original plan had been foiled and wanted the immediate release of the hostages. They promised to retreat in return for their safe release, to which the Plataeans agreed. But as soon as the

Theban army left, the Plataeans went against their word and executed every single one of the hostages.

This, of course, did not go down well. The Thebans were beyond furious. Outraged, they launched a full-scale attack on the city with siege engines and battering rams. The Plataeans were fully expecting this reaction and were well prepared so they fought them off, each attack being effectively rebutted. For two years, the Thebans fought on their own in vain to take the city.

After all this time with no sign of success, yet unwilling to give up, the Spartans arrived on the scene to help their Theban allies (part of the confederate). The Spartans suggested another approach.

First, they built another wall around the city to protect themselves from any Athenian armies that might arrive to rescue the Plataeans.

Next, they built a giant mound of earth outside the city wall from which they planned to mount an attack by climbing and entering over the top of the wall. But the higher they built the mound, the higher the Plataeans inside the city built the defending wall. The Plataeans laughed at their pathetic attempt. This made the Thebans and Spartans even more enraged.

Next, the Thebans and Spartans brought in their big battering rams, but these were rendered useless by the Plataeans, who used large beams on chains swung from the walls that were so effective that they smashed the rams. Again, the Plataeans jeered and shouted insults at the attackers from the ramparts of the city wall.

Seething with rage and undeterred, the Thebans then tried to burn and smoke them out.

They waited until the wind was in the right direction then took huge bales of hay up to the top of the mound they had built earlier and hurled them over. The Plataeans saw what they were up to and were ready with buckets of water and beaters to put out the flames. A large part of the city was destroyed, but still the Plataeans would not surrender.

The Plataeans seemed able to outwit their every move. The Thebans and Spartans were now weary; they had used up all their best weapons and had got nowhere. But they were still furious at the slaughter of the hostages, they were determined to beat the Plataeans somehow. They would not give up.

With no effective weapons left at their disposal, the decision was taken to sit it out and wait, to starve them into submission. The plan was to keep them captive. No food would be allowed to enter, and no-one was to escape the city.

This was a strategy that required much patience, but the Theban troops camped outside the city walls for a further two years and just remained there in readiness to pick off anyone attempting to flee.

Eventually, in 427 BC, four years after the start of this battle, the Plataeans, weak, hungry, and reduced in number, eventually decided to surrender on the promise that they should be given a fair trial. The Spartans agreed.

Were they shown any mercy as promised? Or a fair trial? After they had brutally slaughtered the Theban hostages? Certainly not!

In a mock trial they were asked a single question by five Spartan judges:

'Have you done anything to help the Spartans and their allies in the present war?'

As each soldier could only answer 'no', inevitably they were led away to their execution. Horrified, the surviving women looked on as their menfolk were murdered, before they themselves were taken away and sold into slavery.

The city of Plataea, once so strong and indestructible, was razed to the ground.

Lessons:

1. Weaken the Enemy.
Attacking an enemy when they are in a position of strength is a waste of resources and effort. You risk losing troops and allies in the fight and there will be lots of collateral damage. With the most difficult, seemingly invincible foe, one who is quickly adaptable, it is easiest to kill him when he is weak and defenseless.

2. Starve the Enemy.
It is a simple and effective tactic still used by warring factions today.

A cancer cell needs constant sources of energy, predominantly glucose and access to proteins and fat, to keep on making more copies of itself. Think of it like building a new house. You cannot create a home using tools and a workforce alone. You need the bricks and mortar. Likewise, cancer needs proteins and fat for biomass and glucose for the energy to build new cells. If you starve a cancer cell of its energy from glucose alone, it redirects to other sources of energy instead like glutamine and fat. The trick is to starve it of its critical fuel pipelines.

3. Patience.
Weakening and starving may not shrink tumours overnight. It may take many months to use this method, but once the cancer is weak, then other treatments like chemotherapy, radiotherapy, intravenous vitamin

C and other drugs like NSAIDs and statins can be employed far more effectively. Crucially, they can be used at less toxic levels to pick off the remaining cancer cells by triggering apoptosis.

4. Combine Forces.

Starving cancer by maintaining a very strict diet alone is not a feasible or realistic option for most patients. So combining other approaches – off label low toxicity drugs, a personalised (but not extreme) diet, specific supplements and timely exercise will all work synergistically. Once starved, triggering apoptosis by less toxic methods, the caspase cascade and low dose chemotherapy, will be far more effective if you have already made the cancer weak and vulnerable. If you only target fast dividing cells, as current conventional cancer protocols dictate, yet ignore the stem cell, you allow the cancer to continue to flourish and become more aggressive.

Where to Start?

All the metabolic processes in the cell are either a breakdown (lysis) – like glycolysis, glutaminolysis (catabolic reactions), or they are a re-building (anabolic) process to make new cell components.

The Warburg Effect (Glycolysis) and Reverse Warburg Effect (OXPHOS)

An increase in aerobic glycolysis is one of the most common properties of cancer cells, detected by glucose PET scans in around 80-90% of all tumours, which means it is the prime target for most types of cancer. But in a few cancers, glycolysis is in fact very low.[120] For example, in prostate cancer the Warburg Effect is only present at late stages after many mutational events. Prostate cancer instead relies on lipogenesis (energy from fat) and glutaminolysis (energy from glutamine).

---

120 Eidelman E, Twum-Ampofo J, Ansari J, Siddiqui MM. The Metabolic Phenotype of Prostate Cancer. Frontiers in Oncology. 2017;7: 131. doi: 10.3389/fonc.2017.00131.

Other cancers (such as certain melanomas) upregulate oxidative phosphorylation (OXPHOS) in the mitochondria rather than glycolysis in the cytosol right from the beginning.[121] Also, the numbers of mitochondria reaccumulate in a great many different cancer cells as a cancer progresses, making it more resistant to being killed off by oxygen free radicals and by glycolysis inhibition alone.[122] This is why it is imperative to know what kind of fuel your cancer is demanding and to target that as a priority. Targeting the wrong fuel could make the situation worse by making the cancer yet more resistant. Generally, it helps to remember that the majority of cancers use glycolysis first, then they switch to glutamine/fat pathways as they become more advanced. More aggressive cancers like ovarian make this switch earlier in their progression, which makes them behave in a more aggressive way – the more aggressive the cancer, the more pathways need to be blocked.

Aerobic Glycolysis, the 'Warburg Effect,' is the switch from making ATP – the energy currency – efficiently in the mitochondria to an inefficient fermentation process in the cytoplasm even in the presence of oxygen (which is why it is called aerobic even though it is an anaerobic process – most confusing). This unusual metabolic feature of cancer has been well documented and is the most understood of all the abnormal metabolic pathways. This makes glycolysis the prime target for most types of cancer.

The process of glycolysis involves several steps, with each step providing an opportunity to use a drug or a natural compound to block each one. The by-products of glycolysis are used for lipogenesis (the generation of fatty acids) to satisfy the increased demand for energy and the macromolecules (nucleotides, cell membranes, enzymes etc.) needed for growth and proliferation, so by blocking glycolysis you can start to block the fat

---

121 Francisca Vazquez et al, PGC1α Expression Defines a Subset of Human Melanoma Tumors with Increased Mitochondrial Capacity and Resistance to Oxidative Stress Cancer Cell, Volume 23, Issue 3, 18 March 2013, Pages 287-301

122 Maiuri, Maria Chiara *et al.* Essential Role for Oxidative Phosphorylation in Cancer Progression. Cell Metabolism, Volume 21, Issue 1, 11-12

pathways too. The focus on this pathway is so extreme that it is often targeted to the exclusion of the other pathways. Using a combination of DCA, 2-deoxyglucose, 3BP and ketogenic diets can achieve remarkable remissions, but it may be too extreme a method if it fails to tackle other pathways concurrently. Dr Nasha Winters, a Naturopath specialising in the metabolism of cancer, has witnessed patients ultimately having a rebound effect. This is most likely because the cancer learns to scavenge extracellular nutrients and use glutamine pathways, so ultimately it returns more aggressively than ever. Achieving remission is good but staying there is another thing altogether. Targeting glycolysis alone in my view is not a good long-term strategy. I am convinced that extremes need to be avoided and that a slower, safer reduction in tumour size and metabolic activity is a better path to tread.

Lactate, a by-product of glycolysis can, become a fuel in a 'Reverse Warburg' effect, leading to an upregulation in the oxidative phosphorylation (OXPHOS) pathway. Lactate is not only a by-product in the cancer cell, but it can also be manufactured by the surrounding fibroblasts in the connective tissue around the cancer cell. The fibroblasts are instructed by their neighbouring cancer cell to destroy their mitochondria (mitophagy), so that they too obtain their energy from the fermentation of glucose, glycolysis, the product of which is lactate. The increase in lactate in the tumour microenvironment is then shuttled back into the cancer cell where it is converted to pyruvate. Pyruvate then re-enters the Kerbs cycle (OXPHOS) in the mitochondria in the cancer cell. This is known as the 'Reverse Warburg Effect'. Many mitochondria show an increase in activity in cancer cells, contrary to the belief that these energy powerhouses in the cells are all 'switched off' or damaged in cancer cells. With more advanced disease, it is not imperative to turn the mitochondria back on, as many suggest, as this could make the situation worse.

What **is** imperative is to starve each source of fuel that the cancer demands. So, whilst many mitochondria may be damaged, others are working overtime with a surge in numbers to maintain the fuel supply.

How should you target these highly activated mitochondria? I was to learn the antibiotic doxycycline is highly effective as it breaks down these mitochondria, the energy-giving organelles found in super-charged cancer cells.[123] Mitochondria are ancient bacteria that were engulfed by a single cell over a billion years ago to help facilitate its adaptation to an oxygen environment, resulting in one of the most successful partnerships ever. All our cells (bar our red blood cells) are descendants of this endosymbiotic arrangement. Berberine, with its antibiotic effect, can also reduce the upregulated cancer OXPHOS pathway, as can niclosamide; an old drug for tapeworms.

This 'Reverse Warburg' concept is hard for many to grasp as it is hard enough to get your head around the glycolytic metabolic shift. The cancer cell will adapt to meet its changing nutrient circumstances, and it can use almost anything it can get hold of. Even in nutrient poor circumstances, like in pancreatic cancer, the cancer cell cleverly develops a process called macropinocytosis, a ruffling of the cell membrane to engulf extracellular protein and fat to feed itself.[124] The environmental constraints on the pancreatic cancer, including hypoxia (a lack of oxygen), only serves to enhance the tumour's aggressiveness. Sarcomas, melanomas, lymphomas, mesothelial and hepatocellular carcinomas behave a little differently and use the amino acid arginine for fuel, so depriving arginine in these specific cancers may be a useful target if shutting down the other pathways is not enough.

123 Fares M, Abedi-Valugerdi M, Hassan M, Potacova Z. DNA damage, lysosomal degradation and Bcl-xL deamidation in doxycycline and minocycline-induced cell death. Biochem Biophys Res Commun 463, 268-274 (2015).

124 Kamphorst JJ, Nofal M, Commisso C, *et al*. Human pancreatic cancer tumors are nutrient poor and tumor cells actively scavenge extracellular protein. Cancer research. 2015;75(3): 544-553. doi: 10.1158/0008-5472.CAN-14-2211.

These metabolic pathways feed the cancer with either amino acids (protein – e.g., glutamine, serine, arginine), glucose or fatty acids, and if one of these becomes depleted (e.g., glucose on a ketogenic diet) then the stem cell switches to another pipeline. The important message is that it is targeting several, not just one or two of the stem cell 'metro' fuel lines, which is vital to achieve a lasting remission and avoid rewiring your cancer to a more aggressive phenotype.

I have included a few other pathways that I personally didn't target like the macropinocytosis (e.g., upregulated in pancreatic cancer, HER2 breast, triple negative breast) and fatty acid oxidation (upregulated in Myc overexpressing Triple Negative Breast cancer, PC3 prostate cancer and diffuse large B-cell lymphoma, Burkitts lymphoma and GBM[125]), because there is little point in just copying what I did if your cancer is metabolically different to mine. If you have a more aggressive cancer, you will need to add more to your armoury to starve it, possibly adding the glutaminase inhibiting drugs.

By blocking or reducing several fuel sources at the same time, I had weakened my cancer and made it more vulnerable to the normal cell suicide process of 'apoptosis'. Once starved, it only took a small change, either through lowering the glutathione (antioxidant) or increasing the levels of free radicals (ROS) to make it vulnerable to being killed.

This multiple hit approach is shared by Professor Michael Lisanti in Salford, Manchester in the UK. In 2017, he published a paper in the journal *Oncotarget*, which showed that gradually increasing levels of doxycycline, a common antibiotic, over several weeks, blocks OXPHOS (glutamine, lactate or glucose fuelled) and fatty acid oxidation. This creates drug resistance to the doxycycline (metabolic rewiring) and

---

125 Camarda R, Zhou Z, Kohnz RA, *et al*. Inhibition of fatty acid oxidation as a therapy for MYC-overexpressing triple-negative breast cancer. Nature medicine. 2016;22(4): 427-432. doi: 10.1038/nm.4055.

forces the stem cell to convert its metabolism from OXPHOS to a more glycolytic phenotype. This was then followed by the addition of oral vitamin C, which blocks step 6 of glycolysis. This starved the cancer and caused remaining cells to die in ER positive breast cancer which rely heavily on OXPHOS to maintain their energy stores. This two-pronged approach of attacking two pathways together proved lethal to many different cancer cell types.[126] Lisanti also discovered that the addition of berberine enhanced his results. This was no surprise to me!

This ability of the cancer stem cell to shift its metabolism and adapt to a new environment is applicable to **all** types of cancer stem cells.

This flexibility to switch to an alternative fuel pipeline is easy to spot once you are aware that it happens, when you too scour the current medical literature – which you are going to do of course! This is the reason cancer develops drug resistance, not just because of 'genes'; the genes are a result of altered metabolism, and the cancer evading treatment by scurrying down another Metro line.

As I read the research, I learned that:

- If you block mTOR, the cancer cell upregulates a process called 'autophagy' (self-eating).[127]
- If you block glycolysis (in the cytoplasm) the cancer cell upregulates oxidative phosphorylation (OXPHOS) in the mitochondria.[128]

---

126 Ernestina Marianna De Francesco, Gloria Bonuccelli, Marcello Maggiolini, Federica Sotgia, and Michael P. Lisanti; Vitamin C and Doxycycline: A synthetic lethal combination therapy targeting metabolic flexibility in cancer stem cells (CSCs) Oncotarget. 2017 Sep 15; 8(40): 67269-67286.

127 Cancers (Basel). 2018 Jan 12;10(1). pii: E18. doi: 10.3390/cancers10010018. mTOR Pathways in Cancer and Autophagy. Paquette M1,2, El-Houjeiri L3,4, Pause A5,6.

128 Energy metabolism of cancer: Glycolysis versus oxidative phosphorylation (Review) J Zheng – Oncology letters, 2012

- If you block mevalonate with a statin, the cell can upregulate the cholesterol pathway through SREBP-2.[129]

- Certain cancers, for example. sarcomas, lymphomas, hepatocellular, melanomas, prostate, AML, pancreatic and a subset of GBM, rely on arginine as fuel. When they are deprived of it, some cancers use an alternative pathway (autophagy) to acquire glutamine and other amino acids.[130] With other cancers, concurrent arginine deprivation and glutaminase inhibition (reducing glutamine) caused the cancer cells to use serine.[131] If you block fatty acid synthesis the cancer cell can upregulate ketone metabolism and glutaminolysis.[132]

- If you block fatty acid oxidation the cancer cell upregulates aerobic glycolysis.[133]

- If you block glutaminolysis your cancer can upregulate macropinocytosis.[134]

- If you block ATP citrate lyase (ACLY), the stem cell increases the SREBP1, SREBP2 and acetate pathways.[135]

129 Pandyra A, Penn LZ. Targeting tumor cell metabolism via the mevalonate pathway: Two hits are better than one. Molecular & Cellular Oncology. 2014;1(4): e969133. doi: 10.4161/23723548.2014.969133.

130 Arginine Deprivation Inhibits the Warburg Effect and Upregulates Glutamine Anaplerosis and Serine Biosynthesis in ASS1-Deficient Cancers. Cell Reports 2017. *https://www.sciencedaily.com/releases/2017/01/170124140803.htm*

131 Reiss C 10,1159/000495

132 Juri G Gelovani *et al.* Metabolic shifts induced by Fatty Acid Synthase Inhibitor Orlistat in NSCLC Mol Imaging Biol. 2013 Apr; 15(2): 136-147. Using orlistat, a diet pill, to block FASN will mess up your metabolism! This is a pretty blunt tool in my opinion.

133 Qu Q, Zeng F, Liu X, Wang QJ, Deng F. Fatty acid oxidation and carnitine palmitoyltransferase I: emerging therapeutic targets in cancer. Cell Death & Disease. 2016;7(5): e2226-. doi: 10.1038/cddis.2016.132.

134 Recouvreux MV, Commisso C. Macropinocytosis: A Metabolic Adaptation to Nutrient Stress in Cancer. Frontiers in Endocrinology. 2017;8: 261. doi: 10.3389/fendo.2017.00261.

135 Nousheen Zaidi, Ines Royaux, Johannes V. Swinnen and Karine Smans ATP Citrate Lyase Knockdown Induces Growth Arrest and Apoptosis through Different Cell- and Environment-Dependent Mechanisms. Mol Cancer Ther September 1, 2012 (11) (9) 1925-1935; DOI: 10.1158/1535-7163.MCT-12-0095

If you look at the way these paths reroute by mapping them out on the Metro Map, you will see that generally the cancer will reroute up the same side of the triangle. In other words, if it can't access fat one way it will use another fat pathway. The knowledge that this metabolic shift occurs has huge implications for treatment. It is essential to take a comprehensive cocktail of drugs and supplements, and it is best to take them together rather than one at a time to prevent the cancer from rerouting at all. Taking a little metformin just isn't going to work, wonder drug though it is. Timing and dosage of each is also important and is best worked out by a doctor who understands the metabolic nature of your disease and who has experience in this area. The Care Oncology Clinic would be my first port of call even though they don't use all the drugs I suggest. You can always add more, and I have a list of doctors to contact on my website.

At the very least I would target the following pathways with every cancer: NF-kB, JAK2, STAT3, Glut1, Aerobic Glycolysis (cover each enzyme in this pathway), OXPHOS, Reduce Insulin, IGF-1/2, mTOR, Mevalonate, SREBP-2, Fatty Acid Synthesis, Glutaminolysis (use several modalaties), xCT antiporter and block lactate, fat (FABP) and glutamine transporters. The Pin1 can be very important with some cancers like gliomas and breast whereas the proteasome is more important with myeloma.

How to Starve Cancer of Glucose

Insulin – PI3k, Akt pathway is strongly correlated to insulin – the most dangerous hormone in the body (no, it's not oestrogen!). Insulin is reduced by a low glycaemic diet, metformin, berberine, appropriate and timely exercise (15-30 mins after eating), good quality sleep, chromium picolinate, gymnema sylvestre, stevia, naringenin, danshen, baicalin (from Chinese skullcap). Improving insulin sensitivity is important, you need insulin to remove glucose from the blood into muscles. You do not want excess levels of insulin as this helps cancer cells access glucose.

PI3K and AKT are strongly related to excess glucose uptake by tumours. Nimbolide will naturally help prevent this.[136] Amiloride has been found to be very effective for pancreatic cancer[137] and ritonavir, a HIV protease inhibitor can stop this pathway in several cancer lines including ovarian.[138]

Glut (Glucose transport receptor) 1 – Glucose transport receptors 1,2,3,4,5 – Known as Glut Receptors. The Glut receptor moves to the surface of the cell in cancer (in healthy tissues and muscle cells it is Glut 4) to accept more glucose into the cell. Glut1 is the main glucose transporter in cancer – It can be inhibited by Statins, mebendazole, silibinin and Quercetin. [139]

Natural inhibitors

Glut1 – Quercetin, phloretin, oxymatrine, silibinin

Glut2 – Quercetin, EGCG (liver cancer)

Glut3 – Kaempferol (breast, ovarian, colorectal, rhabdomyosarcoma)

Glut4 – ritonavir (myeloma)

Glut5 – apigenin, rubus chingii (breast, prostate, renal cell)

---

136 Sophia, J., Kowshik, J., Dwivedi, A. et al. Nimbolide, a neem limonoid inhibits cytoprotective autophagy to activate apoptosis via modulation of the PI3K/Akt/GSK-3β signalling pathway in oral cancer. Cell Death Dis 9, 1087 (2018). https://doi.org/10.1038/s41419-018-1126-4

137 Zheng, Yt., Yang, Hy., Li, T. et al. Amiloride sensitizes human pancreatic cancer cells to erlotinib in vitro through inhibition of the PI3K/AKT signaling pathway. Acta Pharmacol Sin 36, 614–626 (2015). https://doi.org/10.1038/aps.2015.4

138 Kumar, Sanjeev et al. "Ritonavir blocks AKT signaling, activates apoptosis and inhibits migration and invasion in ovarian cancer cells." Molecular cancer vol. 8 26. 22 Apr. 2009, doi:10.1186/1476-4598-8-26

139 Ana Filipa Brito *et al.* New Approach for Treatment of Primary Liver Tumors: The Role of Quercetin, Nutrition and Cancer Volume 68, 2016

Glut 5 – specifically transports fructose so be aware that fruit is not a 'safe' form of sugar.

Pentose Phosphate Pathway – The first step of the oxidative pentose phosphate pathway is catalyzed by the enzyme glucose-6-phosphate dehydrogenase (G6PD). DHEA (not for hormone driven cancers), polydatin, physcion (parietin).[140] These will all reduce NADPH – needed to make new DNA. Leflunamide is being investigated for pancreatic cancer as it blocks Dihydroorotate Dehydrogenase, another enzyme in this pathway.

Oxidative Phosphorylation (OXPHOS) – This is how normal cells make ATP (Krebs cycle) but it is dysfunctional in cancer cells – modulated by Berberine, PEITC (in watercress) Metformin, Lonidamine, Ivermectin and Niclosamide. Doxycycline is highly effective but many worry about its antibiotic effects. A new derivative, myristoyl amide, which does not have antibiotic effects will be available in the near future. Blocking both glycolysis enzymes and OXPHOS together can be a highly synergystic combination.

Metformin virtually abolishes Complex I function.[141]

---

140 Antonina I. Frolova, Kathleen O'Neill, Kelle H. Moley; Dehydroepiandrosterone Inhibits Glucose Flux Through the Pentose Phosphate Pathway in Human and Mouse Endometrial Stromal Cells, Preventing Decidualization and Implantation, Molecular Endocrinology, Volume 25, Issue 8, 1 August 2011, Pages 1444-1455, https://doi.org/10.1210/me.2011-0026

141 Owen MR, Doran E, Halestrap AP Evidence that metformin exerts its anti-diabetic effects through inhibition of complex 1 of the mitochondrial respiratory chain. Biochem J. 2000 Jun 15; 348 Pt 3(): 607-14.

Berberine causes mitochondrial fragmentation and depolarisation,[142] and alters mitochondrial membrane permeability.[143]

Doxycycline suppresses mitochondrial function.129[144]

Niclosamide affects the inner membrane potential of the mitochondria, resulting in the uncoupling of **oxidative phosphorylation** from electron transport, which inhibits the production of ATP.

There is an unfounded fear of switching off excess ATP production. People believe that this will cause instant death but switching off excess ATP also happens when people take antibiotics, and these have a long history of safety.

Aerobic Glycolysis – The abnormal fermentation of glucose (Warburg Effect). This process involves several enzymes. Because this is a key metabolic difference to healthy cells, all cancers need one drug or supplement for blocking each of the following enzymes: LDH, PKM2, PDK, HK-2.

G6PDH – Fermented wheat germ, vitamin C.[145]

LDH (lactate dehydrogenase) – fermented wheat germ, fisetin, cardamonin, vitamin D

---

142 Pereira GC *et al.*Mitochondrially targeted effects of berberine on K1735-M2 mouse melanoma cells: Comparison with direct effects on isolated mitochondrial fractions
143 Cláudia V. Pereira Nuno G. Machado Paulo J. Oliveira. Mechanisms of Berberine – Induced Mitochondrial Dysfunction: Interaction with the Adenine Nucleotide Translocator Toxicological Sciences, Volume 105, Issue 2, 1 October 2008, Pages 408-41
144 Lamb, R. *et al.* Antibiotics that target mitochondria effectively eradicate cancer stem cells, across multiple tumor types: treating cancer like an infectious disease. Oncotarget 6, 4569-4584 (2015).
145 Jihye Yun, Lewis C. Cantley et al Vitamin C selectively kills KRAS and BRAF mutant colorectal cancer cells by targeting GAPDH Science. 2016 Dec 11.

PKM2 (Pyruvate Kinase M2) – oxymatrine, fisetin, quercetin, shikonin

PDK (Pyruvate Dehydrogenase Kinase) – melatonin, DCA, 2-DG

HK-2 – metformin, lonidamine, chrysin, fermented wheat germ

Short Term Fasting[146,147] will slow down glycolysis. It is offten viewed as 'dangerous' for cancer patients, but what is more dangerous: terminal cancer, or one day off eating twice a week? Alternatively, you can try stopping at 3pm and not eating until the next day. I would suggest that a good quality extra virgin olive oil with danshen is safe to consume even during a 'fast' because of all its beneficial properties, not least calories.

2 Deoxy-d-Glucose (2-DG) is similar in structure to glucose, so it blocks the cell from taking up normal glucose molecules, like putting water in a car's gas tank rather than petrol. It has shown to work synergistically with metformin. 2-DG is being used by Professor Thomas Seyfried and the ChemoThermia clinic in Istanbul.[148]

Dichloroacetate (DCA) is a pyruvate dehydrogenase kinase (PDK) inhibitor which enhances the oxidative activity of cells by activating pyruvate dehydrogenase (PDH), the enzyme of glucose oxidation in mitochondria.

At high doses it causes neuropathy and inflammation. Because it fosters the conversion of pyruvate into acetyl-CoA and activates mitochondrial OXPHOS, best combined with OXPHOS inhibitors, especially in advanced cancers that use mitochondrial respiration.

146 Marini C, Bianchi G, Buschiazzo A, *et al.* Divergent targets of glycolysis and oxidative phosphorylation result in additive effects of metformin and starvation in colon and breast cancer. Scientific Reports. 2016;6: 19569. doi: 10.1038/srep19569.
147 Raffaghello L, Lee C, Safdie FM, Wei M, Madia F, Bianchi G, Longo VD Starvation-dependent differential stress resistance protects normal but not cancer cells against high-dose chemotherapy. Proc Natl Acad Sci USA. 2008 Jun 17; 105(24): 8215-20.
148 Ben Sahra I, Laurent K, Giuliano S, Larbret F, Ponzio G, Gounon P, Le Marchand-Brustel Y, Giorgetti-Peraldi S, Cormont M, Bertolotto C, et al Targeting cancer cell metabolism: the combination of metformin and 2-deoxyglucose induces p53-dependent apoptosis in prostate cancer cells. Cancer Res. 2010 Mar 15; 70(6): 2465-75. Epub 2010 Mar 9

Metformin virtually abolishes Complex I function[149] and inhibits Hexokinase 2.[150]

3 Bromopyruvate (3BP) – a powerful glycolysis inhibitor that may be too extreme. Currently there lots of arguments about patent rights flying around it, and it is not without side effects. I believe less aggressive cocktails are equally successful.

Remember that using extreme glycolytic inhibition (including ketogenic diets) without blocking other 'metro' routes concurrently may cause a rebound effect through a different pathway and lead to a more aggressive tumour phenotype further down the road.

Lactate Transport – lactate is a by-product of glycolysis, originally just thought of as a waste product, it is now recognised as another source of fuel. Pumped out of one cell, it is transported into neighbouring cells through MCT transporters to be converted back to pyruvate to re-enter the OXPHOS pathway. Although N-Acetyl Cysteine blocks this in stage 0 DCIS, it can create treatment resistance in most cancers so is best avoided. A better option is to use Haritaki. Syrosingopine is effective (it works well with metformin) but is difficult to get hold of.

How To Starve Cancer of Fat

Fat is ignored by a great many people in the cancer field.[151] Alterations in fat metabolism are now considered an important feature of cancer cells because lipids are a store for energy, they are essential components of cellular membranes, and they act as signaling molecules and a source

---

149 Viollet B, Guigas B, Sanz Garcia N, Leclerc J, Foretz M, Andreelli F. Cellular and molecular mechanisms of metformin: an overview. Clinical Science (London, England : 1979). 2012;122(6):253-270. doi:10.1042/CS20110386.

150 Marini C, Salani B, Massollo M, *et al.* Direct inhibition of hexokinase activity by metformin at least partially impairs glucose metabolism and tumor growth in experimental breast cancer. Cell Cycle. 2013;12(22): 3490-3499. doi: 10.4161/cc.26461.

151 Currie E, Schulze A, Zechner R, Walther TC, Farese RV. Cellular Fatty Acid Metabolism and Cancer. Cell metabolism. 2013;18(2): 153-161. doi: 10.1016/j.cmet.2013.05.017.

of fuel for cancer cells. Cancers upregulate the LDL receptor on their surface to acquire more circulating low-density lipoprotein (LDL – bad cholesterol) from the circulation. Statins will help to prevent this nutrient uptake by reducing the amount of LDL in circulation. Remember, the more pathways you can block effectively, with the least amount of toxicity, the better. You will need less of the really toxic drugs like chemotherapy or other targeted drugs.

All cancer cells upregulate fat metabolism for the manufacture of new cell membranes, through fatty acid synthesis (SREBP-1 and FAS) and the cholesterol pathways (Mevalonate and SREBP-2). Blocking all these pathways means that the cancer cell will struggle to make new cell membranes. You can slow growth markedly.

Treatments:

SREBP-1 (sterol regulating end binding protein 1) – The master regulator of lipogenesis – **Fibrates, xanthohumol, black chokeberry, niacin, silibinin, berberine.**[152,153]

SREBP-2 (sterol regulating end binding protein 2) – another cholesterol pathway – **Dipyridamole**[154], **Luteolin, Delta Tocotrienol,** and **Betulin (chaga mushroom).**

---

152 Xia X., Yan J., Shen Y. Berberine improves glucose metabolism in diabetic rats by inhibition of hepatic gluconeogenesis (2011) PLoS ONE, 6 (2), art. no. e16556.

153 SREBP-1 inhibitors may raise the risk of rhabdomyolysis when used in addition to statins, a very rare condition which affects 3 people in a million. If treated promptly it is curable. Look out for sudden pain and weakness (not just cramps which are common with statins).

154 Pandyra, Aleksandra & Z Penn, Linda. (2014). Targeting tumor cell metabolism via the mevalonate pathway: Two hits are better than one. Molecular & Cellular Oncology. 1. e969133. 10.4161/23723548.2014.969133.

ACLY (ATP citrate lyase) – **Hydroxycitrate** from Garcinia Cambogia is highly effective at blocking this pathway.[155] **Cucurbitacin B.**[156]

F.A.S. (Fatty Acid Synthesis)[157] – **Metformin/berberine + aspirin**[158], **sea buckthorn oil, black chokeberry extract**.

Metformin or **Berberine** reduces the availability of glucose to the cancer.

The 'acetyl' part of **aspirin** (acetyl salicylic acid) binds to the amino acid serine.

Fatty Acid Synthase is upregulated in many cancers and is strongly associated with metastases in breast, prostate and lung cancer. This is partly why aspirin is associated with lower recurrence rates. The addition of metformin or berberine with low dose aspirin would improve survival rates significantly as it is important to block both glucose and serine uptake together. Aspirin should not be used at the same time as a stronger NSAID because this raises the risk of gastric problems significantly. It is over activation of this FAS pathway that leads to activation of the HER1/HER2 tyrosine kinase receptors in breast cancer.[159]

Mevalonate – the lipophilic (fat-loving) statins – **lovastatin, atorvastatin** and **simvastatin** block the cells' ability to make cholesterol for

155 ACLY is a cross-link between glucose metabolism and fatty acid synthesis/mevalonate pathways controlled by SREBP-1. Potently inhibited by hydroxycitrate. Xu-Yu Zu Qing- Hai Zhang, Jiang-Hua Liu et al; ATP Citrate Lyase Inhibitors as Novel Cancer Therapeutic Agents Recent Patents on Anti-Cancer Drug Discovery, 2012, 7, 154-167

156 Gao Y, Islam MS, Tian J, Lui VW, Xiao D. Inactivation of ATP citrate lyase by Cucurbitacin B: A bioactive compound from cucumber, inhibits prostate cancer growth. Cancer Lett. 2014 Jul 10;349(1):15-25. doi: 10.1016/j.canlet.2014.03.015. Epub 2014 Mar 29. PMID: 24690568.

157 Menendez JA, Lupu R Fatty acid synthase and the lipogenic phenotype in cancer pathogenesis. Nat Rev Cancer. 2007 Oct; 7(10): 763-77

158 Ford RJ, Fullerton MD, Pinkosky SL, *et al.* Metformin and salicylate synergistically activate liver AMPK, inhibit lipogenesis and improve insulin sensitivity. The Biochemical journal. 2015;468(1): 125-132. doi: 10.1042/BJ20150125.

159 Overexpression of fatty acid synthase gene activates HER1/HER2 tyrosine kinase receptors in human breast epithelial cells.[Cell Prolif. 2008]

new cell walls. Hydrophilic (water loving) statins may make cancer worse as these statins target the liver, triggering a rise in mevalonate in other tissues in the body to compensate. Pravastatin (hydrophilic) has been shown to make cancer worse in lung cancer,[160] whereas simvastatin (lipophilic) has potent beneficial effects.[161] **Bisphosphonates**, prescribed for osteoporosis also help block the mevalonate pathway and every breast cancer and myeloma patient should insist on having these prescribed at diagnosis. Both cancers have a strong proclivity for bone metastases, an event that can be prevented by taking bisphosphonates.[162]

Fatty Acid Oxidation – Upregulated in many resistant cancers like prostate cancer,[163] MYC driven TNBC[164] melanoma and GBM, it is critical for stem cell renewal and chemotherapy resistance.[165]

Doxycycline[166] alters fatty acid oxidation.

---

160 Michael J. Seckl Allan Hackshaw *et al.* Multicenter, Phase III, Randomized, Double-Blind, Placebo-Controlled Trial of Pravastatin Added to First-Line Standard Chemotherapy in Small-Cell Lung Cancer (LUNGSTAR) Journal of Clinical Oncology 2017 DOI: 10.1200/ JCO.2016.69.7391 Journal of Clinical Oncology 35, no. 14 (May 2017) 1506-1514.

161 Michael J Seckl A Arcaro et al, Potent inhibition of small-cell lung cancer cell growth by simvastatin reveals selective functions of Ras isoforms in growth factor signalling. Oncogene volume 25, pp 877-887 (09 Feb 2006)

162 Goldvaser H, Amir E. Role of Bisphosphonates in Breast Cancer Therapy. Curr Treat Options Oncol. 2019 Mar 14;20(4):26. doi: 10.1007/s11864-019-0623-8. PMID: 30874905.

163 Liu Y. Fatty acid oxidation is a dominant bioenergetic pathway in prostate cancer (2006) Prostate Cancer and Prostatic Diseases, 9 (3), pp. 230-234.

164 Camarda R, Zhou Z, Kohnz RA, *et al.* Inhibition of fatty acid oxidation as a therapy for MYC-overexpressing triple-negative breast cancer. Nature medicine. 2016;22(4): 427-432. doi: 10.1038/nm.4055.

165 JAK/STAT3-Regulated Fatty Acid β-Oxidation Is Critical for Breast Cancer Stem Cell Self-Renewal and Chemoresistance Wang, Tianyi *et al.*Cell Metabolism, Volume 27, Issue 1, 136-150.e5

166 De Francesco EM, Maggiolini M, Tanowitz HB, Sotgia F, Lisanti MP. Targeting hypoxic cancer stem cells (CSCs) with Doxycycline: Implications for optimizing anti-angiogenic therapy. Oncotarget. 2017;8(34): 56126-56142. doi: 10.18632/oncotarget.18445.

Mildronate – a drug used by many sporting athletes to 'cheat' and enhance their metabolism (Maria Sharapova was banned because of the use of this drug). It is also used in Silicon Valley as a 'nootropic' to enhance cognitive abilities. This is an old forgotten FAO inhibitor. There was no research to back up my theory of mildronate in cancer when I first published in 2018, but since then two research papers back up its use for both TNBC and GBM. It has virtually no toxicity.[167,168] The more toxic FAO inhibitor etomoxir was shown to reduce ATP, reduce glutathione and increase ROS in Glioblastoma cells and cause cancer cell death.[169]

Fat Transporters – There are three fat transporters involved in cancer. The first is the MCT transporter which also transports lactate. Taking **Haritaki** should help inhibit transport of both fuels. The second is the low density lipoprotein receptor (LDLR) which is targeted by **statins**. The third is called the CD36 which is inhibited by **danshen**.[170] This fat transporter is responsible for resistance to a ketogenic diet and it also imports oleic acid. Oleic acid is a monounsaturated fatty acid which helps inhibit HER2 cancer, but can help other cancers progress such as breast and cervical cancer. It needs to be inhibited when activating ferroptosis.[171]

---

167 UT Southwestern Medical Center. "Triple negative breast cancer meets its match: BBOX1 enzyme could serve as a drug target for the deadly subset of breast cancer." ScienceDaily. ScienceDaily, 22 July 2020.

168 Juraszek, B, Czarnecka-Herok, J, Nałęcz, KA. Glioma cells survival depends both on fatty acid oxidation and on functional carnitine transport by SLC22A5. J. Neurochem. 2021; 156: 642– 657. https://doi.org/10.1111/jnc.15124

169 Lisa S. Pike, Amy L. Smift, Nicole J. Croteau, David A. Ferrick, MinWu Inhibition of fatty acid oxidation by etomoxir impairs NADPH production and increases reactive oxygen species resulting in ATP depletion and cell death in human glioblastoma cells Biochimica et Biophysica Acta (BBA) – Bioenergetics Volume 1807, Issue 6, June 2011, Pages 726-734

170 Yang J, Park KW, Cho S. Inhibition of the CD36 receptor reduces visceral fat accumulation and improves insulin resistance in obese mice carrying the BDNF-Val66Met variant. J Biol Chem. 2018;293(34):13338-13348. doi:10.1074/jbc.RA118.002405

171 Li, Zm., Xu, Sw. & Liu, Pq. Salvia miltiorrhizaBurge (Danshen): a golden herbal medicine in cardiovascular therapeutics. Acta Pharmacol Sin 39, 802–824 (2018). https://doi.org/10.1038/aps.2017.193

Fatty Acid Binding Protein (FABP family) – These proteins are linked to storage and incorporation of fat in membranes and transport of fat.

FABP3. In some cancers expression of FABP3 is linked to progression (e.g., NSCLC, melanoma, GIST) and in other cancers FABP3 acts as a tumor suppressor (e.g. breast).

FABP4 is strongly associated with ovarian cancer and bladder cancer progression. Reduction of FABP4 may be as simple as taking **omega 3 fatty acids**[172] or by taking **THC** and **CBD**. Because of FABP3 acting as a tumour suppressor, this might be why there are variable results using cannabinoids in breast cancer.[173]

FABP5 is associated with many cancers including prostate, colorectal, cervical, TNBC, uveal melanomas, cholangiocarcinoma. With castration resistant prostate cancer the inhibition of FABP5 led to a massive reduction in tumour size and stopped progression. **Truxillic acid**, the main component of the herbal medicine incarvillea sinensis, in an inhibitor of this pathway. Incarvillea sinensis is also exceptionally good as an anti inflammatory and pain reliever, traditionally used for rheumatism.[174]

172 Furuhashi, Masato et al. "Reduction of circulating FABP4 level by treatment with omega-3 fatty acid ethyl esters." Lipids in health and disease vol. 15 5. 12 Jan. 2016, doi:10.1186/s12944-016-0177-8

173 Elmes MW, Kaczocha M, Berger WT, Leung K, Ralph BP, Wang L, Sweeney JM, Miyauchi JT, Tsirka SE, Ojima I, Deutsch DG. Fatty acid-binding proteins (FABPs) are intracellular carriers for Δ9-tetrahydrocannabinol (THC) and cannabidiol (CBD). J Biol Chem. 2015 Apr 3;290(14):8711-21. doi: 10.1074/jbc.M114.618447. Epub 2015 Feb 9. PMID: 25666611; PMCID: PMC4423662

174 Al-Jameel W, Gou X, Jin X, et al. Inactivated FABP5 suppresses malignant progression of prostate cancer cells by inhibiting the activation of nuclear fatty acid receptor PPARγ. Genes Cancer. 2019;10(3-4):80-96. doi:10.18632/genesandcancer.192

FABP7 is involved in renal cell cancer and gliomas in particular. A high level of **DHA omega 3** oil will prevent the detrimental effects of arachidonic acid.[175]

Starving the tumour of Glutamine and other amino acids

Direct glutamine inhibitors rapidly cause necrosis (cell death) of the intestinal mucosa and problems in the nervous system, so inhibiting glutamine should be approached indirectly, avoiding powerful inhibiting drugs like acivicin or DON.

Every cancer cell needs glutamine for growth, and cancer cells seem to be particularly addicted to glutamine if they have a MYC mutation. Glutamine is the most abundant amino acid in the human bloodstream. Levels are maintained through a combination of dietary uptake, *de novo* synthesis, and the breakdown of muscle protein (catabolism). Glutamine is needed for the manufacture of DNA, organelles, fatty acids and enzymes, and to produce glutathione. In 2012, Harvard University showed that glutamine consumption is higher than other amino acids in tumours and many become glutamine-addicted. Glutamine starvation interferes with metabolism which inhibits proliferation and triggers cancer cell death.

After glutamine enters the cancer cell, it is broken down by glutaminase to form glutamate. Glutamate is then either converted to glutathione or broken down to alpha ketoglutarate, which is then taken into the Krebs cycle for OXPHOS. Mitochondria can convert the broken-down glutamine into lactate very rapidly to support fatty acid synthesis. By simultaneously making glutathione (the master antioxidant), the tumour can neutralise the excess lactic acid produced during this process.

---

175 Mita R, Beaulieu MJ, Field C, Godbout R. Brain fatty acid-binding protein and omega-3/omega-6 fatty acids: mechanistic insight into malignant glioma cell migration. J Biol Chem. 2010 Nov 19;285(47):37005-15. doi: 10.1074/jbc.M110.170076. Epub 2010 Sep 12. PMID: 20834042; PMCID: PMC2978629.

IGF-1 – Stopping this is critical. If you have any doubt about this, investigate Laron Syndrome. This syndrome affects a tiny population in Ecuador. These people have a genetic defect in the liver that prevents them from being able to bind the IGF-1 hormone. This means they do not grow higher than four feet tall, but as a trade-off, they are protected against cancer, diabetes and Alzheimer's. Methods to reduce IGF-1 are:

Metformin.[176]

Dietary restriction of protein and dairy.[177]

Tamoxifen, raloxifene, nimbolide, indole 3 carbinol.

IGF-2 – In some cancers IGF-2 can be of equal importance if not more than IGF-1. IGF-2 is used by rhabdomyosarcoma, osteosarcoma, CRC, breast, prostate, lung, bladder, ovarian, liver and Wilms tumours.

To inhibit IGF-2 take **baicalin** from scutellaria baicalensis. It is powerful stuff but needs to be stopped for ferroptosis.

---

176 Sarfstein R, Friedman Y, Attias-Geva Z, Fishman A, Bruchim I, Werner H. Metformin Downregulates the Insulin/IGF-I Signaling Pathway and Inhibits Different Uterine Serous Carcinoma (USC) Cells Proliferation and Migration in p53-Dependent or -Independent Manners. Nadal A, ed. PLoS ONE. 2013;8(4): e61537. doi: 10.1371/ journal. pone.0061537.
177 Fontana L, Adelaiye RM, Rastelli AL, *et al.* Dietary protein restriction inhibits tumor growth in human xenograft models of prostate and breast cancer. Oncotarget. 2013;4(12): 2451-2461.

mTOR (Mammalian Target of Rapamycin)

Metformin/Berberine – both raise the master metabolic regulating enzyme AMPK, which in turn lowers mTOR.[178] Dihydroartemesinin and niclosamide also suppress mTOR.[179,180]

AMPK is an anti-ageing enzyme present in every cell. mTOR is an enzyme that gathers proteins together just prior to the cell dividing. Reducing the number of cell divisions slows both cancer and ageing. Hence both metformin and berberine's anti-ageing effects.

Serine – an amino acid used as fuel by some breast cancer, also used for making fatty acids with glucose and serine. In 2016 the Cantley lab discovered that disulfiram, a drug first approved in 1948 for chronic alcoholism by making the body sensitive to ethanol (if you ingest any alcohol, even vinegar, it gives you a nasty hangover). Disulfiram inhibits both the enzyme ALDH and phosphoglycerate dehydrogenase (PHGDH), the first and limiting step of the so-called serine synthetic pathway assisted by dietary depletion of serine and glycine. The dietary addition of copper gluconate can enhance its effects. It may also assist ferroptosis and is also a proteasome inhibitor. Sertraline a commonly prescribed antidepressant can also stop serine/glycine synthesis. Check before adding any medications as the liquid form of sertraline contains alcohol and is contraindicated. Another enzyme in this pathway PSAT-1 can be inhibited by regorafenib in glioblastoma. PSAT-1 is also a

178 Ming Ming, James Sinnett-Smith,Jia Wang, Heloisa P. Soares, Steven H. Young, Guido Eibl, Enrique Rozengurt Dose-Dependent AMPK-Dependent and Independent Mechanisms of Berberine and Metformin Inhibition of mTORC1, ERK, DNA Synthesis and Proliferation in Pancreatic Cancer Cells. PLOS December 10, 2014

179 Odaka, Yoshinobu et al. "Dihydroartemisinin the mammalian target of rapamycin-mediated signaling pathways in tumor cells." Carcinogenesis vol. 35,1 (2014): 192-200. doi:10.1093/carcin/bgt277

180 Pan JX, Ding K, Wang CY. Niclosamide, an old antihelminthic agent, demonstrates antitumor activity by blocking multiple signaling pathways of cancer stem cells. Chin J Cancer. 2012 Apr;31(4):178-84. doi: 10.5732/cjc.011.10290. Epub 2012 Jan 9. PMID: 22237038; PMCID: PMC3777479.

target for NSCLC. Regorafenib is structurally similar to sorafenib – so unsurprisingly it can also assist ferroptosis as they help block the xCT antiporter when used in combination with a GPX4 enzyme inhibitor.

Aspirin,[181] **Disulfiram,**[182] **Regorafenib,**[183] and **Sertraline.**[184]

Nucleoside Salvage (Autophagy) –

Dipyridamole. Salvianolic acid (danshen)

The cancer cell will grab nucleosides (which are hard work for it to make), fatty acids and other proteins from the surrounding microenvironment rather than make them from nothing (de novo). After chemotherapy when there are lots of dead cell fragments left behind in the tumour microenvironment, the cancer cell quickly learns how to recycle and reuse them, becoming more aggressive in the process. Chemotherapy is more effective (cytotoxic) in combination with dipyridamole[185] and with danshen.[186] This is because both dipyridamole and danshen prevent nucleosides being salvaged.[187]

181 Tóth, L; Muszbek, L; Komáromi, I (2013). 'Mechanism of the irreversible inhibition of human cyclooxygenase-1 by aspirin as predicted by QM/MM calculations'. Journal of Molecular Graphics and Modelling. 40: 99-109. doi: 10.1016/j.jmgm.2012.12.013. PMID 23384979

182 Disulfiram might not require the addition of copper when used for ferroptosis.

183 Jingwen Jiang, Canhua Huang et al (2020) Regorafenib induces lethal autophagy arrest by stabilizing PSAT1 in glioblastoma, Autophagy, 16:1, 106-122, DOI: 10.1080/15548627.2019.1598752

184 Geeraerts SL, De Keersmaecker K et al. Repurposing the Antidepressant Sertraline as SHMT Inhibitor to Suppress Serine/Glycine Synthesis–Addicted Breast Tumor Growth Mol Cancer Ther January 1 2021 (20) (1) 50-63; DOI: 10.1158/1535-7163. MCT-20-0480

185 Jean L. Grem and Paul H. Fischer. Augmentation of 5-Fluorouracil Cytotoxicity in Human Colon Cancer Cells by Dipyridamole. Cancer Res July 1 1985 (45) (7) 2967-2972;

186 Salvianolic acid A inhibits nucleoside transport and potentiates the antitumor activity of chemotherapeutic drugs August 2004Yao xue xue bao = Acta pharmaceutica Sinica 39(7):496-9)

187 Weber G, Lui MS, Natsumeda Y, Faderan MA. Salvage capacity of hepatoma 3924A and action of dipyridamole. Adv Enzyme Regul. 1983;21: 53-69

Macropinocytosis (Autophagy) –

Chloroquine, Loratadine, Pyrvinium Pamoate. Natural substances that will help inhibit autophagy are **oleacanthol** (found only in high quality olive oil – see my website for recommended products), **thymoquinone** (found in black seed oil) and **oxymatrine** (Kushen)

This mechanism enables cancer cells to scavenge extracellular nutrients if they are in short supply or if demand is high. Macropinocytosis is a process where the cell membrane 'ruffles' and engulfs extracellular fluid, pulling in proteins and fats from outside the cell to supply itself. The antimalarial Chloroquine and antihistamine Loratadine (Claritin) both work by disturbing the pH of the lysosomes that are breaking down the engulfed extracellular fat and protein.[188] In later stages, cancer is able to make nearby adipocytes release their stored fat into the circulation (this is a cause of cachexia) making it available for the lysosome on the surface of the cancer cell to engulf. Fortunately, cancer lysosomes are fragile, so this makes them an attractive target. Cancer lysosomes are involved in the metastasis and progression of most tumours, e.g. breast, lung, brain, head and neck, ovarian, melanoma, uterine, colorectal and prostate. Lysosomes are the most acidic parts of a cell and the enzymes inside these organelles become even more acidic as cancer progresses, encouraging further oncogenic changes.

Targeting the disturbance in their pH is an Achilles heel in the abnormal cancer metabolism. Loratadine and Chloroquine have both been shown to alter the pH and function of the cancer lysosome, effectively putting a spanner in the works of the metastasis machinery. Loratadine can increase survival in NSCLC and ER positive breast cancers, especially in combination with chemotherapy,[189] whilst also boosting the immune system by targeting myeloid suppressor cells. However, Loratadine fails to cross the blood-

---

188 Chloroquine inhibits lysosomal enzyme pinocytosis and enhances lysosomal enzyme secretion by impairing receptor recycling. The Journal of Cell Biology. 1980;85(3): 839-852.

189 Ellegaard A-M, Dehlendorff C, Vind AC, *et al.* Repurposing Cationic Amphiphilic Antihistamines for Cancer Treatment. *EBioMedicine*. 2016;9:130-139. doi:10.1016/j.ebiom.2016.06.013.)

brain barrier, so in instances where the brain is involved, chloroquine or pyrvinium pamoate would be a better choice.[190] To trigger ferroptosis all these autophagy inhibitors must be stopped, except perhaps oxymatrine.

Macropinocytosis occurs when glutamine and cholesterol levels are insufficient to meet demand. It happens early in some strongly Ras-dependent cancers[191] like pancreatic cancer,[192] melanomas,[193] bladder cancer, colon cancer, Leukaemias, and nearly a third of lung adenocarcinomas. Approximately 30% of all cancers contain a mutation to the Ras family of genes. Commisso et al. demonstrated that starving a tumour of glutamine stimulates (upregulates) macropinocytosis. This scavenging process might be used by a great many Ras-driven cancers, upregulating this pathway as the tumour progresses. Glioblastoma (GBM), the most lethal of the primary tumours, uses this pathway. Professor Thomas Seyfried, Ahmed Alsekka and others have been using chloroquine sulphate successfully as part of a cancer-starving combination to treat GBM.[194] Chloroquine (or the safer hydroxychloroquine), in my view, should be part of many cancer's treatment from diagnosis. It was also found that blocking macropinocytosis with chloroquine overcomes resistance to

190 Deng, Longfei & Lei, Yunlong & Liu, Rui & Li, Jingyi & Yuan, Kefei & Li, Yi & Chen, Yi & Liu, Yi & Lu, You & Edwards III, Carl & Huang, Canhua & Wei, Yuquan. (2013). Pyrvinium targets autophagy addiction to promote cancer cell death. Cell death & disease. 4. e614. 10.1038/cddis.2013.142.

191 Commisso C, et al. Macropinocytosis of protein is an amino acid supply route in Ras-transformed cells. Nature. 2013;497: 633-637

192 Kamphorst JJ, Nofal M, Commisso C, et al. Human pancreatic cancer tumors are nutrient poor and tumor cells actively scavenge extracellular protein. Cancer research. 2015;75(3): 544-553. doi: 10.1158/0008-5472.CAN-14-2211.

193 Inhibition of autophagy with chloroquine is effective in melanoma Egger M.E., Huang J.S., Yin W., McMasters K.M., McNally L.R. (2013) Journal of Surgical Research, 184 (1), pp. 274-281.

194 Ahmed M. A. Elsakka, Mohamed Abdel Bary, Eman Abdelzaher, Mostafa Elnaggar, Miriam Kalamian, Purna Mukherjee, Thomas N. Seyfried *Management of Glioblastoma Multiforme in a Patient Treated With Ketogenic Metabolic Therapy and Modified Standard of Care: A 24-Month Follow-Up Front. Nutr., 29 March 2018

EGFR inhibitors[195] (e.g. Erlotinib) and HER2 inhibitors[196] (Herceptin), which suggests the inclusion of a macropinocytosis inhibitor may be essential for cancers that express these genes.

The downside with chloroquine is that it inhibits a gene called Bcl-xl and caspase 3, which are both important in triggering apoptosis, so perhaps it is best used cyclically and stopped just before (24 hours prior to) a 'kill phase' if starving the tumour alone is insufficient. Loratadine may also increase the possibility of muscle pain when used in combination with a statin. This should always be discussed with your doctor who can adjust dosages.

The combination of chloroquine and dipyridamole or pyrvinium and dipyridamole have not yet been investigated, but I have a hunch they would enhance each other synergistically when used together. If so, this combination may be extremely useful for more aggressive Ras-driven cancers like pancreatic cancer, where dipyridamole has been shown to inhibit 70-90% of liver metastases as part of a multimodal drug cocktail.[197] Dipryridamole is also synergistic with mTOR inhibitors and MEK inhibitors for treating KRAS tumours.[198]

195   Zou Y, Ling Y-H, Sironi J, Schwartz EL, Perez-Soler R, Piperdi B. The autophagy inhibitor chloroquine overcomes the innate resistance to erlotinib of non-small cell lung cancer cells with wild-type EGFR. Journal of thoracic oncology: official publication of the International Association for the Study of Lung Cancer. 2013;8(6): 10.1097/JTO.0b013e31828c7210. doi: 10.1097/JTO.0b013e31828c7210.

196   L. Masuelli, M. Granato, M. Benvenuto, R. Mattera, R. Bernardini, M. Mattei, G. d'Amati, G. D'Orazi, A. Faggioni, R. Bei, M. Cirone. Chloroquine supplementation increases the cytotoxic effect of curcumin against HER2/neu overexpressing breast cancer cells in vitro and in vivo in nude mice while counteracts it in immune competent mice Oncoimmunology. 2017; 6(11): e1356151. Published online 2017 Jul 31. doi: 10.1080/2162402X.2017.1356151

197   George N. Tzanakakis M.D. Kailash C. Agarwal Ph.D. Michael P. Vezeridis M.D. Prevention of human pancreatic cancer cell-induced hepatic metastasis in nude mice by dipyridamole and its analog RA-233 Cancer Volume 71, Issue 8 15 April 1993 Pages 2466-2471

198   Sheng Zhou, Feng Bi et al. Dipyridamole Enhances the Cytotoxicities of Trametinib against Colon Cancer Cells through Combined Targeting of HMGCS1 and MEK Pathway Mol Cancer Ther January 1 2020 (19) (1) 135-146; DOI: 10.1158/1535-7163. MCT-19-0413)

Glutamine/Amino Acid transport – It is possible to starve tumours very effectively by preventing the import of the amino acids they need to thrive such as glutamine, glutamate and cysteine. The transporters involved include the xCT antiporter, ASCT2, AMPA and NMDA.

xCT cysteine-glutamate antiporter – Starving tumours by blocking the import of cysteine through this channel is one of the most exciting methods to eradicate cancer and yet it is virtually unknown in the clinic because this is a new discovery. It can be used both in the starve phase to deplete cysteine and in the kill phase to trigger ferroptosis. I have dedicated a new chapter on this subject, as I truly believe it is going to be the solution for triple negative breast cancer, pancreatic, GBM and metastatic tumours that have become treatment resistant. I suggest using some of the following in your starve phase to block the xCT but when it comes to ferroptosis, you will require a unique set of drugs and supplements to activate this cancer killing option.

Sulfasalazine, Sorafenib, Erastin, Piperlongumine, Parthenolide, Sodium Selenite. Sulfasalazine and sodium selenite might be best 'pulsed' with artemisinin and intravenous vitamin C as part of a a kill phase. Longer term use may suppress the immune system.

ASCT2 Glutamine Transporter – The ASCT2 is the primary transporter on the cell surface to import glutamine. Blocking this can have a strong anti-tumour effect, particularly in strongly glutamine and leucine driven cancers such as NSCLC, pancreatic, prostate, melanoma, AML, neuroblastoma. Blocking ASCT2 and LAT1 also stops glutamine being used for making fatty acids through reductive carboxylation in hypoxic (low oxygen) conditions, very common in cancer. ASCT2 is also linked to the androgen receptor and inhibition stopped metastasis in prostate cancer.[199] Curcumin can help to block this pathway, this is probably one of its major anti-cancer effects. Blocking the heat shock protein HSP90 with radicicol prevented the transporter from reaching the cell surface. Delta tocotreniol was highly

199 Wang, Q., Hardie, Holst, J. et al (2015), Targeting ASCT2-mediated glutamine uptake blocks prostate cancer growth and tumour development. J. Pathol., 236: 278-289. https://doi.org/10.1002/path.4518

effective in NSCLC and may be why Joe Tippens did so well with his cocktail.[200] This is also probably why vitamin D is so critical for breast cancer.[201]

Radicicol (antibiotic), Delta-tocotrienol, Curcumin, vitamin D, Gambogic Acid, Celastrol. A combination of **ursolic acid** and **resveratrol** or **ursolic acid combined with curcumin** prevents glutamine uptake by the cancer cell.[202]

The NMDA and AMPA Receptors – These import glutamate.

The NMDA is upregulated in gliomas, prostate, breast, lung, melanoma, liver, CRC, larynx, thyroid and SCLC. **Memantine** (a treatment for Alzheimer's)[203] **dizocilpine, magnesium, CBD, theanine** can inhibit this receptor.

The AMPA is more relevant for gliomas, and neuroblastomas.

Telampanel, a drug developed for ALS, helps block excess glutamate in newly diagnosed GBM patients in combination with radiotherapy and the chemotherapy drug temozolomide. [204]

---

200 Rajasinghe LD, Hutchings M, Gupta SV. Delta-Tocotrienol Modulates Glutamine Dependence by Inhibiting ASCT2 and LAT1 Transporters in Non-Small Cell Lung Cancer (NSCLC) Cells : A Metabolomic Approach. Metabolites. 2019; 9(3):50. https://doi.org/10.3390/metabo90300500

201 Zhou, Xuanzhu et al. "1,25-Dihydroxyvitamin D inhibits glutamine metabolism in Harvey-ras transformed MCF10A human breast epithelial cell." The Journal of steroid biochemistry and molecular biology vol. 163 (2016): 147-56. doi:10.1016/j.jsbmb.2016.04.022

202 Stefano Tiziani et al Combinatorial treatment with natural compounds in prostate cancer inhibits prostate tumor growth and leads to key modulations of cancer cell metabolism Precision Oncology volume 1, Article number: 18(2017)

203 NMDA and AMPA glutamate receptor antagonists in the treatment of human malignant glioma xenografts Ranjit K. Goudar, Stephen T. Keir, Darell D. Bigner and Henry S. Friedman Cancer Res April 1 2004 (64) (7 Supplement) 1053-1054;

204 Grossman SA, Ye X, Chamberlain M, et al. Talampanel with standard radiation and temozolomide in patients with newly diagnosed glioblastoma: a multicenter phase II trial. J Clin Oncol. 2009;27(25):4155-4161. doi:10.1200/JCO.2008.21.6895

Pin1 Pathway (Prolyl Isomerase) – Pin1 drives many of the hallmarks of cancer and is highly expressed in many cancers, especially in the cancer stem cells.[205]

Especially relevant for Li Fraumeni, GBM, prostate, lung, ovary, breast (inc TNBC), cervical, melanoma, AML.

Juglone (black walnut)[206], **ATRA** and **arsenic trioxide** (TNBC).[207]

The Proteasome and Cancer – The proteasome is a cellular dustbin or shredder. Proteins that are misfolded or damaged are tagged with ubiquitin then taken to the proteasome for 'shredding' down to their amino acids. This needs inhibiting in cases where tumour suppressors have been degraded and are deleted or mutated. e.g. P53, p21, BRCA, APC, VHL, PTEN.

In myeloma Bortezomib is a conventional treatment. Proteasome inhibitors are now being explored for other cancers such as colon, lung, prostate, melanoma, breast, mesothelioma and renal cancer. Pentoxifylline is an old drug for poor circulation (intermittent claudication) in the legs.

Disulfiram[208], Pentoxifylline.[209]

---

205 Chen, Y., Wu, Yr., Yang, Hy. et al. Prolyl isomerase Pin1: a promoter of cancer and a target for therapy. Cell Death Dis 9, 883 (2018). https://doi.org/10.1038/s41419-018-0844-y

206 Chao, S H et al. "Juglone, an inhibitor of the peptidyl-prolyl isomerase Pin1, also directly blocks transcription." Nucleic acids research vol. 29,3 (2001): 767-73. doi:10.1093/nar/29.3.767

207 Kozono, S., Lin, YM., Seo, HS. et al. Arsenic targets Pin1 and cooperates with retinoic acid to inhibit cancer-driving pathways and tumor-initiating cells. Nat Commun 9, 3069 (2018). https://doi.org/10.1038/s41467-018-05402-2

208 Boris Cvek, Zdenek Dvorak, The value of proteasome inhibition in cancer: Can the old drug, disulfiram, have a bright new future as a novel proteasome inhibitor? Drug Discovery Today, Volume 13, Issues 15–16, 2008, https://doi.org/10.1016/j.drudis.2008.05.003

209 Cai, W., Mastrandrea, N., Tham, K., Monks, T. and Lau, S. (2014), Pentoxifylline induces GSK-3β-independent proteasomal degradation of cyclin D1 and arrests renal cancer cells in the G1 phase (616.5). The FASEB Journal, 28: 616.5. https://doi.org/10.1096/fasebj.28.1_supplement.616.5

Glutaminolysis

This important pathway breaks down glutamine, an amino acid, so that it can be used to make new proteins, enzymes and nucleotides. Glutamine addiction and reliance on glutaminolysis is common in most cancers, to break down glutamine for fuel to enter the TCA cycle (OXPHOS). Like the glycolysis pathway, the glutaminolysis pathway also involves steps that can each be targeted, the enzymes glutamate dehydrogenase and glutaminase. Glutaminase can have two isoforms, kidney type glutaminase (KGA) and glutaminase C (GAC). As prostate cancer progresses from androgen dependent to androgen independent, it changes the glutaminase fuel from one glutaminase (KGA) to the other (GAC).[210] Glutaminolysis is highly active in many aggressive forms of human cancers, including triple-negative breast cancer (TNBC), pancreatic cancer, lung cancer, lymphoma and glioblastoma, as well as prostate cancer. It is a general feature of metastatic cancer as these are more aggressive than the primary.

Glutamate Dehydrogenase/Ketoglutarate Dehydrogenase – EGCG (green tea), **Stevia**

Glutaminase inhibitors – The harder a cancer is to treat, the more you will need to add. Particularly aggressive cancers may need the following glutaminase inhibitors:

Natural inhibitors – Physapubescin A. Brachyantheraoside A8, Morin and **esculetin**.

BPTES – clinically it was not shown to be that effective until recently. A new version has been developed, emulsifying the drug into nanoparticles to help absorption. This has improved its efficacy and importantly it had no effect on the plasma levels of liver enzymes. As it starves glutamine, it encourages

---

210 Lingfan Xu, Jiaoti Huang et al. A glutaminase isoform switch drives therapeutic resistance and disease progression of prostate cancer Proceedings of the National Academy of Sciences Mar 2021, 118 (13) e2012748118; DOI: 10.1073/pnas.2012748118

glycolysis, so when used in combination with a glycolysis and glycogen inhibitor it becomes even more effective. It has been tested on pancreatic cancer patients in combination with metformin, and this combination showed significantly enhanced results than either treatment alone. The more pathways blocked, the more effective the combination. Other glutaminase inhibitors developed from BPTES are **CB-839** and **compound 968**, currently in several clinical trials. If you can locate a trial it may be worth enrolling.

L-asparaginase – this drug is used for childhood leukaemia (ALL). Described in textbooks as anti-metabolite 'chemotherapy', this is not true! It is in fact a metabolic enzyme that starves not just the amino acid asparagine but also glutamine. Childhood Acute Lymphoblastic Leukaemia is one cancer that the medical profession claim can be completely cured, so if you need any proof that starving cancer is the answer, here it is! Natural asparaginase inhibitors are **Ashwagandha** and **capsaicin** (from chilli peppers).

We have been tripping over the truth! The cure rate of acute lymphoblastic leukaemia increased from 5% in the 1950's to the present 90% when doctors began using multimodal chemotherapy regimens containing L-asparaginase. No surprise then that is being 'rediscovered' after being around for nearly 60 years, returning as a treatment for other glutamine-driven cancers like Triple Negative Breast cancer and Pancreatic cancer. This drug is also being reformulated to be less toxic (side effects include hepatitis, pancreatitis, coagulopathy and neurotoxicity, which can occur at high dose). The new version is being encapsulated inside red blood cells to avoid the allergic reactions and to stop it from being broken down by enzymes to extend its action.

Dietary restriction of asparagine – If you have one of these aggressive cancers it is a good idea to deplete asparagine from your diet. It is found in many foods, including asparagus, beef, poultry and potatoes. Asparagus also has high levels of glutathione so definitely avoid this innocuous looking vegetable. Removing these foods has been shown to reduce metastases.[211]

Leucine, a branched chain amino acid has been linked to prostate cancer, breast cancer and pancreatic cancer, a result of excessive amounts of protein in the diet which stimulates mTOR. Intermittent fasting is especially important for these amino acid driven cancers.

211 60-Year-Old Drug May Hold Clues to Stopping Spread of Breast Cancer *https://www. forbes.com/sites/victoriaforster/2018/02/07/sixty-year-old-drug-may-hold-the-key-to-stopping-spread-of-breast-cancer/#7355a0d2423e*

Chapter Twenty-Three:

How to Stop Dangerous Metastases

Starving the cancer is good, adding ways to prevent its spread is even better, as it is the migration of cancer to areas like the brain, liver and lungs that almost always kills, not the primary site. Here are yet more additions to your cocktail to manage growth factors. Fortunately, you are already controlling some of these with your drug cocktail already.

Managing Growth Factors and MMPs (matrix metalloproteinases)

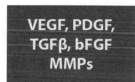

The metabolic changes in the cell trigger changes in the surrounding tumour microenvironment. Rapid cell division creates lots of lactic acid, the acidic by-product of glycolysis, which is damaging to the surrounding tissues. So, to protect itself, the body attempts to remove the lactic acid by making new blood vessels (angiogenesis), with an increase in vascular endothelial growth factor. The increase in blood vessels also has the downside of supplying more nutrients to the tumour so the result is an ongoing cascade of further growth. Other key growth factors that are secreted are Platelet derived growth factor (PDGF), Transforming Growth Factor beta (TGF-β) and Fibroblast Growth Factor.

There is also an increase in enzymes called matrix metalloproteinases (MMPs), which break down the surrounding stromal tissue (scaffold around the cell), allowing the cancer cells to break off and spread. Metastasis, the spread to distant organs, can happen very early in cancer, contrary to previous medical thinking. Blocking MMPs and other growth factors are an essential part of treatment alongside 'starving' the cancer and should be instigated from diagnosis.

Treatments to Stop Abnormal Growth factors (FGF, VEGF, PDGF, MMP2, 3, 9)

To explain the importance of blocking these growth factors, especially the MMP's, I describe my 'Great Fire of London' theory to cancer patients.

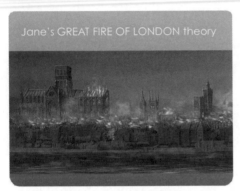

Stage one cancer is akin to a house fire. By stage IV it is like the Great Fire of London. It will devour everything in its path and is virtually unstoppable. Throwing buckets of water from the Thames was not enough to put out the flames in the summer of 1666, but what did eventually work was the destruction of houses in its path, using explosives to clear areas to create 'fire breaks', blocking its ability to jump from house to house and depriving the fire of its fuel.

In the same way, cancer needs to be stopped from spreading by creating 'fire breaks.' Metastases (secondary cancers) are the cause of over 80% of deaths from cancer.

To support its growth, the cancer cell sends signals to the surrounding area (microenvironment). These signals change three main structures:

Fibroblasts in the connective tissue. The fibroblasts eat their own mitochondria (mitophagy) and convert to using the glycolytic pathway (Warburg Effect) to create lactate. Metastases are observed to behave in a

374

metabolically different way to the primary tumour, possibly because they can more readily use lactate and ketones.

- **Immune cells (macrophages)** – The immune cells become transformed into tumour associated macrophages – TAMs.
- **Blood vessels (angiogenesis)** – Hypoxia, a lack of oxygen, triggers a protein called HIF (hypoxia inducible factor) which then stimulates the release of vascular endothelial growth factor (VEGF), leading to the proliferation of blood vessels.
- **HIF-1alpha** – caused by hypoxia can be suppressed by **chrysin**, acetogenins from **paw paw, baicalein, apigenin, catalpol**. These can help stop malignant transformation and angiogenesis (VEGF).

It is a release of growth factors from the fibroblasts that triggers a breakdown of the extracellular matrix by enzymes called matrix metalloproteinases (MMPs) which allows the cancer to spread. MMPs are currently completely overlooked by oncology. They were all the rage in research decades ago, but, having failed to find patentable drugs, Big Pharma decided to try new approaches like targeting vascular endothelial growth factor (VEGF), the growth signal for the cancer to form new blood vessels to feed itself. Avastin (Bevacizumab), a drug which stops VEGF, was hailed as a new 'game changer' when it launched in 2004 but, on its own, it did not have the expected results everyone had hoped for and it came with nasty side effects. However, in combination with other modalities, its value may be more beneficial.

Unknowingly, I had inhibited vascular endothelial growth factor (VEGF), Platelet Derived Growth Factor (PDGF) and transforming growth factor β (TFGβ) with my combination of aspirin and dipyridamole, but I had also stopped the extracellular matrix changes too. My cocktail had targeted all the growth factors and MMPs. Other drugs also work on these growth factors, including mebendazole, pimozide, propranolol, pentoxifylline, nifuroxazide and doxycycline:

- **MMP-1** – Pimozide, Xanthohumol, Andrographis
- **MMP-2** – chito-oligosaccharides (chitin), Mebendazole,[212,213] Propranolol,[214] and THC,[215] Catalpol, Baicalein, Danshen, Andrographalide, Xanthohumol, Saikosaponnin, Maitake-D-Fraction.
- **MMP-3** – Glucosamine sulphate, Kaempferol, Quercetin.[216]
- **MMP-7** – Triptolide, Poria cocos.
- **MMP-9** – Dipyridamole,[217] Doxycycline,[218] Propranolol,[219] Pentoxifylline, Ritonavir, Danshen, Xanthohumol, Maitake-D-Fraction.
- **MMP-10** – chrysin
- **MMP-11** – Andrographolide
- **MMP-13** – Danshen, Catalpol
- **MMP-14** – Pimozide, Curcumin

212 Moon-MooKimaSe-KwonKimab Chitooligosaccharides inhibit activation and expression of matrix metalloproteinase-2 in human dermal fibroblasts. FEBS Letters

213 Pinto, Laine & Soares, Bruno & Pinheiro, João & J Riggins, Gregory & Assumpcao, Paulo & Burbano, Rommel & Carvalho Montenegro, Raquel. (2015). The anthelmintic drug mebendazole inhibits growth, migration and invasion in gastric cancer cell model. Toxicology in vitro: an international journal published in association with BIBRA. 29. 10.1016/j.tiv.2015.08.007.

214 Pantziarka P, Bouche G, Sukhatme V, Meheus L, Rooman I, Sukhatme VP. Repurposing Drugs in Oncology (ReDO) – Propranolol as an anti-cancer agent. ecancermedicalscience. 2016;10: 680. doi: 10.3332/ecancer.2016.680.

215 THC helps cancer in this regard but beware its immunosuppressive effect and avoid THC use with immunotherapies.

216 Pohlig F1*et al.* Glucosamine sulphate suppresses the expression of matrix metalloproteinase-3 in osteosarcoma cells in vitro. BMC Complement Altern Med. 2016 Aug 25;16(1): 313

217 Massaro M1 et al Dipyridamole decreases inflammatory metalloproteinase-9 expression and release by human monocytes. Thromb Haemost. 2013 Feb;109(2): 280- 9

218 Zhang C, Gong W, Liu H, Guo Z, Ge S. Inhibition of matrix metalloproteinase-9 with low-dose doxycycline reduces acute lung injury induced by cardiopulmonary bypass. International Journal of Clinical and Experimental Medicine, 2014;7(12): 4975-4982.

219 Guo K, *et al.* Norepinephrine-induced invasion by pancreatic cancer cells is inhibited by propranolol. Oncol Rep. 2009;22(4): 825-30

- **VEGF** – Aspirin,[220] Propranolol, Cimetidine, Itraconazole, Thalidomide, Modified Citrus Pectin, Artemesinin, Baicalin, Honokiol, Withaferin A
- **FGF** – Propranolol, Leflunamide, Stilbenes, Shark Liver Oil
- **PDGF** – Dipyridamole,[221] Aspirin, Pentoxifylline, Indole 3 Carbinol, Apigenin, Ellagic acid, Luteolin, Piperlongumine
- **TGFβ** – Dipyridamole,[222] Pentoxifylline, Hesperidin, Cryptotanshinone (danshen), Withaferin A, Cinnamomum cassia, Celastrol

Chitin is found in the exoskeleton of shellfish like shrimps (which I love, and I make a point of eating some of the shell) and it is also found in abundance in mushrooms, which I ate every day. This is one of the reasons why mushrooms are so beneficial for cancer prevention and treatment: they help to keep the extracellular matrix intact and in turn stop the transformation of macrophages. They also contain naturally high levels of aromatase inhibitors, the plain button ones being the best. Chitin is also helpful for renal failure and problems with creatinine kinase.

When conventional VEGF inhibitors fail (sutent, avastin) the reason is often because the cancer is using fibroblast growth factor as an alternative route. Dual inhibition would be a better strategy.

I had taken glucosamine sulphate, not for cancer but for my damaged knee, not realising that it would help stop my cancer spreading. This may in part explain why I was 'lucky' and only had one lung metastasis, despite an appalling diet following my first diagnosis for a couple of years. And

220 X. Zhang, Z. Wang, Y. Zhang, Q. Jia, L. Wu, and W. Zhang, 'Impact of acetylsalicylic acid on tumor angiogenesis and lymphangiogenesis through inhibition of VEGF signaling in a murine sarcoma model,' Oncology Reports, vol. 29, no. 5, pp. 1907-1913, 2013
221 Takehara K, Igarashi A, Ishibashi Y, Dipyridamole Specifically Decreases Platelet-Derived Growth Factor Release from Platelets Pharmacology 1990;40: 150-156
222 Tun-Jun Tsai et al. Dipyridamole inhibits TGF-β – induced collagen gene expression in human peritoneal mesothelial cells. Kidney International Volume 60, Issue 4, October 2001, Pages 1249-1257

dipyridamole is a powerful MMP-9 inhibitor, which is the reason why it is so effective at stopping the cancer spreading to other parts of the body. I occasionally now take the beta blocker drug propranolol, which is both a powerful MMP-2 and MMP-9 inhibitor, but it cannot be used at the same time as dipyridamole as both can cause drops in blood pressure. Propranolol can also affect my Raynaud's (poor circulation in my fingers and toes), so I avoid it in cold weather, whereas the combination of dipyridamole and a statin improves my Raynaud's. Doxycycline, which is not only useful for starving cancer, is another powerful MMP-9 inhibitor. Pentoxyfylline can replace dipyridamole in many instances. Dipyridamole is becoming hard to get hold as Boehringer Ingelheim are withdrawing it slowly, despite knowing it has huge anticancer effects. (Legal action anyone?)

Note that MMP expression is different for every type of cancer, e.g. ovarian cancer uses MMP-1, 2, 7, 9, 10, 13. Triple negative breast cancer uses MMP-1, 2, 7, 8, 9, 10, 13. Multiple myeloma uses MMP-1, 2,7,9,14. A bit of research will reveal which combination of growth blockers will be best for you.[223]

---

223 Wang Y, H, Wang Q et al. Saikosaponin A Inhibits Triple-Negative Breast Cancer Growth and Metastasis Through Downregulation of CXCR4. Front Oncol. 2020 Jan 28;9:1487. doi: 10.3389/fonc.2019.01487. PMID: 32047724; PMCID: PMC6997291.

Chapter Twenty-Four:

How to Reboot the Immune System

Cancer is the result of abnormalities in white blood cells (macrophages), which become altered. Because these are 'self,' the body does not recognise them as the enemy. This allows the cancer to spread unchecked.

 Macrophages are converted to tumour associated macrophages (TAMs) because of a combination of hypoxic (lack of oxygen) conditions, the presence of the abnormal growth factor 'transforming growth factor-β' (TGF-β), immunosuppressive inflammatory cytokines (IL-1, and IL-10), PGE2 (bad prostaglandin) and exposure to Th2 (the humoural immune response).[224] These factors convert ordinary macrophages into tumour-associated macrophages, and it is these little blighters that allow the cancer to grow unchecked by our immune system. These macrophages break away from the original tumour with the help of the matrix metalloproteinases (MMPs) and can travel throughout the circulation to seed new tumours.

With growth factors and MMPs put on hold, inflammation quelled, and hypoxia improved, you can reduce the transformation of tumour associated macrophages ('TAMs'). Those naughty TAMs in my body had sought to evade detection and eradication by the rest of my immune system by traveling around the blood hidden in a clump of platelets and saturated fat (another reason to avoid saturated fat if you have metastatic

---

224 Quatromoni JG, Eruslanov E. Tumor-associated macrophages: function, phenotype, and link to prognosis in human lung cancer. American Journal of Translational Research. 2012;4(4): 376-389.

cancer). Aspirin and dipyridamole, which are both antiplatelet drugs, synergistically serve to break down the platelet clumps and expose the abnormal macrophages to the rest of the immune system. Statins help lower the amount of fat available for these metastatic clumps in the circulation, making them more vulnerable to eradication. Berberine and niacin also lower triglyceride levels.

My magic cocktail had been very successful for beating cancer, but another problem remained: I still had a suppression of my Th1 (pathogen response which includes Natural Killer cells) and a raised Th2 response (humoral immune response). In other words, the few Natural Killer cells I had in my system were suppressed, so I could not mount the necessary attack to finish the cancer off once and for all.

It took me until 2007 to discover how to rectify this by using the antihistamine cimetidine to reverse the Th1:Th2 imbalance. This, I believe, was the biggest boost to my immune system, but other 'big guns' were shark liver oil (alkylglycerols), Chinese mushrooms (e.g., shitake, maitake and turkey tail), correcting my gut microbiome, eliminating any parasites, taking pre and probiotics, especially bifidobacteria, along with the berberine and metformin which both favourably alter the gut flora. All of these were key to my immune improvement during this 'recovery phase' after the onslaught of not just cancer but the after effects of all the treatment. I have no doubt that the intravenous vitamin C gave my immune system a huge kick, along with the ultraviolet blood irradiation before I was given the dendritic vaccine, which may have had little effect in reality. I will never know. Vaccines were seen as the Holy Grail of cancer treatment, but despite all that promise, they were spectacularly unsuccessful. This was before the realisation that abnormal cell signalling, growth factors and the abnormal metabolism were to blame, and that vaccines wouldn't work if these were not switched off first. Success would always be elusive without those measures first. Even then, I am convinced the immune system needs to be enhanced and

vaccine. I wonder whether I would have had a better response if I had used cimetidine before my dendritic vaccine. Perhaps, in the future, they will try vaccines again with a more holistic approach.

I am also sceptical of the new immunotherapy drugs for the same reasons. I overcame stage IV cancer long before the invention of the new 'mabs' or 'nibs', or any new PDL-1 inhibiting immunotherapies. Without addressing any of the preceding reasons for the immune system to be malfunctioning, the use of these new drugs, in my view, is ultimately futile.[225] It is no surprise that the use of many of the drugs in my metabolic cocktail and correcting the gut are being shown to overcome resistance to immunotherapy drugs. It is the metabolic rewiring of the stem cell that is both the problem and the answer. Starve your cancer!

Your immune system competes with cancer cells for fuel, glucose, glutamine, arginine, fats and an amino acid called tryptophan. There are several metabolic check points that switch off the immune system:

- Toll like Receptors, IL-1, IL-6, microbiome
- STAT3 (kynurenine pathway), NF-kB, glycolysis, lactate.

The kynurenine pathway, which degrades tryptophan, can be highly expressed in cancer. L-tryptophan is an essential amino acid that is a prerequisite for protein biosynthesis and the production of melatonin and serotonin hormones.

---

225 The following articles all point to the importance of the right bacterial balance in the gut. Whilst many patients focus on boosting lactobacilli with fermented foods, it may be increasing the levels of the bifidobacteria that may be more important.
IMMUNOTHERAPY. *Could microbial therapy boost cancer immunotherapy?* [Science. 2015]
Tumour immunology: Intestinal bacteria are in command. [Nat Rev Immunol. 2016]
Immunotherapy Not Working? Check Your Microbiota. [Cancer Cell. 2015]

is best combined with a Stat3 inhibitor (e.g. metformin, nifuroxazide, lithium orotate).

Low dose pimozide, an old antispychotic drug, or cimetidine, can help normalise myeloid derived suppressor cells and assist immune suppressive tumour associated macrophages (M2) transform back to anticancer macrophages (M1).[226]

Normalising Tregs, which are responsible for autoimmune issues when on PD-1 inhibitors, can be achieved by the addition of pentoxifylline, an old drug used to treat poor circulation, an exciting recent discovery. It additionally improved the cancer fighting levels of T cells. Combining check point inhibitors with pentoxifylline may eventually be adopted for every conventional immunotherapy treatment.[227]

Normalising the immune system also requires:

- **Arginase-1 inhibitors** such as picetannol, Gingerol-6 PDE5 inhibitors like Cilalis, Viagra.
- **Cox2 inhibitors** such as boswellia, curcumin, aspirin, siegsbeckia glabrescens.
- **iNOS inhibitors** such as quercetin, siegsbeckia glabrescens, danshen.

The immune system is complicated as some immune cells acutally assist cancer (TAMs, MDSCs, Tregs), whereas others fight it (NK cells, cytotoxic T cells). You may find it easier to watch the videos in my on-line course.

---

226 Shuangshuang Yang, Qing Yang et al. Discovery of Tryptanthrin Derivatives as Potent Inhibitors of Indoleamine 2,3-Dioxygenase with Therapeutic Activity in Lewis Lung Cancer (LLC) Tumor-Bearing Mice: J. Med. Chem. 2013, 56, 21, 8321–8331 Publication Date:October 7, 2013 https://doi.org/10.1021/jm401195
227 Targeting the c-Rel Subunit of NF-κB Inhibits Treg Function in Melanoma Cancer Discov November 1 2017 (7) (11) OF13; DOI: 10.1158/2159-8290.CD-RW2017-175

Chapter Twenty-Five:

How to Kill Cancer

 You've stopped the abnormal cell signalling. You've starved it. You've stopped the growth factors. You've addressed your gut issues.

This may be enough to make many early or less aggressive cancers disappear, although this approach may take longer to achieve (it can take up to 7 or 8 months for the metabolic drugs to show effects). But what if your cancer is aggressive, a stage three or four, and not under control? You need to reduce the fast-dividing cells too, not just the stem cells, by triggering 'apoptosis' or 'ferroptosis', both will cause cancer cell suicide.

Remember that tumours contain two different sets of cancer cells: fast-dividing cells and stem cells. Whilst starving your cancer you are targeting both stem cells and fast dividing cells, whereas conventional medicine focuses on removing fast dividing cells. Chemotherapy and radiotherapy leave behind the stem cells. Combine the two approaches and you can more than double the results (see my graphs on the following pages).

Fast division is the last event to occur in the steps leading to transformation. These fast-dividing cells are the progeny of the stem cells but not stem cells themselves.

Seeds for Cancer's Survival

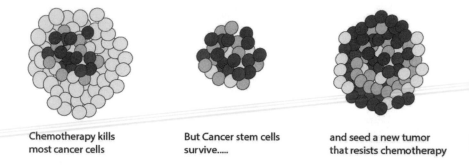

Chemotherapy kills most cancer cells

But Cancer stem cells survive.....

and seed a new tumor that resists chemotherapy

Figure 23.2. *Stem cells survive chemotherapy.*

So, which less toxic drugs stop the fast cell division?

Many of my drugs and supplements target several processes at the same time; they are termed 'pleiotropic'. The more targets a drug or supplement has (or the more pleiotropic it is), the more useful I believe the drug or supplement to be. Mebendazole, the antihelminth (deworming) drug has multiple targets and its most recognised benefit in cancer is for slowing down fast cell division. It is a fantastic low toxicity drug that works in the same way as the chemotherapy drug vincristine, but without the toxicity, making it ideal for paediatric use. Exactly like vincristine, it works by fatally disrupting the microtubule formation in cancer cells that occurs as the cell is attempting to divide, a process that all cancer cells undergo.[228] However, mebendazole also helps reduce abnormal cell signalling (something called Sonic Hedgehog), it stops glucose accessing the cancer cell by inhibiting the glucose receptors, it is an MMP-2 inhibitor and there is also evidence it helps to destroy the tumour-associated macrophage cells that suppress immunity when

---

228 Sasaki J, Ramesh R, Chada S, Gomyo Y, Roth JA, Mukhopadhyay T. The anthelmintic drug mebendazole induces mitotic arrest and apoptosis by depolymerizing tubulin in non-small cell lung cancer cells. Mol Cancer Ther 2002;1: 1201-9.

combined with low dose chemotherapy.[229] Mebendazole also activates caspases to promote apoptosis through the 'caspase cascade'. It is a wonder drug! It has low absorption in the gut but taking it with some fat will help. Piperine from black pepper, which you can buy as a supplement, will increase plasma levels too.

Most chemotherapy drugs are acidic (which encourages tumour growth), and the result is a lot of tiny fragments of broken up cells, like DNA pieces, that the metabolically flexible cancer stem cells can learn to scoop up and re-use (autophagy). To outwit the cancer cells, it is essential to target both fast dividing cells and stem cells at the same time. If you kill too much of the tumour with a high dose of chemotherapy, this provides lots of potential nutrients for the remaining stem cells. Reducing both together in a controlled fashion must surely be the best approach? Too often I see patients killed by too much chemotherapy.

To demonstrate this dual approach, this chart shows the cancer kill rate of metformin (targeting the stem cell) and temozolomide (a chemotherapy drug targeting the fast-dividing cell) when used individually and then when they are used together:

229 Doudican NA, Pennell R, Byron S, Pollock P, Liebes L, Osman I *et al.* Mebendazole in the treatment of melanoma: The role of Bcl-2 in predicting response and enhancing efficacy. Presented at the 2010 American Society of Clinical Oncology Annual Meeting, Chicago, IL, USA.

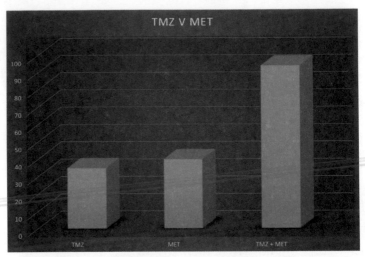

Figure 23.3. *Comparison of temozolide and metformin for brain cancer (Data from the Care Oncology Clinic, UK)*

Note that metformin (at 40%), a cheap off-patent drug with few side effects, has a greater cancer kill than the chemotherapy temozolomide (at 35%)! Note the synergistic effect of adding both together – 35% and 40% creating a 94% cancer kill rate, greater than the sum of each part individually; there is powerful synergy at play.[230] Imagine the potential of adding other synergistic low toxicity metabolic drugs that penetrate the blood brain barrier. Who says brain cancer can't be cured?

This next graph is a comparison of another chemotherapy drug for brain cancer (this time carmustine, aka BCNU) which works on the fast-dividing cell, compared with berberine:

230 YU Z, ZHAO G, LI P, *et al.* Temozolomide in combination with metformin act synergistically to inhibit proliferation and expansion of glioma stem-like cells. Oncology Letters. 2016;11(4): 2792-2800. doi: 10.3892/ol.2016.4315.

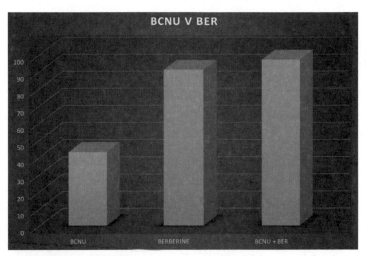

Figure 23.4. *Comparing carmustine and berberine for brain cancer*

This 1990 study tested the tumour-killing powers of berberine and BCNU (carmustine) in vitro and in vivo (cell culture and in rodents). Berberine alone produced a staggering 91 per cent kill rate in glioma cell cultures, more than double the effect of metformin. 91%! Stunning. At this rate of fatality, berberine must surely target both types of cells, the fast-dividing cells and the stem cells. This graph is sadly not the same for every cancer as each has a different metabolic profile. But wow. Combining berberine with BCNU yielded a massive kill rate of 97 per cent![231]

As both metformin and berberine have different stem cell targets, despite many similarities, it would be wise not to rely on berberine and chemotherapy alone. Lower doses of chemotherapy would reduce the terrible side effects of these harsh treatments if the right cocktails were used. For example, mebendazole shows great promise as a chemotherapy enhancer, which could be especially useful for childhood brain cancers as

---

231 Zhang, RX *et al* 1990. Laboratory studies of berberine used alone and in combination with 1,3-bis(2-chloroethyl)-1-nitrosourea to treat malignant brain tumors. Chin Med J (Engl). 1990 Aug;103(8): 658-65.

it has virtually no toxicity.[232] Intravenous vitamin C, when used regularly and at high enough doses, also acts like a chemotherapy drug; it too can cross the blood brain barrier.

Combining Chemotherapy with Non-Steroidal Anti-Inflammatory Drugs (NSAIDs)

NSAIDS are powerful anti-cancer drugs, but exactly how they work eluded researchers for years as it was known that they had greater effects on cancer cells than just COX2 inhibition alone. We have since discovered that they don't 'starve' cancer, instead they trigger apoptosis when used at high enough doses. Non-aspirin NSAIDs disrupt the 'S' phase of cell division, the point when the cell manufactures new DNA, replicating its genetic material. This is the phase of cell division that is the most receptive to conventional chemotherapy drugs and is the phase when cancer cells are most resistant to radiotherapy.[233] It would make sense, then, to sensitise these resistant cells by combining the treatments together, but this is not current clinical practice, despite studies showing that irradiation used with a concurrent high dose NSAID was not associated with an increased level of side effects.[234]

'The real debate comes down to use of these compounds in two settings: cancer prevention, which involves long term use of a drug and cancer treatment involving short-term, focused use of the drug,' said Douglas Trask, M.D., Ph.D., University of Iowa Associate Professor of

---

232 Gregory Riggins at Johns Hopkins is doing sterling work investigating the use of mebendazole in paediatric cancer. It receives little funding and support which is tragic given the potential. Gregory is one of my heroes.

233 University of Iowa. 'Combining NSAIDs With Chemotherapy, Radiation May Improve Cancer Treatment.' ScienceDaily. ScienceDaily, 18 May 2007. <www.sciencedaily.com/releases/2007/05/070517101745.htm>.

234 Ganswindt U, Budach W, Jendrossek V, Becker G, Bamberg M, Belka C. Combination of celecoxib with percutaneous radiotherapy in patients with localised prostate cancer – a phase I study. Radiation Oncology (London, England). 2006;1: 9. doi: 10.1186/1748-717X-1-9.

Otolaryngology in an online report from Science Daily. 'Published studies show that heart and kidney problems occur with long-term use, especially when used for more than one year. While there appear to be cardiorenal effects of NSAIDs even with short-term use, these risks may be minor compared to the potential benefit to treat cancer more effectively.'

Concurrent use of a statin and dipyridamole would also help mitigate any cardio effects and enhance efficacy. If these and intravenous vitamin C, berberine, mebendazole, a non-aspirin NSAID (used short term or 'pulsed') were used in a cocktail alongside chemotherapy, could the maximum tolerated dose be dramatically lowered? Chemotherapy is useful, there is no doubting that, but the maximum tolerated dose is far too much, particularly for the stage IV patient when the toxicity and level of immune suppression often kills the patient faster than if they had been given no chemo at all. My insistence on a lower dose, whilst I also took the berberine and other cancer-starving drugs, dropped my markers into normal range very quickly, but it required a full Oscar-winning performance to get it. At sequentially lower doses, given judiciously, chemotherapy can be immune **stimulating**, a fact that many natural and alternative therapy protagonists will deny. It is a knee jerk reaction to cut it out completely because of its reported inefficacy for stage IV patients, but do not automatically rule it out if your oncologist is willing to give you a low dose.

Metronomic (short, pulsed regular intervals) low dose chemotherapy given every 4 to 8 days, compared to the blasting a patient with the maximum tolerated dose every 21 days, was shown to boost anti-tumour T cell immunity.[235]

---

235 Miki Tongu • Nanae Harashima • Hiroyuki Monma • Touko Inao • Takaya Yamada Hideyuki Kawauchi • Mamoru Harada Metronomic chemotherapy with low-dose cyclophosphamide plus gemcitabine can induce anti-tumor T cell immunity in vivo Cancer Immunol Immunother (2013) 62: 383-391

Triggering apoptosis of cancer cells beyond chemotherapy

This in a nutshell, is my protocol to starve and defeat cancer:

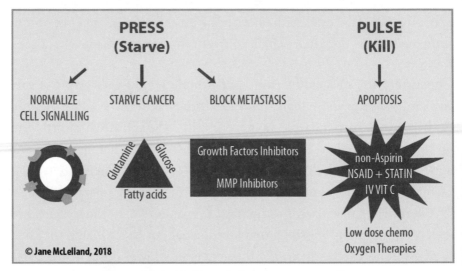

Figure 23.5. *My 'Press Pulse' strategy to eradicate both fast dividing cells and stem cells.*

Apoptosis refers to active, programmed single cell death and it is different to necrosis, which is a passive process. Ferroptosis is yet another programmed cell death which I believe could be even better, I will describe how to achieve this in the next section.

In cancer, the apoptotic process is regulated by:

1. **Caspases** (cysteine-dependent aspartate-directed proteases). These carry out cell death duties with minimal effect on surrounding tissues. These are activated in the mitochondria.

2. **Bcl-2/bax** these regulate apoptosis and can either promote apoptosis or rescue the metabolic function of the mitochondria and prevent apoptosis.

3. **Fas** (first apoptosis signal receptor) is a death receptor on the surface of cells that leads to programmed cell death (apoptosis)

leading to a triggering of caspase 8. Metformin uses this route to cause apoptosis.[236]

Death by Caspases

Caspase activation is an under-utilised and safer option for promoting cancer cell death, although it might take longer to achieve. The natural 'caspase cascade' is activated when the antioxidant (redox) status (glutathione: oxidant balance) of the cancer cell is altered in the mitochondrial membrane. Activation of apoptotic 'caspases' results in the generation of a cascade of signalling events and the **controlled** demolition of cellular components, a less damaging approach than using chemotherapy alone which causes free radical release by sheer damage to the DNA. Mebendazole, which acts like the chemotherapy drug vincristine (but is much safer), destroys fast-dividing cells by disrupting the alignment of spindles in dividing cancer cells. It also triggers the caspase cascade by inactivating Bcl-2 and the release of cytochrome C. All these processes will promote apoptosis in cancer cells.[237] At the beginning of cell transformation, a rise in ammonia and lactic acid levels initially fuels further growth, but after this the cancer needs to tightly control its redox status, or homeostatic regulation of its oxidant level, to ensure its immortality.

Cancer cells survive by keeping glutathione, the master antioxidant, at a high enough level to keep the cancer cell from self-destruction. Reducing levels makes these fast-dividing cells defenceless. If glutathione is lowered

236 GAO Z-Y, LIU Z, BI M-H, *et al.* Metformin induces apoptosis via a mitochondria-mediated pathway in human breast cancer cells in vitro. Experimental and Therapeutic Medicine. 2016;11(5): 1700-1706. doi: 10.3892/etm.2016.3143.

237 Doudican NA, Pennell R, Byron S, Pollock P, Liebes L, Osman I *et al.* Mebendazole in the treatment of melanoma: The role of Bcl-2 in predicting response and enhancing efficacy. Presented at the 2010 American Society of Clinical Oncology Annual Meeting, Chicago, IL, USA.

and ROS or reactive oxygen species levels are increased, the cancer cell becomes unstable and unable to sustain itself and apoptosis results.

How to raise ROS – oxygen free radicals

Intravenous vitamin C

I have witnessed people complaining that intravenous vitamin C made them worse. This is indeed likely to be true in some cancers as intravenous vitamin C blocks glycolysis (glucose), so it will push glutamine-driven cancers to be even more aggressive if the patient has failed to block off other glutamine fuel lines first.[238] This was demonstrated by Professors Lisanti and Sottgia in Salford, Manchester, who found that blocking key pathways (glutamine and glucose OXPHOS and fatty acid oxidation) with doxycycline before administering vitamin C (orally) with berberine was many more times effective and a 'synthetically lethal' combination across many cell lines. On its own, intravenous vitamin C is 10 times more lethal to cancer stem cells than chemotherapy. When this is combined with doxycycline, the synergy multiplied its effects to being 100 times more effective!

Delivering intravenous vitamin C on its own is a risky strategy. However, cancers with RAS and BRAF mutations are particularly sensitive to its therapeutic effects, as these cancers can take up a lot of glucose through the Glut receptors. In 2000, I had used aspirin, berberine and intravenous vitamin C together which had blocked many pathways (you can now work out which ones by checking my Metro Map). It was during this period that my antigen markers dropped to a level of only 40, the lowest they ever reached. It would be wise to use piperlongumine and niclosamide alongside the intravenous vitamin C to prevent glutamine

---

238 De Francesco EM, Bonuccelli G, Maggiolini M, Sotgia F, Lisanti MP. Vitamin C and Doxycycline: A synthetic lethal combination therapy targeting metabolic flexibility in cancer stem cells (CSCs). Oncotarget. 2017;8(40): 67269-67286. doi: 10.18632/oncotarget.18428.

driven OXPHOS becoming upregulated. But ferroptosis is an even better and exciting new approach to use intravenous vitamin C effectively.

Another mistake is that the intravenous vitamin C is not delivered at a high enough dose or given often enough to produce hydrogen peroxide and reduce glycolysis. Many complementary practitioners like to administer it at least three times a week. Once a week is not enough, as shown by the Danish study on prostate cancer[239] which used intravenous vitamin C once a week as a monotherapy at 60g, and probably pushed the cancer into a more aggressive glutamine/fat driven phenotype. As prostate cancer uses glycolysis the least, it is no surprise that this study failed to show any benefit. However ferroptosis may be the solution to making vitamin C work.

Pre-treatment with niclosamide, sensitises cells to apoptosis with hydrogen peroxide (intravenous vitamin C).[240] Given its many other targets (Stat3, Notch, OXPhOS, NF-κB, Wnt/β-catenin, mTOR), this old worming drug has risen to become one of my top drug choices, especially for more aggressive glutamine cancers, if you can get hold of it.

How to Lower Glutathione

Glutathione is made from glutamate (from glutamine), glycine and cysteine. The trick is to lower cysteine as the body has ready access to glycine and glutamate. To lower cysteine, avoid L-cysteine and NAC supplements, whey protein and asparagus. Possibly even avoid bone

239 Nielsen TK, Højgaard M, Andersen JT, *et al*. Weekly ascorbic acid infusion in castration-resistant prostate cancer patients: a single-arm phase II trial. Translational Andrology and Urology. 2017;6(3): 517-528. doi: 10.21037/tau.2017.04.42.

240 Sae-lo-oomLee, A-RangSonabJiyeonAhn, Jie-YoungSong Niclosamide enhances ROS-mediated cell death through c-Jun activation Biomedicine & Pharmacotherapy, Volume 68, Issue 5, June 2014, Pages 619-624. Kai Yu et al Niclosamide induces apoptosis through mitochondrial intrinsic pathway and inhibits migration and invasion in human thyroid cancer in vitro Biomedicine & Pharmacotherapy, Volume 92, 2017, pp. 403-41

broth during a 'kill phase'. Certain antioxidants also need to be avoided, as CoQ10, low dose vitamin C and vitamin E will all neutralise the free radicals you need. Sulphoraphane, despite its other beneficial effects on cancer, reduces the activity of caspase-3 while upregulating Bcl-2 which puts the brakes on apoptosis, so this needs to be stopped during a 'kill' phase,[241] as does luteolin. However, pre-treatment with chloroquine (stopped 12-24 hours prior to chemo) showed that it sensitised cells to apoptosis through mitochondrial caspases.[242] Sulphoraphane and luteolin might also sensitise the cells to the caspases.

1. **Statins** get a bad rap for their glutathione-lowering effect in other diseases (e.g. cardiovascular), but this is a huge benefit for cancer patients,[243] as I discovered in 2003; statins increase the cancer kill of non-steroidal anti-inflammatory drugs by five times.

   Sadly, the 'dangers' of statin therapy are everywhere you look nowadays with grim predictions of dementia, sore muscles and an increased risk of type 2 diabetes. These effects take mostly years to develop, if they have any effect on you at all (I had no side effects). And these side effects can be stopped or reduced by the addition of resveratrol, metformin, berberine and a few supplements like omega-3 oils, squalene (shark liver oil or olive oil) and vitamin D (avoid CoQ10 as this will help the cancer cell recycle glutathione – no good if you want to cause apoptosis through the caspase cascade). It is a fact that many cancer patients are now refusing a statin because of the hype of side effects, yet

241 An-Shi Wang, Yan Xu, Xiao-Hong Zhang et al Sulforaphane protects MLE-12 lung epithelial cells against oxidative damage caused by ambient air particulate matter, Food and Function issue 12, 2017

242 Arnab Ganguli, Diptiman Choudhury, Satabdi Datta, Surela Bhattacharya, Gopal Chakrabarti Inhibition of autophagy by chloroquine potentiates synergistically anti-cancer property of artemisinin by promoting ROS dependent apoptosis Biochemie 19th July 2014

243 Chapman-Shimshoni D, Yuklea M, Radnay J, Shapiro H, Lishner M. Simvastatin induces apoptosis of B-CLL cells by activation of mitochondrial caspase 9. Exp Hematol. 2003 Sep; 31(9): 779-83.

still allowing themselves to undergo high dose chemotherapy. These are worlds apart when it comes to toxicity. Treating cancer is completely different to treating cardiovascular disease and I see many patients failing to grasp the unrealistic fear of statins when compared to the nature and prognosis of their disease, such is the level of scaremongering in the media.

2. **Feverfew:** (parthelonide)[244] a natural botanical, lowers glutathione, generates reactive oxygen species, and activates caspase 7, -8, and -9.

3. **Sulfasalazine:** Some cancers like pancreatic are very hard to treat with chemotherapy; they are a mass of extremely resistant and metabolically adapted cells. Lowering glutathione and re-sensitising the cancer to chemotherapy with sulfasalazine has been shown to be helpful,[245] which might be the extra nudge it needs to send it into a death spiral.

The Press: Pulse Strategy

Professor Thomas Seyfried, author of *Cancer as a Metabolic Disease*, likes the press-pulse approach. He believes the cancer environment needs to be stressed by reducing nutrient availability, using the ketogenic diet and a glycolysis inhibitor (2-deoxyglucose) combining with EGCG, hyperbaric oxygen therapy (HBOT) and the macropinocytosis inhibitor chloroquine sulphate.[246]

---

244 Oxidative Stress-mediated Apoptosis THE ANTICANCER EFFECT OF THE SESQUITERPENE LACTONE PARTHENOLIDE The Journal of Biological Chemistry277, 38954-38964. October 11, 2002
245 Lo M, Ling V, Low C, Wang YZ, Gout PW. Potential use of the anti-inflammatory drug, sulfasalazine, for targeted therapy of pancreatic cancer. Current Oncology. 2010;17(3): 9-16.
246 Kazuhito Sasaki, Nelson H Tsuno, Eiji Sunami et al Chloroquine potentiates the anti-cancer effect of 5-fluorouracil on colon cancer cells BMC Cancer, 2010, Volume 10, Number 1, Page 1

He is achieving some success in glioblastoma patients with this cocktail, which shows proof of this multi-pronged 'starving' concept.[247] If you look at my Metro Map you can see which routes are blocked with this combination. He tried pulsing DON, the powerful glutamine inhibitor in animals, but he found that this was too toxic with the risk of serious gut and brain damage. He is a firm advocate of ketogenic diets, which seem to be more successful for brain tumours. This is a mystery to me as these tumours appear to have an appetite for ketones,[248] but perhaps it is the cocktail that is the answer. If you try this diet, which does benefit some patients, it would be wise, in my view, to add other starving modalities (like berberine, which targets the acetate/ketone pathway by blocking SREBP-1),[249] to prevent the cancer becoming more aggressive and harder to treat in the longer term. In my experience, many patients who try this diet for treating their cancer find it hard to achieve ketosis for long periods anyway, but the diet at least encourages a low glycaemic intake. It might be best to 'pulse' the ketosis (for one or two days) if you choose this diet rather than follow it strictly for extended periods. However, if you get epilepsy as a result of a brain tumour, the ketogenic diet can be very beneficial for reducing seizures, but perhaps berberine might achieve the same effect.[250]

Valter Longo, gerontologist at the University of Southern California and author of the Longevity Diet, has also proved the 'cancer-starving' principle. He has shown enhanced cancer kill with a five day 'fasting

247 Ahmed M. A. Elsakka1, Mohamed Abdel Bary2, Eman Abdelzaher3, Mostafa Elnaggar4, Miriam Kalamian5, Purna Mukherjee6 and Thomas N. Seyfried6*Management of Glioblastoma Multiforme in a Patient Treated With Ketogenic Metabolic Therapy and Modified Standard of Care: A 24-Month Follow-Up Front. Nutr., 29 March 2018

248 Tomoyuki Mashimo et al Acetate Is a Bioenergetic Substrate for Human Glioblastoma and Brain Metastases Cell, Volume 159, Issue 7, 18 December 2014, Pages 1603-1614

249 Schug ZT, Peck B, Jones DT, et al. Acetyl-CoA Synthetase 2 Promotes Acetate Utilization and Maintains Cancer Cell Growth under Metabolic Stress. Cancer Cell. 2015;27(1):57- 71. doi:10.1016/j.ccell.2014.12.002.

250 Tzu-Yu Lin, Yu-Wan Lin, Cheng-Wei Lu, Shu-Kuei Huang, Su-Jane Wang Berberine Inhibits the Release of Glutamate in Nerve Terminals from Rat Cerebral Cortex

mimicking diet' where specific foods and calories are withheld, then followed by low dose chemotherapy. Not only did it show enhanced cancer kill, but also an increase in tumour infiltrating lymphocytes (cancer killing white blood cells), so an increase in the immune response.[251] Sadly, Longo seems to be of the impression that statins reduce life span and he discourages their use. I can only assume he has been looking at reported cardiovascular effects, without consideration to the synergy and potential of the statin and dipyridamole combination or the benefits of statins for cancer patients – they are spectacularly effective in increasing survival times.[252]

251 Di Biase, Stefano *et al.* Fasting-Mimicking Diet Reduces HO-1 to Promote T Cell-Mediated Tumor Cytotoxicity Cancer Cell, Volume 30, Issue 1, 136-146

252 Wang A, Aragaki AK, Tang JY *et al.* Statin use and all-cancer mortality: Prospective results from the Women's Health Intiative. Presented at the 2015 American Society of Clinical Oncology Annual Meeting, Chicago, IL, USA, 29 May – 2 June 2015.

Chapter Twenty-Six

The Ferroptosis Protocol
– A new way to Kill Cancer

Starving cancer has proven successful for many patients, but if your tumours seem to be treatment resistant, continue to metastasise and refuse to be killed by the starving protocol, even when combined with conventional treatments, then you should consider trying a relatively unknown form of treatment called ferroptosis. This literally means 'death by iron' and it involves starving the cell of the amino acid cystcine and using oxygen. It is fundamentally different to apoptosis and it is a new and powerful weapon in the fight against cancer.[253]

Iron is the most abundant metal and it is used by every cancer cell to fuel its prolific growth. It is a vital element for many fundamental biological functions because it can readily donate and accept electrons to participate in oxidation–reduction reactions. When "free" labile iron is present in the cell it can react with oxygen, releasing free radicals. It is this property that enables it to destroy cancer cells by oxidation during a process called the Fenton Reaction. This process of ROS (reactive oxygen species) generation is created by the interaction between iron ($Fe2+$) and hydrogen peroxide ($H2O2$) to produce iron free radicals and hydroxyl free radicals ($OH \cdot + OH$) that accumulate in cell membranes.

---

253 Dixon SJ, Lemberg KM, Lamprecht MR, et al. Ferroptosis: an iron-dependent form of nonapoptotic cell death. Cell. 2012;149(5):1060-1072. doi:10.1016/j.cell.2012.03.042

If you want the chemistry, this is the Fenton reaction:

$$Fe^2+ + H_2O_2 \rightarrow Fe^3+ + OH\cdot + OH-$$

This means that the more aggressive cancers like triple negative breast cancer, gliomas, pancreatic cancers, renal cell, ovarian and tricky cancers like sarcomas can respond to ferroptosis especially well, as the faster the growth, the more they rely on iron. However, all cancers will respond to ferroptosis with the right combination of drugs and supplements. It is also a viable option for rarer cancers like mesothelioma and rhabdomyosarcoma, as well as cancers that have a naturally high affinity for iron. RAS mutated cancers (H-, N-, K- RAS) including aggressive colorectal phenotypes (about 40 to 50 percent of colon cancers have a mutation in the RAS pathway) and also YAP-driven cancers are particularly sensitive. Melanoma cancer cells can evade apoptosis through the process of epithelial to mesenchymal transition, an event that can happen early in oncogenesis and a process that makes melanoma so potentially difficult to treat. But while melanoma is resistant to programmed cell death by apoptosis, these cells are far more sensitive to ferroptosis.

Starving a cancer cell by depriving it of nutrients is a slow, passive way to kill cancer cells by the process of apoptosis. For more aggressive cancers, this might not reduce the tumour fast enough to suppress its growth, therefore it is best to include treatments that create oxygen free radicals or ROS (reactive oxygen species). Any treatment that creates these oxygen free radicals is what I consider to be a Kill Phase therapy, so targeted drugs and immunotherapy are not included, but treatments that create oxygen free radicals can, in most cases, be added to immunotherapy and targeted drugs to enhance their effects. Chemotherapy, radiotherapy and regular aerobic exercise will oxidise tumours and these will help debulk the fast dividing cells, but often treatment resistance develops to conventional therapies as they do not target the stem cell, leading to recurrence and progression. The more aggressive a cancer, the more pulsed Kill Phases with ROS you may need to eradicate it.

Ferroptosis combines starving the cell (depriving it of cysteine by blocking the xCT antiporter) with a kill phase as it produces oxygen free radicals, oxidising iron and creating hydroxyl radicals to destroy cell membranes and eradicate cancer cells. Although it is not essential to stimulate ferroptosis, the addition of intravenous vitamin C to release hydrogen peroxide will further oxidise the tumour microenvironment improving the effectiveness of this treatment. IVC also blocks glycolysis, so this addresses both the fast dividing cells and the stem cells, whereas generating free radicals through chemotherapy alone merely addresses fast dividing cells.

Starve and Kill Phases generally act as a kind of Yin and Yang, they each need specific combinations of supplements to trigger cell death and it is best to try and time the Kill Phase for when cancer is at its weakest. The starve phase is a prolonged stress, slowly weakening the cancer over time and many of the supplements listed in this ferroptosis protocol will also be useful during a starve phase, such as piperlongumine, PEITC and artemisinin, as these all appear on my Metro Map. The drug sulfasalazine which also inhibits the xCT antiporter to starve the cell of cysteine can have some side effects, so I am suggesting short term use over a few weeks (perhaps only a few days over the period when you have IVC), to coincide with the COC protocol, alternate months while taking mebendazole. If you can tolerate it and the ferroptosis protocol is working, then this could be extended. It will be up to your doctors to evaluate your progress.

The kill phase is normally an acute 'pulse' of free radicals given over one or two days (sometimes over a few days) but with ferroptosis the aim is to deliver a low dose of oxidative therapy over a longer period, enhanced when possible, with a pulse of intravenous vitamin C. Some patients receive daily low dose chemotherapy which merges the starve and kill phases together, but you can still safely add intravenous vitamin C on top for an extra burst of ROS.

A recent study by Edward and George Mathews into the effects of glucose deprivation found that cancer is at its weakest roughly 28 days after starting a glucose restricted diet.[254] This might then be the best time to try ferroptosis. After that time the tumour slowly learns to adapt using other nutrients and pathways for fuel until around 90 days, when it has gained resistance to glucose restriction alone. This is why it is a mistake to rely on a ketogenic diet as a monotherapy and why a combination approach works best.

Ferroptosis is a unique and independent form of programmed cell death, where the cell's membranes fail, including those of the mitochondria, so that energy production is impaired and the cancer starves to death. For decades researchers assumed apoptosis, a regulated process of cell suicide, was the only way to kill cancer cells, either by activating the 'caspase cascade' in the cell machinery or by creating ROS. Autophagy and necrosis as other forms of cell death were added, but since the more recent discovery of ferroptosis by Stockwell and Dixon in 2012, the realisation of its great potential for cancer therapy has led to a growing number of articles and excitement in the research field.

Programmed cell death is an integral part of life and it is involved in shaping the proper structure and function of organs; in immune cells it enables the appropriate response without triggering autoimmune disease. Programmed cell death is a homeostatic process found in every cell and there are theories that ferroptosis may even be a normal process for healthy cells to eradicate cancer as it is heavily influenced by the p53 gene, which is a tumour suppressor.

---

254 Edward Henry Mathews, George Edward Mathews, In vitro quantification: Long-term effect of glucose deprivation on various cancer cell lines, Nutrition, Volume 74, 2020, https://doi.org/10.1016/j.nut.2020.110748.

Using this vulnerability, we can sabotage cancer's desire to hog iron and turn it into a potent anticancer weapon. Ferroptosis is characterised by an overwhelming, iron-dependent accumulation of oxidised polyunsaturated fats (PUFA) and reactive oxygen species (ROS).

Ferroptosis can occur when

- cysteine import into the cell is blocked (preventing the manufacture of the antioxidant glutathione)
- and/or with inhibition of the glutathione peroxidase 4 enzyme (GPX4) that repairs lipid peroxides, preventing repair of fatty membranes.

As a result of ferroptosis, membranes of mitochondria are altered by oxidation and the cristae inside are damaged, lowering the ability of the cancer cell to make energy and replicate. The consequence is death of the cancer cell.

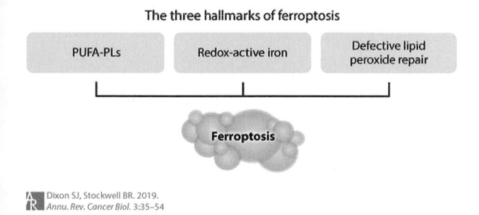

The three hallmarks of ferroptosis

Dixon SJ, Stockwell BR. 2019.
Annu. Rev. Cancer Biol. 3:35–54

Cancer, as we know, is a wily, metabolically flexible beast. To survive and reprogram its metabolism against conventional treatment, cancer relies on maintaining a delicate balance of oxidants to antioxidants, also known as the 'redox' balance. Tumours produce far more by-products than healthy cells as they are more metabolically active, e.g. metabolism creates ammonia and lactic acid. Consequently, these cells need more antioxidants than healthy cells (glutathione and cysteine) to quench the excess free radicals (ROS) that they produce. To acquire more antioxidants, most, if not all, chemo-resistant cancers have an overexpressed xCT cystine-glutamate antiporter system, also known as system Xc which features on the glutamine side of my Metro Map. This transporter is situated on the surface of the cell to pump extra cystine inside the cell to make glutathione, while exchanging the import of cysteine for the export of glutamate. Adding sulfasalazine, which blocks the xCT antiporter, to chemotherapy in hard to treat cancers like triple negative breast cancer, gliomas and pancreatic cancer can cause a marked inhibition of growth. Sulfasalazine also helps to stop seizures, a common side effect of both a primary or a secondary cancer in the brain.[255]

While chemo resistant cancers have an active ability to pump in extra supplies of the antioxidant cysteine (to make glutathione), they also actively pump out chemotherapy drugs (via an efflux pump), known as the P-glycoprotein or Multi Drug Resistance protein (MDR1). Fortunately this can be suppressed by the addition of the anti-parasitic drug mebendazole. Mebendazole also behaves like the chemotherapy drug vincristine, increasing ROS in the cell, which makes it a very useful low toxic addition to this Kill Phase. If you are on the COC protocol, which alternates mebendazole monthly with doxycycline, it might be worth combining ferroptosis drugs and supplements with mebendazole, before returning to a starve phase with the doxycycline. This is only a suggested approach, how long or how much you choose will depend on the aggressiveness of you cancer and how it responds.

255 Sontheimer H, Bridges RJ. Sulfasalazine for brain cancer fits. Expert Opin Investig Drugs. 2012 May;21(5):575-8. doi: 10.1517/13543784.2012.670634. Epub 2012 Mar 12. PMID: 22404218; PMCID: PMC3644176.

Varying the levels of ROS, the free radicals produced when a cell metabolises nutrients, can have different effects, so these can be divided into three stages.

- Low levels of ROS are normal, they are needed for healthy cellular signalling and metabolism.
- Then there is a narrow middle band where cancer cells survive with a raised level of ROS, neutralised by importing cysteine (through xCT antiporter).
- If the levels of ROS exceed this narrow band, the cancer defences are overwhelmed, and the excess ROS then causes cancer cell death as it cannot import cysteine in enough quantity to neutralise the free radicals. This is a key metabolic vulnerability of cancer, and it doesn't take too much extra ROS to trigger cancer cell death.

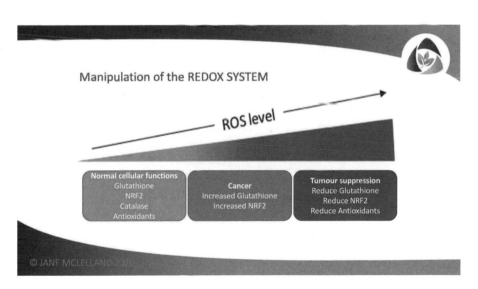

So, at higher doses, ROS can tip cancer into programmed cell death. Activating excess free radical levels is the way in which many chemotherapy drugs and radiotherapy work, but it is not a very selective treatment as it also targets healthy fast dividing cells as well. Ferroptosis is much more selective as the requirement for iron, cysteine and glutathione is that much greater in cancer cells. Depriving cancer of these vital nutrients makes their cells defenceless. Interestingly, they have recently discovered cisplatin, a commonly used chemotherapy drug, helps reduce cysteine and glutathione peroxidase activity so it could be a good partner for ferroptosis. Researchers discovered the combination of cisplatin and erastin (an inducer of ferroptosis), was found to be effective for colorectal and lung tumours.[256]

Since 2012 there has been an explosion of articles about ferroptosis with nearly a thousand on PubMed, yet only a handful of doctors use this vulnerability of cancer effectively. Many doctors use artemisinin with intravenous vitamin C, but this can be enhanced by suppressing the xCT antiporter or inhibiting the GPX4 enzyme by some of the drugs and supplements I have listed below.

As previously mentioned, intravenous vitamin C (IVC) used on its own to kill cancer has been highly controversial, and not very successful. It won't activate ferroptosis unless combined with the right combination of drugs and supplements. IVC is still only proven useful in a handful of cancers when used as a single agent, such as in KRAS and BRAF driven colorectal cancers and these cancers are also more sensitive to ferroptosis (Yang et al., 2014). Ever since the original trials by Pauling and Cameron using both IV and oral ascorbate were repeated by the Mayo clinic using oral only, IVC has been viewed with scorn and derision by the medical establishment. Given its potential for stimulating ferroptosis as a complementary cancer treatment, doctors are finally going to have to accept that high dose vitamin C really does work for cancer after all![257]

256 Guo J, Xu B, Han Q, Zhou H, Xia Y, Gong C, Dai X, Li Z, Wu G. Ferroptosis: A Novel Anti-tumor Action for Cisplatin. Cancer Res Treat. 2018 Apr;50(2):445-460. doi: 10.4143/crt.2016.572. Epub 2017 May 10. PMID: 28494534; PMCID: PMC5912137.

257 Liangfu Zhou, Lixiu Zhang, Shenghang Wang, Bin Zhao, Huanhuan Lv & Peng Shang (2020) Labile iron affects pharmacological ascorbate-induced toxicity in osteosarcoma cell lines, Free Radical Research, 54:6, 385-396, DOI: 10.1080/10715762.2020.1744577

The Riordan clinic use IVC the day after chemotherapy to reduce the toxicity of the chemotherapy drugs and to further boost and extend the free radical burst needed to kill off more tumour cells, the vitamin C specifically targeting cancer stem cells that the chemotherapy has left behind.[258]

In the same way that cancer is metabolically flexible to avoid being starved, it can also rewire its metabolism to avoid being killed by ferroptosis. There are several systems in place to block ferroptosis such as the FSP1/CoQ10/NAD(P)H that run parallel to the two key ferroptosis channels (xCT and the GPX4). It is important to acknowledge that failure to block these parallel routes in addition to the xCT and GPX4 may result in a less than satisfactory result. The FSP1 pathway creates CoQ10 and if you are taking this supplement don't even think about trying ferroptosis! Fortunately being on the H2SC (How To Starve Cancer) and COC protocol will prepare you for ferroptosis nicely as statins block CoQ10. The statins lovastatin, simvastatin and fluvastatin appear to have the best research so far for ferroptosis, but atorvastatin is likely a good candidate too as it is also lipophilic (fat loving).

Blocking all of the salvage routes below may not be necessary, but it is easy to add many of the ferroptosis supplements into your protocol. You can knock these back with a smoothie including watercress (PEITC) and cucumber (cucurbitacin B) alongside apple, carrot and beetroot to make it more palatable.

Note that many natural supplements are given the broad term 'antioxidants', but this does not mean you should necessarily cut these out during chemotherapy. Many supplements work on specific pathways that starve the cancer or reduce inflammation – these properties far outweigh their 'antioxidant' property. For example, green tea lowers

---

258 Combining vitamin C with antibiotics destroys cancer stem cells (medicalnewstoday.com)

catalase, which is far more important than its antioxidant property in controlling cancer and makes it a perfect partner for chemotherapy. Green tea's iron binding properties are very strong, so it needs to be stopped before you try ferroptosis, however its metabolite EGCG can be continued to be taken (at low dose) as this stimulates endoplasmic reticulum stress, triggering more ROS.

When you chelate iron, which removes the availability of free iron for ferroptosis, it prevents the formation of reactive radical species, protecting cancer cells from ferroptosis. A great many natural supplements and drugs chelate iron, including curcumin, so in order to induce ferroptosis, some of your cancer-starving supplements will need to be stopped, reduced or pulsed. Almost all polyphenols bind iron or prevent lipid peroxidation e.g. quercetin, IP6, baicalein, luteolin, and genistein, so these will need to be stopped during a ferroptosis phase.[259] Melatonin will also inhibit the process of ferroptosis, so avoid taking it during a ferroptosis phase. However I cannot sleep well without it, so perhaps pulse it during a ferroptosis phase if, like me, you cannot do without it.

Alpha lipoic acid is a strong antioxidant and I have seen it work very well in some people to starve their cancers as it can block a metabolic pathway (PDK) particularly when given IV. But for ferroptosis it needs to be stopped as it strongly chelates (binds) with iron and also has the potential to neutralise any free radicals, the opposite of what you want to achieve.

It is crucial to understand the process of inducing ferroptosis is unique and it requires a complete change of tack, not only to starving cancer but also to other methods of triggering ROS for a Kill Phase. It is important to know what to take and what to leave out if you want to try this

---

259 Cai Q, Rahn KO, Zhang R. 1997. Dietary flavonoids, quercetin, luteolin and genistein, reduce oxidative DNA damage and lipid peroxidation and quench free radicals. Cancer Letters 119:99-107.

approach. To ensure effective ferroptosis, it might be best to err on the safe side and stop all supplements and drugs not listed in this section other than conventional chemotherapy, radiotherapy, immunotherapy and targeted drugs.

Instead of blocking most of the pathways on the Metro Map as you would when starving cancer in combination with chemotherapy and radiotherapy, with ferroptosis you want to leave some pathways open and unblocked, specifically glutaminolysis and autophagy. Glutaminolysis may contribute to lipid peroxidation by providing precursors for fatty acid or lipid synthesis. Autophagy is required for ferritinophagy, the degradation of ferritin in the lysosome, an enclosed digestive sack-like organelle. So not only do you need a totally different set of supplements and drugs during this phase, your diet will need to change too.

The Ferroptosis Diet

In some ways it is restrictive, but in other ways you can be permitted some foods you may otherwise avoid.

- Methionine can be converted to cysteine through the transsulfuration pathway, so a methionine and cysteine-free diet for a couple of weeks may be advantageous before you start. If you are not already doing so, this means a switch to a vegan diet. Avoid meat, fish and eggs. Eat mainly vegetable proteins.
- Increase glutamate during ferroptosis days as this blocks cysteine import into the cell. Glutamate is the 'umami' flavour in foods and is found in mushrooms, tamari, miso, soy sauce, tomato paste, and parmesan cheese (in moderation – it also contains beneficial buytrate). Do not take MSG.

- A ketogenic diet may not be helpful as nutrient starvation may actually hinder ferroptosis, but you should still stick to low glycaemic foods.[260]

- Even the fats you consume will need to be different, with a big emphasis on PUFA fats - omega 3 oils like flaxseed and walnut oil which oxidise easily (peroxidation). Monounsaturated fatty acid (MUFA) oleic acid found in many oils, especially olive oil, can inhibit ferroptosis by competing with PUFAs for incorporation into the phospholipid fatty membrane.[261] To avoid MUFA oils on Ferroptosis days, avoid olives and olive oil, avocados, nuts (e.g. almonds, cashews, pecans and macadamias) and nut butters and peanut oil.

- Omega 3 PUFA oils DHA and EPA will help activate ferroptosis but supplements are almost always combined with tocopherol (vitamin E), a very powerful inhibitor of ferroptosis. Instead, for this phase it might be best to use cod liver oil rather than traditional omega 3 oils as cod liver oil is stabilised by vitamin A and D rather than vitamin E.[262]

- Selenium also needs to be given a wide berth, so no brazil nuts, as these contain naturally high amounts. Both vitamin E and selenium inhibit lipid peroxidation.[263] As selenium is a heavy metal, it is best pulsed in your treatment protocol in any case, and perhaps should be stopped at least a week before a ferroptosis phase.

- As with all Kill Phases, the avoidance of NAC (N-acetyl cysteine) is paramount. NAC is naturally present in most meat, fish, chicken and bone broth, lentils, peas and asparagus. Pre-

260 Energy Stress Inhibits Ferroptotic Cell Death via AMPK Activation Cancer Discov April 1 2020 (10) (4) 485; DOI: 10.1158/2159-8290.CD-RW2020-023

261 Magtanong, L. et al. Exogenous monounsaturated fatty acids promote a ferroptosis-resistant cell state. Cell Chem. Biol. 26, 420–432.e429 (2019).

262 Dyck MC, Ma DW, Meckling KA. The anticancer effects of Vitamin D and omega-3 PUFAs in combination via cod-liver oil: one plus one may equal more than two. Med Hypotheses. 2011 Sep;77(3):326-32. doi: 10.1016/j.mehy.2011.05.006. Epub 2011 May 31. PMID: 21632182.

263 BIERI, J. An Effect of Selenium and Cystine on Lipide Peroxidation in Tissues Deficient in Vitamin E. Nature 184, 1148–1149 (1959). https://doi.org/10.1038/1841148a0

treatment with NAC prevents ferroptosis. Sadly articles on the internet from doctors and biochemists claiming this amino acid will 'starve cancer' has led to many patients failing treatment. Yes, it may affect lactate transport, but it also drives resistance by boosting cancer's cellular defence, as mentioned above. You really need to know what you are doing if you add it into your programme. NAC may block lactate transport in Stage 0 DCIS, but this is hardly cancer at all compared to other cancers and I have witnessed many cancers metastasise and spread after being given NAC by well-meaning doctors. The same can be said of CoQ10. I am repeating myself, but this is important. For a Kill Phase, especially when inducing ferroptosis, you need to block CoQ10 formation with a statin and avoid supplementation. Exceptions to this will be people highly sensitive to statins, but during your starve phase you can lower statin intake if you combine it with delta tocotrienol. Lovastatin and delta tocotrienol is a particularly good combination for bone metastases and osteoporosis (they synergistically block cholesterol pathways).[264]

- Some supplements can activate a powerful detox pathway called NRF2, a cellular protector. This is the NRF2 paradox, activators of this pathway show wonderful results for starving and protecting against cancer, but these also protect cancer from the levels of ROS necessary to destroy them. Taking sulforaphane, milk thistle, indole 3 carbinol, DIM and resveratrol will all activate NRF2 and prevent ferroptosis. NRF2 has been linked to reactivating dormant breast cancer cells after treatment, which is another reason to try this ferroptosis protocol to thoroughly eradicate the chances of it returning, even if you are NED (no evidence of disease).[265] This means no broccoli sprouts the day before or on the days of ferroptosis treatment either.

264 Abdul-Majeed S, Mohamed N, Soelaiman IN. Effects of tocotrienol and lovastatin combination on osteoblast and osteoclast activity in estrogen-deficient osteoporosis. Evid Based Complement Alternat Med. 2012;2012:960742. doi: 10.1155/2012/960742. Epub 2012 Aug 13. PMID: 22927884; PMCID: PMC3425381.

265 Fox, Douglas B et al. "NRF2 activation promotes the recurrence of dormant tumour cells through regulation of redox and nucleotide metabolism." Nature metabolism vol. 2,4 (2020): 318-334. doi:10.1038/s42255-020-0191-z

- Pomegranate is to be avoided too. Not only does pomegranate juice contain vitamin E, it activates NRF2 as it contains both ellagic acid and luteolin, and if you have prostate cancer you need to be aware that if you drink pomegranate juice before you exercise you cancel out any of the beneficial effects of either![266] Despite each having tremendous benefits for cancer individually, together they fail to work at all! This shows the importance of defining a starve phase and a kill phase.

- Trigonelline, a NRF2 inhibitor, is the major compound of fenugreek, which enhances both ferroptosis and the effects of exercise, increasing muscle size and power. Despite stimulating growth in muscles through mTOR, its anti-cancer potential outweighs this growth effect because of its NRF2 inhibition. For prostate cancer patients on ADT, dismayed at your diminishing muscles, this is just what you need. Forget the pomegranate juice on exercise days, add some ground fenugreek to your meals. On starve phase days cinnamon helps with erectile function as well as blocking mTOR, but avoid on ferroptosis days as it may block the lipid peroxidation. Note that fenugreek activates the oestrogen receptor, but predominantly ER beta which is protective for both breast and prostate cancer.[267]

- Consume lots of watercress which contains phenethyl isothiocyanate (PEITC) and cucumber or bitter melon (Cucurbitacin B) on ferroptosis days.

- Anaemia is a common problem amongst cancer patients, caused by either the disease or by bone marrow suppression following chemotherapy. The result is hypoxia (oxygen is not delivered to the tissues) which can stimulate the formation of

266 Jordan Gueritat, Françoise RannouBekono, Amélie Rebillard et al Exercise training combined with antioxidant supplementation prevents the antiproliferative activity of single treatment in prostate cancer through inhibition of redox adaptation, Free Radical Biology and Medicine, http://dx.doi.org/10.1016/j.freeradbiomed.2014.09.009

267 Yusharyahya SN, Bramono K, Hestiantoro A, Edwar SQ, Kusuma I. Fenugreek (Trigonella foenum-graceum) increases postmenopausal fibroblast-associated COL1A1 and COL3A1 production dominantly through its binding to estrogen receptor beta. J Appl Pharm Sci, 2020; 10(04):022–027.

hypoxia-inducible factor 1-alpha (HIF-1α) which can then drive further cancer. Holo-lactoferrin significantly enhanced erastin treatment (ferroptosis) in triple negative breast cancer and prevented the hypoxic environment. Holo-lactoferrin is an iron-saturated form of lactoferrin which is synergistic with ferroptosis inducers whereas apo-lactoferrin inhibits ferroptosis. The hypoxic environment can also be helped by taking extracts of pawpaw (Asimina triloba) and/or chrysin, as both inhibit hypoxia-inducible factor-1 (HIF-1) signaling. Take both for a few weeks before commencing ferroptosis, but this may reduce lipid peroxidation so they need to be stopped 24-48 hours before starting ferroptosis.[268] Noscapine, a drug found in many over the counter cough medicines with a mild analgesic effect can also help stop unwanted HIF-1 and could be continued through the ferroptosis phase. Red and pinto beans contain kaempferol which inhibits iron absorption, even with the addition of vitamin C. However eating white beans can help increase iron levels, despite containing lower iron levels as they have more bioavailable iron. Yellow Dock or Burdock root can help raise ferritin levels before commencing ferroptosis but stop during treatment as these can inhibit lipid peroxidation. Parietin, a compound that inhibits 6GPD, an important pathway to block for both starving and killing cancer, and chrysophanol which helps inhibit glutathione peroxidase can both be found in Syrian Rhubarb.

The two main ways to trigger Ferroptosis are:

1. By blocking the xCT cystine-glutamate antiporter which imports cystine to convert it to cysteine to create the antioxidant glutathione (see illustration below). At the same time it pumps out glutamate, raising extracellular glutamate levels which also helps trigger ferroptosis.

268 Lirdprapamongkol, K., Sakurai, H., Abdelhamed, S., Yokoyama, S., Maruyama, T., Athikomkulchai, S. ... Saiki, I. (2013). A flavonoid chrysin suppresses hypoxic survival and metastatic growth of mouse breast cancer cells. Oncology Reports, 30, 2357-2364. https://doi.org/10.3892/or.2013.2667

2. Blocking the glutathione peroxidase enzyme (GPX4).

Diffuse large B cell lymphomas and renal cell carcinomas are particularly susceptible to GPX4-regulated ferroptosis, so the primary focus for these two cancers should be on this pathway, whereas all other cancers rely more on the xCT antiporter. The antiporter is expressed in many resistant tumours and is associated with tumour proliferation, invasion, metastasis and drug resistance.

To activate ferroptosis you require

1. A lowering of cellular glutathione(GSH) levels by inhibiting xCT antiporter.
2. The presence of phospholipids containing polyunsaturated fatty acids; these are the substrates for peroxidation.
3. The accumulation of iron-dependent ROS. Iron needs to be present both in the labile iron pool in the cytoplasm of the cell and as iron-dependent lipoxygenases, to drive the peroxidation process.
4. Glutathione peroxidase 4 (GPX4) inhibitors which prevent the complex repair system that eliminates lipid peroxidation products.

It is only when all these are met, that conditions are ripe for ferroptosis.

The xCT Cystine Glutamate Antiporter

The xCT pathway is the main route for tumours to recruit cysteine, drawing it into the cell while pushing out glutamate. Once inside the cell, the cystine is converted to cysteine, which is then combined with glutamate and converted into glutathione. This pathway is under the control of NRF2 which is a major cellular detox pathway, activated by compounds like sulforaphane in broccoli sprouts. Sulforaphane is a wonderful detoxifying agent, great during a Starve Phase, but stop 48 hours before a Kill Phase as it will activate NRF2 and prevent ferroptosis.

Results blocking the xCT on its own in vitro looked fantastic, but when these were repeated in vivo, there was an initial drop in progression, but then the cancer learnt to compensate by using other salvage pathways to recruit cysteine and cancer growth returned.

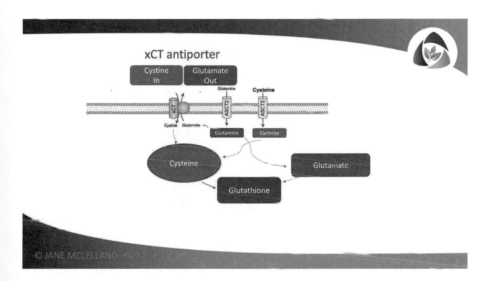

The Treatment Protocol

One of the most experienced doctors in this field is Dr Ahmed Elsakka, an oncologist in Cairo who has been using ferroptosis for several years using daily sulfasalazine to block the xCT antiporter. He also prescribes lipososmal artemisinin and withaferin A, nitazoxanide, EGCG and he pulses intravenous vitamin C to stimulate the oxidative stress. He also adds leflunomide (a DHODH inhibitor) at low dose as it synergistically helps prevent cancer defence against upregulation the GPX4 enzyme. Dihydroorotate dehydrogenase (DHODH) an enzyme in the pentose phosphate pathway operates in parallel to mitochondrial GPX4 to produce CoQ10 which inhibits ferroptosis. He often adds hyperbaric oxygen therapy (HBOT) and exercise with oxygen to increase the effects. Dr Elsakka uses quite a high dose of sulfasalazine (4-8g a day) which needs to be given in divided doses every six hours to be effective. The addition of other xCT inhibitors such as piperlongumine, feverfew or sodium selenite (the latter is compounded by some doctors for medical use) could reduce the dosage of sulfasalazine.

Before starting ferroptosis, Dr Elsakka checks certain parameters are met as this will improve the chances of success. To evaluate patient suitability before commencing treatment, Dr Elsakka checks the following:

- Ferritin level
- Total Iron Profile
  - Serum ferritin
  - Transferrin saturation (FESA)
  - Total iron and unsaturated binding capacity
- Homocysteine level
- ESR – Erythrocyte Sedimentation Rate
- MTHFR status. If positive this will reduce homocysteine clearance and the trans-sulphuration pathway which will affect effectiveness. 70% of cancer patients have this mutation which affects folate levels and homocysteine.
- Lactate to pyruvate ratio
- NADH levels (this can recycle glutathione)

The iron profile is the best way to tell the difference between iron deficiency (not enough iron in your blood) and anaemia. Iron deficiency anaemia is more prevalent in babies, children, young teenagers, and pregnant women. The iron profile is also helpful for discovering iron overload (having too much iron in your blood).

Patients receiving blood transfusions will have higher than normal ferritin levels. The ratio of ESR to Ferritin levels will help determine whether it is appropriate to attempt ferroptosis.

If you divide the Ferritin level by the ESR, a normal level should be less than 11.5.

A high ESR to ferritin ratio indicates inflammation or autoimmune disease. If this is the case Dr Elsakka uses LDN and mistletoe as a primary approach to help normalise levels prior to ferroptosis.

Dr Elsakka repeats the ESR:Fe ratio every two weeks and if the ferritin level is higher and ESR drops, then he commences ferroptosis.

To prevent the activation of salvage pathways where cancer cells replenish their stores of cysteine, Dr Elsakka recommends inhibiting the transsulfuration pathway before commencing ferroptosis. This pathway creates homocysteine from methionine and then homocysteine becomes an alternative source of cysteine for cancer cells. He looks for a homocysteine level of less than 15 micromoles per litre (mcmol/l) and as close to 10 mcmol/l as possible before starting treatment.

To normalise homocysteine

- Eat a methionine and cysteine free diet
- Take Betaine Anhydrase 50mg/kg bid (e.g. if you weigh 60kg take 3g bid) or TMG
- 5-methyltetrahydrofolate
- Vitamin B6
- Methylcobalamin
- Choline

Dr Elsakka measures homocysteine levels once a fortnight – if it is high, then it may not be worth trying ferroptosis until levels are lower.

The xCT antiporter is considered to be the main transporter of cystine in cancer to create glutathione and a key regulator of ferroptosis. The xCT is controlled by nuclear factor erythroid 2-related factor 2 (NRF2), a master regulator of the cellular redox state so this needs to be inhibited in concert with the xCT to ensure ferroptosis is stimulated adequately. Cancer strongly resists attempts to lower glutathione to survive and there are several escape routes it uses to replenish its stores by importing or creating cysteine from other sources. How many of the following pathways or which combination may be best will vary between cancer types.

To achieve ferroptosis, blocking these routes is essential, so add at least one of each:

- **Increase concentration of iron in cells:** dihydroartemisinin or artesunate, ironomycin (salinomycin)[269] The addition of extra **iron is not recommended and may end up fuelling further cancer.**
- **Produce H2O2 free radicals:** IV vitamin C, dihydroartemisinin or artesunate

269 Mai TT, Hamaï A, Hienzsch A, Cañeque T, Müller S, Wicinski J, Cabaud O, Leroy C, David A, Acevedo V, Ryo A, Ginestier C, Birnbaum D, Charafe-Jauffret E, Codogno P, Mehrpour M, Rodriguez R. Salinomycin kills cancer stem cells by sequestering iron in lysosomes. Nat Chem. 2017 Oct;9(10):1025-1033. doi: 10.1038/nchem.2778. Epub 2017 May 16. PMID: 28937680; PMCID: PMC5890907

- **To inhibit xCT/lower glutathione (GSH):** Sulfasalazine, sodium selenite, erastin or sorafenib. Also assisted by Piperlongumine,[270] Parthenolide[271]

- **To inhibit GPX4:** PEITC[272], Dihydrotanshinone (danshen)[273,] lipophilic statins, Heteronemin, RSL3, Cucurbitacin B,[274] Withaferin A (Ashwagandha), Chrysophanol (oral cancer), Altretamine (a treatment for ovarian cancer),

- **FPSP1 (ferroptosis suppressor protein – regenerates CoQ10):** Statins

- **DHODH (Dihydroorotate dehydrogenase – regenerates Coq10):** Brequinaar, Leflunomide[275]

- **Protect neurons with HDAC inhibitors:** beta hydroxybutyric acid or sodium valproate[276]

270 Yamaguchi Y, Kasukabe T, Kumakura S. Piperlongumine rapidly induces the death of human pancreatic cancer cells mainly through the induction of ferroptosis. Int J Oncol. 2018 Mar;52(3).1011-1022. doi: 10.3892/ijo.2018.4259. Epub 2018 Jan 31. PMID: 29393418.

271 Pei S, Minhajuddin M, Callahan KP, Balys M, Ashton JM, Neering SJ, Lagadinou ED, Corbett C, Ye H, Liesveld JL, O'Dwyer KM, Li Z, Shi L, Greninger P, Settleman J, Benes C, Hagen FK, Munger J, Crooks PA, Becker MW, Jordan CT. Targeting aberrant glutathione metabolism to eradicate human acute myelogenous leukemia cells. J Biol Chem. 2013 Nov 22;288(47):33542-33558. doi: 10.1074/jbc.M113.511170. Epub 2013 Oct 2. PMID: 24089526; PMCID: PMC3837103

272 Lv H, Zhen C, Liu J, Shang P. β-Phenethyl Isothiocyanate Induces Cell Death in Human Osteosarcoma through Altering Iron Metabolism, Disturbing the Redox Balance, and Activating the MAPK Signaling Pathway. Oxid Med Cell Longev. 2020 Apr 4;2020:5021983. doi: 10.1155/2020/5021983. PMID: 32322335; PMCID: PMC7160723.

273 Tan S, Hou X and Mei L: Dihydrotanshinone I inhibits human glioma cell proliferation via the activation of ferroptosis. Oncol Lett 20: 122, 2020

274 Huang, S., Cao, B., Zhang, J. et al. Induction of ferroptosis in human nasopharyngeal cancer cells by cucurbitacin B: molecular mechanism and therapeutic potential. Cell Death Dis 12, 237 (2021). https://doi.org/10.1038/s41419-021-03516-y

275 Mao, C., Liu, X., Zhang, Y. et al. DHODH-mediated ferroptosis defence is a targetable vulnerability in cancer. Nature (2021). https://doi.org/10.1038/s41586-021-03539-7

276 Zille M, Kumar A, Kundu N, Bourassa MW, Wong VSC, Willis D, Karuppagounder SS, Ratan RR. Ferroptosis in Neurons and Cancer Cells Is Similar But Differentially Regulated by Histone Deacetylase Inhibitors. eNeuro. 2019 Feb 15;6(1):ENEURO.0263-18.2019. doi: 10.1523/ENEURO.0263-18.2019. PMID: 30783618; PMCID: PMC6378329.

- **Inhibit glutathione-s-transferase:** artesunate, nitazoxanide[277]

Sulfasalazine, which is a disease-modifying antirheumatic drug (DMARD), has long been used to treat rheumatoid arthritis and ulcerative colitis and is now being repurposed for cancer treatment. Leflunomide, another DMARD is a dihydroorotate dehydrogenase (DHODH) inhibitor, an enzyme of the pentose phosphate pathway, which been shown to synergise with sulfasalazine to promote ferroptosis. Other DMARDs are also included in my list of drugs to induce ferroptosis - methotrexate and auranofin. These provide alternative options for you, but make sure you choose combinations that are not toxic by seeking professional advice.

Salinomycin is an old antibiotic, used in chicken feed and now being repurposed for cancer treatment as it was found to kill breast cancer stem cell 100 times more effectively than the chemotherapy drug paclitaxel by triggering ferroptosis but it is potentially toxic at the wrong dose. A derivative, ironomycin is even more effective (ten times stronger than salinomycin with less side effects) but as yet there are no clinical trials for either.[278] Where possible, add the supplement options and if after a month of ferroptosis there is no improvement, then consider adding extra drugs, but check with your doctor first for interactions.

Piperlongumine, an extract from long pepper (Piper longum) has a multitude of benefits for cancer, it can be used both in the starve and kill phase and it enhances the blocking of the xCT antiporter by sulfasalazine. Parthenolide, a compound found in the botanical feverfew, also reduces cysteine and is being investigated for use in several cancers including paediatric leukaemia and colorectal cancer.

---

277 Shakya A, Bhat HR, Ghosh SK. Update on Nitazoxanide: A Multifunctional Chemotherapeutic Agent. Curr Drug Discov Technol. 2018;15(3):201-213. doi: 10.2174/1570163814666170727130003. PMID: 28748751.

278 Zhao, B., Li, X., Wang, Y. et al. Iron-dependent cell death as executioner of cancer stem cells. J Exp Clin Cancer Res 37, 79 (2018). https://doi.org/10.1186/s13046-018-0733-3

The following pathways are the key 'salvage' or escape routes I have discovered so far. Cancer cells upregulate these salvage routes to stop ferroptosis, so just as with blocking the routes on the Metro Map, do not get hung up on exactly what each pathway means, you just need to understand that adding supplements (or drugs) to block these may improve ferroptosis. I have gone overboard here, you won't necessarily need all the supplements and drugs on this list but if you are already on either cisplatin, lapatinib or sorafenib, then you are in luck! Adding some of the following protocol will enhance the anticancer effects. The HER2 targeted drug neratinib was also found to induce ferroptosis, but the mechanism for how it does this is not yet clear, but this could be another synergistic drug with other ferroptosis inducers for this set of breast cancer patients or for other cancers with overexpressed HER2.

- Lower cysteine in the cancer cell.
- Increase uptake of iron in the cancer tissues.
- Inhibit the xCT cystine glutamate antiporter to reduce the import of cystine.
- Lower Glutathione peroxidase (GPX4) the enzyme that protects against lipid peroxidation.
- Block DHODH, upregulated when GPX4 is inhibited.
- Reduce NRF2 which is a major cellular detox pathway.
- Inhibit thioredoxin reductase 1 (TrxR1) - a selenocysteine-containing antioxidant enzyme.
- Stop intake of antioxidants like vitamin E, CoQ10, ALA.
- Stop taking certain polyphenols and iron chelators like green tea, IP6.
- Inhibit FSP1 (CoQ10) mevalonate pathway.
- Block the transsulfuration pathway which converts methionine to cysteine.
- STAT3 suppresses expression of ACSL4, an enzyme that enriches membranes with long polyunsaturated fatty acids and is required for ferroptosis.

- Modulate haem oxygenase-1 (HO-1).

- Allow glutaminolysis.

- Allow autophagy.

- Increase lysosomal permeabilisation.

- Some chemotherapies e.g. cisplatin, methotrexate are weak inducers of ferroptosis.

- Some TKIs are inducers of ferroptosis e.g. sorafenib, lapatinib.

- Increase glutamate (within reason) as this also helps block the xCT antiporter. Be cautious if you have a brain tumour.

- Block the oestrogen receptor as it inhibits the effect of sulfasalazine.

- Avoid autophagy inhibitors as ferritinophagy is required to breakdown iron.

- Inhibit the gamma-glutamyl cycle –making cysteine from glutathione is one of the main functions of this cycle.

- Block Prominin 2, a pathway using cholesterol and ceramides to form vesicles (exosomes) to remove iron from cells.

- VDAC2/3, opening the voltage dependant anion channel in mitochondria.[279] VDAC proteins regulate the flux of small ions (Cl-, K+, Na+, and Ca2+) which participate in fatty acid transport and cholesterol distribution in mitochondrial membranes.

- Inhibit Stearoyl-CoA Desaturase 1 (SCD1) which is involved in the synthesis of monounsaturated fatty acids for fatty components of cell membranes. This enzyme is regulated by TP53 and BAP1 (tumour suppressor genes). Tumours with these two common mutations might benefit significantly from inhibition of SCD1.

Whilst stimulating ferroptosis is important in cancer cells, it is equally important to prevent damage to healthy cells, especially neurons which are particularly vulnerable to ferroptosis. Over the long term ferroptosis is linked to Alzheimer's and Parkinson's, kidney and liver problems.

---

279 Mathupala SP, Pedersen PL. Voltage dependent anion channel-1 (VDAC-1) as an anti-cancer target. Cancer Biol Ther. 2010;9(12):1053-1056. doi:10.4161/cbt.9.12.12451

Fortunately the addition of histone deacetylase (HDAC) inhibitors not only prevents damage to neurons, but also enhances ferroptosis.[280] The addition of beta hydroxybutyric Acid (BHBA), a ketone and HDAC inhibitor, can prevent damage to neuronal cells, but rather than producing the butyrate endogenously (in the body) by following a strict ketogenic diet during this phase, an exogenous source may be best. In Oxphos-driven cancers or where ketones may fuel cancer (Braf-driven), such as in some types of colon cancer or melanomas, another HDAC inhibitor might be better, valproic acid, which is normally prescribed to prevent brain seizures or bipolar syndrome. [281][282]

The day after IVC treatment you might need to check ferritin levels again. A strong response to IVC can create many dead cancer cells which can then release a lot of iron. This might be taken up by remaining cancer cells, an unwelcome consequence that might fuel cancer growth. If you discover there is a large amount of ferritin released into the blood, it may be worth having an iron chelator to remove the excess. Dr Taufiq Benjemain in Australia has witnessed the effectiveness of IV artesunate and vitamin C, with ferritin levels in the thousands. This is not only potentially dangerous, it makes the patient feel lousy. He often uses deferoxamine, an iron chelator and ferroptosis inhibitor, the day after IV therapy to prevent and limit any side effects of this iron release. Baicalein can also help reverse ferroptosis, even at low doses it has been shown to offer protection to the brain as it strongly inhibits ferroptosis so might

280 Zille M, Kumar A, Kundu N, Bourassa MW, Wong VSC, Willis D, Karuppagounder SS, Ratan RR. Ferroptosis in Neurons and Cancer Cells Is Similar But Differentially Regulated by Histone Deacetylase Inhibitors. eNeuro. 2019 Feb 15;6(1):ENEURO.0263-18.2019. doi: 10.1523/ENEURO.0263-18.2019. PMID: 30783618; PMCID: PMC6378329.
281 Shakery, Azam et al. "Beta-Hydroxybutyrate Promotes Proliferation, Migration and Stemness in a Subpopulation of 5FU Treated SW480 Cells: Evidence for Metabolic Plasticity in Colon Cancer." Asian Pacific journal of cancer prevention : APJCP vol. 19,11 3287-3294. 29 Nov. 2018, doi:10.31557/APJCP.2018.19.11.3287
282 Sodium valproate protects against neuronal ferroptosis in epilepsy via suppressing lysyl oxidase Qin Li, Qiu-Qi Li, Ji-Ning Jia, Zhao-Qian Liu, Hong-Hao Zhou, Wei-Lin Jin, Xiao-Yuan Mao

be a useful addition the day after IVC. Baicalein is extracted from Blue Skullcap and is used extensively in Chinese medicine (Huang Qin) and has many powerful anticancer effects to trigger apoptosis, but it acts in opposition to ferroptosis. It has a short elimination half-life (6.36 ± 5.85 h) but it is important to stop taking it at least 48 hours before recommencing ferroptosis.

To address these pathways, the following list of supplements and drugs will help inhibit the cellular reprogramming. Acetaminophen (Tylenol, paracetamol) is available over the counter, which, when taken at normal dosages on its own, is safe, but be aware that you are also lowering glutathione in other ways and it is notorious for inducing liver failure because of its ability to lower glutathione in the liver.[283] A low dose may be advisable if you choose to add it, but take advice and check for interactions.[284]

Only add extra drugs after consulting with your doctor or pharmacist.[285] Blocking many of these pathways e.g. NRF2, thioredoxin and xCT will also enhance and synergise with chemotherapy treatment:

283 Yamada N, Karasawa T, Takahashi M. Role of ferroptosis in acetaminophen-induced hepatotoxicity. Arch Toxicol. 2020 May;94(5):1769-1770. doi: 10.1007/s00204-020-02714-5. Epub 2020 Mar 16. PMID: 32180037.

284 Benson GD, Koff RS, Tolman KG. The therapeutic use of acetaminophen in patients with liver disease. Am J Ther. 2005 Mar-Apr;12(2):133-41. doi: 10.1097/01.mjt.0000140216.40700.95. PMID: 15767831.

285 Benson GD, Koff RS, Tolman KG. The therapeutic use of acetaminophen in patients with liver disease. Am J Ther. 2005 Mar-Apr;12(2):133-41. doi: 10.1097/01.mjt.0000140216.40700.95. PMID: 15767831.

- To inhibit NRF2: Brutasol,[286] Trigonelline,[287] Ibuprofen (GBM)[288]

- To inhibit Thioredoxin: Piperlongumine, Gambogic Acid,[289] Auranofin, isoforretin A (Rhabdosia rubescens)[290]

- Inhibit Stat3 and increase autophagy: Phenethyl Isothiocyanate (PEITC)

- Inhibit mTOR and increase autophagy: Metformin,[291] Dihydroartemesinin, 6-Gingerol[292]

- Inhibit NADPH-dependent CoQ10: Simvastatin, Lovastatin, Atorvastatin

286 Ren D, Villeneuve NF, Jiang T, Wu T, Lau A, Toppin HA, Zhang DD. Brusatol enhances the efficacy of chemotherapy by inhibiting the Nrf2-mediated defense mechanism. Proc Natl Acad Sci U S A. 2011 Jan 25;108(4):1433-8. doi: 10.1073/pnas.1014275108. Epub 2011 Jan 4. PMID: 21205897; PMCID: PMC3029730

287 Roh, Jong-Lyel et al. "Nrf2 inhibition reverses the resistance of cisplatin-resistant head and neck cancer cells to artesunate-induced ferroptosis." Redox biology vol. 11 (2017): 254-262. doi:10.1016/j.redox.2016.12.010

288 Gao X, Guo N, Xu H, Pan T, Lei H, Yan A, Mi Y, Xu L. Ibuprofen induces ferroptosis of glioblastoma cells via downregulation of nuclear factor erythroid 2-related factor 2 signaling pathway. Anticancer Drugs. 2020 Jan;31(1):27-34. doi: 10.1097/CAD.0000000000000825. PMID: 31490283.

289 Pan H, Jansson KH, Beshiri ML, Yin J, Fang L, Agarwal S, Nguyen H, Corey E, Zhang Y, Liu J, Fan H, Lin H, Kelly K. Gambogic acid inhibits thioredoxin activity and induces ROS-mediated cell death in castration-resistant prostate cancer. Oncotarget. 2017 Aug 24;8(44):77181-77194. doi: 10.18632/oncotarget.20424. PMID: 29100379; PMCID: PMC5652772.

290 Sun X, Wang W, Chen J, Cai X, Yang J, Yang Y, Yan H, Cheng X, Ye J, Lu W, Hu C, Sun H, Pu J, Cao P. The Natural Diterpenoid Isoforretin A Inhibits Thioredoxin-1 and Triggers Potent ROS-Mediated Antitumor Effects. Cancer Res. 2017 Feb 15;77(4):926-936. doi: 10.1158/0008-5472.CAN-16-0987. Epub 2016 Dec 23. PMID: 28011619.

291 Hou Y, Cai S, Yu S, Lin H. Metformin induces ferroptosis by targeting miR-324-3p/GPX4 axis in breast cancer. Acta Biochim Biophys Sin (Shanghai). 2021 Mar 2;53(3):333-341. doi: 10.1093/abbs/gmaa180. PMID: 33522578.

292 Tsai Y, Xia C, Sun Z. The Inhibitory Effect of 6-Gingerol on Ubiquitin-Specific Peptidase 14 Enhances Autophagy-Dependent Ferroptosis and Anti-Tumor in vivo and in vitro. Front Pharmacol. 2020 Nov 13;11:598555. doi: 10.3389/fphar.2020.598555. PMID: 33281606; PMCID: PMC7691590.

- Inhibit NADPH via G6PD and 6PGD inhibition:
  - G6PD: Intravenous vitamin C
  - 6PGD: Ketotifen (antihistamine), Methotrexate, physcion (parietin)[293] found in Syrian Rhubarb. Chrysin and fermented wheat germ also block 6PGD but these may stop the lipid peroxidation which is needed for ferroptosis. Use these during a starve phase.
- Increase PUFA oxidising lipids: Flaxseed, GLA, EPA, DHA, Walnut oil. Avoid MUFAs like oleic acid.
- Increase uptake of iron in the cancer tissues. Lactoferrin, Holo-lactoferrin[294] Haloperidol[295] Pioglitazone[296] (Head and neck cancer)
- Transferrin and ferroportin: Ruscogenin (Butcher's Broom)[297]

293 Niu Y, Zhang J, Tong Y, Li J, Liu B. Physcion 8-O-β-glucopyranoside induced ferroptosis via regulating miR-103a-3p/GLS2 axis in gastric cancer. Life Sci. 2019 Nov 15;237:116893. doi: 10.1016/j.lfs.2019.116893. Epub 2019 Oct 10. PMID: 31606381.

294 Zhang Z, Lu M, Chen C, Tong X, Li Y, Yang K, Lv H, Xu J, Qin L. Holo-lactoferrin: the link between ferroptosis and radiotherapy in triple-negative breast cancer. Theranostics 2021; 11(7):3167-3182. doi:10.7150/thno.52028. Available from https://www.thno.org/v11p3167.htm

295 Tao Bai, Shuai Wang, Yuling Sun et al, Haloperidol, a sigma receptor 1 antagonist, promotes ferroptosis in hepatocellular carcinoma cells. Biochemical and Biophysical Research Communications, Volume 491, Issue 4, 2017,

296 Eun Hye Kim, Daiha Shin, Jaewang Lee, Ah Ra Jung, Jong-Lyel Roh, CISD2 inhibition overcomes resistance to sulfasalazine-induced ferroptotic cell death in head and neck cancer, Cancer Letters, Volume 432, 2018, ISSN 0304-3835, https://doi.org/10.1016/j.canlet.2018.06.018.

297 Song Z, Xiang X, Li J, et al. Ruscogenin induces ferroptosis in pancreatic cancer cells. Oncol Rep. 2020;43(2):516-524. doi:10.3892/or.2019.7425

- Increase lysosomal permeability: Sirasemine[298], Clemastine, Disulfiram[299]

- Increase glutamate (avoid excess intake if you have a brain tumour as you do not want to trigger seizures) – tomato paste, mushrooms, soy or tamari sauce, peas, walnuts. Do not take monosodium glutamate (MSG) as this can have many detrimental effects.

- Reduce cysteine: Cysteinase (PDAC),[300] Cisplatin, Acetaminophen[301]

- Modulate heme oxygenase-1 (HO-1): Lapatanib, Acetaminophen Andrographis[302] (CRC), Ginkgetin (NSCLC),[303] Haloperidol[304]

---

298 Ma S, Dielschneider RF, Henson ES, Xiao W, Choquette TR, et al. (2017) Ferroptosis and autophagy induced cell death occur independently after siramesine and lapatinib treatment in breast cancer cells. PLOS ONE 12(8): e0182921. https://doi.org/10.1371/journal.pone.0182921

299 Qiu C, Zhang X, Huang B, Wang S, Zhou W, Li C, Li X, Wang J, Yang N. Disulfiram, a Ferroptosis Inducer, Triggers Lysosomal Membrane Permeabilization by Up-Regulating ROS in Glioblastoma. Onco Targets Ther. 2020 Oct 20;13.10631-10640 doi: 10.2147/OTT.S272312. PMID: 33116640; PMCID: PMC7585819.

300 Badgley MA, Kremer DM, Maurer HC, DelGiorno KE, Lee HJ, Purohit V, Sagalovskiy IR, Ma A, Kapilian J, Firl CEM, Decker AR, Sastra SA, Palermo CF, Andrade LR, Sajjakulnukit P, Zhang L, Tolstyka ZP, Hirschhorn T, Lamb C, Liu T, Gu W, Seeley ES, Stone E, Georgiou G, Manor U, Iuga A, Wahl GM, Stockwell BR, Lyssiotis CA, Olive KP. Cysteine depletion induces pancreatic tumor ferroptosis in mice. Science. 2020 Apr 3;368(6486):85-89. doi: 10.1126/science.aaw9872. PMID: 32241947; PMCID: PMC7681911

301 Acetaminophen reduces cysteine but can cause liver issues – use with caution.

302 Sharma P, Shimura T, Banwait JK, Goel A. Andrographis-mediated chemosensitization through activation of ferroptosis and suppression of β-catenin/Wnt-signaling pathways in colorectal cancer. Carcinogenesis. 2020 Oct 15;41(10):1385-1394. doi: 10.1093/carcin/bgaa090. PMID: 32835374; PMCID: PMC7566354.

303 Lou JS, Zhao LP, Huang ZH, Chen XY, Xu JT, Tai WC, Tsim KWK, Chen YT, Xie T. Ginkgetin derived from Ginkgo biloba leaves enhances the therapeutic effect of cisplatin via ferroptosis-mediated disruption of the Nrf2/HO-1 axis in EGFR wild-type non-small-cell lung cancer. Phytomedicine. 2021 Jan;80:153370. doi: 10.1016/j.phymed.2020.153370. Epub 2020 Oct 9. PMID: 33113504.

304 Bai, Tao & Wang, Shuai & Zhao, Yipu & Zhu, Rongtao & Wang, Weijie & Sun, Yuling. (2017). Haloperidol, a sigma receptor 1 antagonist, promotes ferroptosis in hepatocellular carcinoma cells. Biochemical and Biophysical Research Communications. 491. 10.1016/j.bbrc.2017.07.136.

- Selenocysteine: stop selenium supplementation (unless selenite), avoid eating brazil nuts.

- Modulate ACSL4: Bromelain[305], Dihydrotanshinone (danshen) Aspirin (HCC)[306]

- Inhibit oestrogen receptor: metformin,[307] Cryptotanshinone (danshen)[308]

- Stimulation of 15-lipoxygenase: Ibuprofen[309] (GBM)

- Block serine synthesis: Disulfiram plus superoxide dismutase (SOD1)

- Inhibit the gamma-glutamyl cycle: Oridonin (Rhabdosia rubescens)[310]

- Inhibit exosomes: CBD[311]

- Activate VDAC2/3: erastin

305 Park S, Oh J, Kim M, Jin EJ. Bromelain effectively suppresses Kras-mutant colorectal cancer by stimulating ferroptosis. Anim Cells Syst (Seoul). 2018 Aug 30;22(5):334-340. doi: 10.1080/19768354.2018.1512521. PMID: 30460115; PMCID: PMC6171431.

306 Xia H, Lee KW, Chen J, Kong SN, Sekar K, Deivasigamani A, Seshachalam VP, Goh BKP, Ooi LL, Hui KM. Simultaneous silencing of ACSL4 and induction of GADD45B in hepatocellular carcinoma cells amplifies the synergistic therapeutic effect of aspirin and sorafenib. Cell Death Discov. 2017 Sep 11;3:17058. doi: 10.1038/cddiscovery.2017.58. PMID: 28900541; PMCID: PMC5592242.

307 Zhang J, Xu H, Zhou X, et al. Role of metformin in inhibiting estrogen-induced proliferation and regulating ERα and ERβ expression in human endometrial cancer cells. Oncol Lett. 2017;14(4):4949-4956. doi:10.3892/ol.2017.6877

308 Yu, H., Yang, C., Jian, L., Guo, S., Chen, R., Li, K., Qu, F., Tao, K., Fu, Y., Luo, F., Liu, S. "Sulfasalazine-induced ferroptosis in breast cancer cells is reduced by the inhibitory effect of estrogen receptor on the transferrin receptor". Oncology Reports 42.2 (2019): 826-838.

309 This effect does not apply to all NSAIDs.

310 Zhang J, Wang N, Zhou Y, Wang K, Sun Y, Yan H, Han W, Wang X, Wei B, Ke Y, Xu X. Oridonin induces ferroptosis by inhibiting gamma-glutamyl cycle in TE1 cells. Phytother Res. 2021 Jan;35(1):494-503. doi: 10.1002/ptr.6829. Epub 2020 Aug 31. PMID: 32869425.

311 Kosgodage US, Mould R, Henley AB, Nunn AV, Guy GW, Thomas EL, Inal JM, Bell JD, Lange S. Cannabidiol (CBD) Is a Novel Inhibitor for Exosome and Microvesicle (EMV) Release in Cancer. Front Pharmacol. 2018 Aug 13;9:889. doi: 10.3389/fphar.2018.00889. PMID: 30150937; PMCID: PMC6099119.

- Inhibit Stearoyl-CoA Desaturase 1 (SCD1): nicotinamide (niacin)[312]

Research into this approach is still in its infancy and each type of cancer has specific nuances, for example blocking both the thioredoxin pathway as well as GPX4 in pancreatic cancer has less effect than just blocking GPX4.[313] However, inhibiting the xCT and GPX4 together is synergistic for pancreatic cancer.[314]

Another drug combination that stimulates ferroptosis is Lapatanib and siramesine which was found to be effective in breast cancer cells, lung cancer and GBM. Siramesine and to a lesser extent clemastine, make the lysosome, the sack which contains the iron, more permeable so that it leeches more of the free iron out into the surrounding cytosol, triggering more ferroptosis.[315] Siramesine was originally developed as an anti-anxiety drug although development was halted after clinical trials showed a lack of efficacy in humans but more recently they have discovered its anticancer potential. Siramesine also synergises with vincristine, a chemotherapy drug, almost identical in action to mebendazole, by modulating tubulin in cancer cells. The synergistic combination of microtubule-disturbing and lysosomal destabilising drugs had a dramatic response in both

312 Michele Carbone and Gerry Melino. Stearoyl CoA Desaturase Regulates Ferroptosis in Ovarian Cancer Offering New Therapeutic Perspectives. Cancer Research Highlights Published October 2019 DOI: 10.1158/0008-5472.CAN-19-2453

313 Modulation of ferroptosis sensitivity by TXNRD1 in pancreatic cancer cells, Luke L. Cai, Richard A. Ruberto, Matthew J. Ryan, John K. Eaton, Stuart L. Schreiber, Vasanthi S. Viswanathan bioRxiv 2020.06.25.165647; doi: https://doi.org/10.1101/2020.06.25.165647 fonc-10-571127-t002.jpg (1458×2155) (frontiersin.org)

314 Chen G, Guo G, Zhou X, Chen H. Potential mechanism of ferroptosis in pancreatic cancer. Oncol Lett. 2020;19(1):579-587. doi:10.3892/ol.2019.11159

315 Clemastine and metformin are another synergistic combination, together they can remyelinate neurons, a wonderful combination for anyone with neuronal damage from chemotherapy (or if you have MS). Remyelination might repair some of the damage and restore any lost function.

breast and cervical cancer that were treatment resistant.[316] Because mebendazole is similarly microtubule disturbing and also promotes autophagy, needed for ferritinophagy, this should be an extremely useful addition.[317] Clemastine, an old low toxicity antihistamine drug, easier to acquire than siramesine, is another lysosomal destabilising drug, so in theory it should also work synergistically with mebendazole to improve ferroptosis, but there is currently no research to support this.

Haloperidol is an antipsychotic medication that has been shown to significantly increase ROS, levels of FE2+ and lipid peroxidation, boosting the effects of xCT inhibitors, so this could be considered as an addition to your protocol if a basic approach is not sufficient to produce results.

The mTOR inhibitors metformin and dihydroartemesinin activate autophagy which will breakdown ferritin in the lysosome (ferritinophagy). To ensure this happens effectively, it is essential that you stop all autophagy inhibitors prior to ferroptosis. This means removing the following drugs and supplements during your ferroptosis phase:

Hydroxychloroquine, chloroquine, pyrvinium pamoate, amiloride, olive oil with oleacanthol, black seed oil. Matrine may assist ferroptosis.

Hydroxychloroquine and chloroquine have a particularly long half-life, but stopping these 24-48 hours prior to a Kill Phase has been shown to enhance the potency of artemisinin, whereas Dr Nai-Di Yang discovered cotreatment with artemisinin was inhibitory, if confirmation

---

316 Groth-Pedersen L, Ostenfeld MS, Høyer-Hansen M, Nylandsted J, Jäättelä M. Vincristine induces dramatic lysosomal changes and sensitizes cancer cells to lysosome-destabilizing siramesine. Cancer Res. 2007 Mar 1;67(5):2217-25. doi: 10.1158/0008-5472.CAN-06-3520. PMID: 17332352.

317 Vincristine Induces Dramatic Lysosomal Changes and Sensitizes Cancer Cells to Lysosome-Destabilizing Siramesine Line Groth-Pedersen, Marie Stampe Ostenfeld, Maria Høyer-Hansen, Jesper Nylandsted and Marja Jäättelä Cancer Res March 1 2007 (67) (5) 2217-2225; DOI: 10.1158/0008-5472.CAN-06-3520

were needed.[318] It might be better to substitute hydroxychloroquine for pyrvinium pamoate as an autophagy inhibitor between ferroptosis sessions to avoid any lingering inhibitory effects. Dipyridamole will also inhibit lipid peroxidation, so this too will need to be stopped, however you can replace it with danshen for the Kill Phase as this has ferroptosis activating properties.

Cordyceps, a medicinal mushroom, can stimulate both glutathione transferase and glutathione, so it may be best to consider lowering intake/pulsing or stopping during a ferroptosis phase.

Celastrol, from the Tripterygium wilfordii (Thunder God Vine) has many potent anticancer effects. As it helps stimulate autophagy and blocks the proteasome, it has been shown to activate ferroptosis with erastin. However, the side effects of celastrol can be severe, but used in combination at low nontoxic concentrations, the unwanted side effects and toxicity can be managed.

Other supplements have potent antioxidant effects and these too will need to be stopped reduced or pulsed e.g. all forms of vit E including gamma and delta tocotrienol, CoQ10, chlorogenic acid which is found in your daily coffee. Doxycycline, part of the Care Oncology Clinic protocol, may not be such a good choice during ferroptosis as it can neutralise hydrogen peroxide radicals.[319]

---

318 Yang ND, Tan SH, Ng S, Shi Y, Zhou J, Tan KS, Wong WS, Shen HM. Artesunate induces cell death in human cancer cells via enhancing lysosomal function and lysosomal degradation of ferritin. J Biol Chem. 2014 Nov 28;289(48):33425-41. doi: 10.1074/jbc. M114.564567. Epub 2014 Oct 10. PMID: 25305013; PMCID: PMC4246098.

319 Saeed M, Arun MZ, Guzeloglu M, Onursal C, Gokce G, Korkmaz CG, Reel B. Low-dose doxycycline inhibits hydrogen peroxide-induced oxidative stress, MMP-2 up-regulation and contractile dysfunction in human saphenous vein grafts. Drug Des Devel Ther. 2019;13:1791-1801 https://doi.org/10.2147/DDDT.S187842

Chelating copper with the drug tetra thiomolybdate is a strategy used by some cancer patients to stay NED, particularly triple negative breast cancer patients (it is only shown to have an effect if you take it when you are already NED), but be aware this drug will inhibit ferroptosis.

Disulfiram (also known as Antabuse) is often said to be more effective for cancer therapy if you add copper, but copper overload may result in damage to normal tissue when activating ferroptosis.

In the case of ferroptosis, disulfiram should be used without additional copper and prescribed at a low dose as there is already a source of ROS from hydrogen peroxide released by intravenous vitamin C and oxygen molecules from artemesinin. Using disulfiram in this way will require a doctor experienced in its use but it could be especially useful for breast and ovarian cancer patients who often have a chromosome 16 mutation in their cancers, making them more sensitive to ferroptosis. Disulfiram decomposes in the lysosome, chelating copper and stimulating copper dependant oxygen free radicals, but it also releases the superoxide anion at the same time. Superoxide is a more powerful oxygen free radical than hydrogen peroxide and it might cause damage to normal tissues. So to prevent any collateral damage from any superoxide anions, you should add SOD1 (superoxide dismutase), an enzyme that can be purchased in supplement form, to break down superoxide into hydrogen peroxide and oxygen. Healthy cells can withstand hydrogen peroxide as they have higher levels of catalase to disarm this, whereas cancer cells are more vulnerable. This will further enhance ferroptosis in the cancer cell.

Improving the response for melanoma can be achieved by adding gambogenic acid to your ferroptosis protocol, found in the Chinese herbal gamboge.[320]

---

320 Wang, Meng; Li, Qinglin. Gambogenic acid induces ferroptosis in melanoma cells undergoing epithelial-to-mesenchymal transition. Toxicol Appl Pharmacol ; 401: 115110, 2020 08 15.

Exosomes and Ferroptosis

One last escape route I have discovered by cancer cells to prevent ferroptosis, is the removal of iron by little micro vesicles produced on the surface of the cell, called exosomes. Exosomes are produced by all cells, we have quadrillions in our bodies at any time, but in cancer these are produced in excess in the tumour microenvironment. These micro vesicles are shed from the budding of the plasma membrane like tiny little bubbles, little smart bombs that carry instructions to neighbouring cells and distant cells to encourage metastasis, drug resistance and they are also responsible for cachexia.

Exosomes taken from the serum of mice with breast cancer can induce cancer when injected into healthy mice. Exosomes carry messages via tiny RNA strands called microRNA and they influence new blood vessel formation (angiogenesis) and the suppression of the immune system.

Exosomes reduce natural killer cells and effector T cells while they expand levels of immunosuppressive cells such as T-regs, myeloid derived suppressor cells, as well as transforming macrophages into M2 or tumour associated macrophages.

Exosomes cause cachexia by delivering messages from the original cancer site through microRNA instructing distant sites to breakdown muscle and adipose tissue to provide more nutrients in the blood. Exosomes also contain survivin, an anti-apoptotic protein. In cells where the GPX4 is inhibited, there is an increase in exosomes containing iron, so it is essential this pathway be inhibited at the same time.

CBD, from cannabis sativa, has been shown to inhibit exosomes in several cancer cell lines, which may be its major anticancer effect.[321] Note this relates to CBD, not THC, the latter may block ferroptosis by preventing lipid peroxidation and increasing glutathione. Also exosomes are dependent on both cholesterol and another waxy lipid called ceramide. Blocking cholesterol with statins combined with gamma tocotrienol was shown to alter the lipid structure in membranes by inhibiting ceramide enzyme DEGS1 after prolonged treatment.[322] As already mentioned, gamma and delta tocotrienol are a form of vitamin E, so they may inhibit ferroptosis, albeit less potently than alpha tocopherol, but it would be prudent to stop, reduce or pulse this during a ferroptosis phase. However taking both gamma and delta tocotrienol in the starve phase have shown to be extremely beneficial in many cancers. Both delta tocotrienol and sulfasalazine are potent inhibitors of NK-kB, a major inflammatory pathway in cancer, which accounts for much of their potent effects.

I realise there are a lot of new pathways, but that is because ferroptosis is almost the opposite of apoptosis, which is what we are striving to achieve with the starve phase. The process of stimulating ferroptosis may seem complicated, but the potential of this kill phase could be the solution to so many cancers.

321 Kosgodage US, Mould R, Henley AB, Nunn AV, Guy GW, Thomas EL, Inal JM, Bell JD, Lange S. Cannabidiol (CBD) Is a Novel Inhibitor for Exosome and Microvesicle (EMV) Release in Cancer. Front Pharmacol. 2018 Aug 13;9:889. doi: 10.3389/fphar.2018.00889. PMID: 30150937; PMCID: PMC6099119.

322 Jang Y, Rao X, Jiang Q. Gamma-tocotrienol profoundly alters sphingolipids in cancer cells by inhibition of dihydroceramide desaturase and possibly activation of sphingolipid hydrolysis during prolonged treatment. J Nutr Biochem. 2017 Aug;46:49-56. doi: 10.1016/j.jnutbio.2017.04.003. Epub 2017 Apr 12. PMID: 28456081; PMCID: PMC5635819.

Summary of my Ferroptosis Protocol:

Preparation Phase:

It is best if you can take a few weeks to prepare yourself before you attempt ferroptosis to

1. Starve and weaken your cancer.
2. Normalise homocysteine levels.
3. Lower CoQ10.
4. Reduce ceramides and cholesterol levels to reduce the production of exosomes. (CBD, Statins and tocotrienols).
5. Inhibit NADPH via G6PD and 6PGD inhibition.
6. Unless you are severely anaemic, supplementing with iron is not recommended to normalise iron levels as this could fuel your cancer.

Ferroptosis Phase:

Key drugs:

Sulfasalazine or other xCT inhibitor (e.g. erastin, sorafenib), lipophilic statins (e.g. simvastatin, atorvastatin), metformin, artesunate or nitazoxanide, mebendazole, clemastine, ibuprofen (GBM).

HDAC inhibitor to protect neurons: sodium valproate (valproic acid, Depakote)

If needed, leflunomide, disulfiram or haloperidol could be added.

Intravenous vitamin C will enhance the effect and can be given if available.

Key supplements:

Artemisinin, Piperlongumine, (Sodium Selenite), Brutasol (Brucea javanica), Bromelain, CBD, Lactoferrin, Withaferin A (Ashwagandha), Trigonelline, Feverfew, Gambogic acid (gamboge garcinia), Syrian Rhubarb, Danshen, PEITC (watercress), Ginkgetin (ginkgo biloba), Cucurbitacin B (cucumber, bitter melon), Andrographis, Rhabdosia rubescens, Ruscogenin (Butcher's Broom), Niacin, Superoxide dismutase.

HDAC inhibitor to protect neurons: Beta hydroxybutyric acid (BHBA)

If your cancer still continues to resist cell death, then you can move to a 'second line' of treatment adding another drug, after consultation with your physician.

Ferroptosis and Immunotherapy

Immunotherapy treatment is currently ineffective for the majority of patients but this could be set to change with the combined treatment of check point inhibitors with ferroptosis inducers. Wang et al. discovered that mice with ovarian or melanoma cancers when given PD-L1 immune check point inhibitors had an increase of lipid peroxidation, a sign that part of its action may be in activating ferroptosis. Wang also discovered that it was the secretion of interferon gamma by CD 8+ cells activated by PD-L1 treatment that had a suppressive effect on the xCT cystine-glutamate antiporter. So the answer to making immunotherapy work in patients may be to further activate ferroptosis in combination with immunotherapy treatments. Perhaps just giving interferon gamma rather than the immunotherapy drugs (which can have serious side effects) in combination with xCT inhibitors may be enough to enhance survival times. This finding could be hugely significant in the future of treatment with immunotherapies.[323] This is an area that is being explored

---

323 Zeng, C., Tang, H., Chen, H. et al. Ferroptosis: a new approach for immunotherapy. Cell Death Discov. 6, 122 (2020). https://doi.org/10.1038/s41420-020-00355-2

in depth as this could have major implications on the cancer industry for treatment resistant cancers. Interferon gamma not only suppressed the xCT transporter but also the amino acid transporter CD98 that is strongly associated with aggressive breast cancer. Surprisingly interferon gamma has not yet been approved for cancer immunotherapy. Conflicting results in the past have led to it being shelved for cancer despite promising results with bladder, melanoma and ovarian cancer. I suspect this may all change with this new finding, as it is all about using the right combination.[324]

Other ROS- forming treatments that synergise and enhance ferroptosis:

Photodynamic Therapy (PDT)

PDT works synergistically with ferroptosis as it provides another source of ROS for the Fenton reaction. It is involves the use of light and a photosensitizing chemical substance, used in conjunction with molecular oxygen to elicit cancer cell death and is currently used in conventional care for melanomas, head and neck, bladder and prostate cancer.

If used together, this could be an option to avoid risky surgery, particularly in cancers where there is a high probability of loss of vocal chords, erectile function or where the tumour is pressing on vital structures.

Magnetic therapy

Magnetic therapy was looked into for cancer therapy as early as 1957, but is not accepted as a standard treatment. How or if it works has been a subject of speculation for years, with most traditional sites suggesting

---

324 Zitvogel L, Kroemer G. Interferon-γ induces cancer cell ferroptosis. Cell Res. 2019 Sep;29(9):692-693. doi: 10.1038/s41422-019-0186-z. PMID: 31160718; PMCID: PMC6796847.

it is of no value. Magnetised mattresses and bracelets have been shown to have no effect.

Theoretically, static magnetic fields (SMFs) alter ion flow, cellular potential, membrane configuration, ion pump activity and have been found to increase ROS and assist both apoptosis and ferroptosis. A study using 50 Hz electromagnetic field modulated by static magnetic field with time-average intensity of 5.1 mT, applied for 2 h daily for over 3 consecutive days led to a persistent activation of ROS and a decrease in growth of many tumours including lung cancer, gastric cancer, pancreatic cancer and nephroblastoma.[325]

BEMER mats might be of value to assist ferroptosis and a medical device based on an EMF of 200 kHz, Optune® (Novocure, Israel), has been approved by the FDA and EU for relapsed and primary glioblastoma.[326]

Hyperbaric Oxygen Therapy (HBOT)

I am lukewarm about HBOT. According to Dominic D'Agostino who has studied this for cancer, it only works if you use it within 15-30 minutes of chemotherapy or radiotherapy (and presumably IVC), unachievable for most people.

Exercise

If you are receiving intravenous vitamin C, remember that it blocks the G6PD, a route for your cells to acquire glucose, so you may put yourself at risk of hypoglycaemia and fainting if you exercise too soon afterwards.

---

325 Yuan LQ, Wang C, Lu DF, Zhao XD, Tan LH, Chen X. Induction of apoptosis and ferroptosis by a tumor suppressing magnetic field through ROS-mediated DNA damage. Aging (Albany NY). 2020;12(4):3662-3681. doi:10.18632/aging.102836

326 Graeb M, Kinzel A, Kirson E. Technical Features of a Medical Device Generating Alternating Electric Fields (Tumor Treating Fields) for the Treatment of Glioblastoma. Neuro-oncol. 2018. (suppl_3); 20:243–243. 10.1093/neuonc/noy139.101

Short hits of high intensity exercise (HIIT) for 30 seconds to one minute with one to two minute rests in between have been found to be effective and safe, they do not cause an immediate drop in blood glucose yet raise the oxygen levels. Twelve weeks of high intensity exercise (total exercise time 40 minutes/week i.e. only for 6 mins/day) improved blood glucose to a similar extent as running at 65% VO2 max for 150 minutes/week.

Warning: Do not attempt HIIT exercise without professional guidance as many cancer patients have cardiac issues after some chemotherapy drugs.

One of the leading researchers in exercise for cancer is Prof Robert Newton of Edith Cowan University, Perth, Western Australia. In 2019 he was awarded Western Australia's Scientist of the Year for his work exploring the benefits of exercise with cancer patients. He suggests

"The factor limiting oxygenation of tumour tissue is not so much the partial pressure of oxygen in the blood but rather the fact that tumours have low blood perfusion, in particular across the transition from incoming blood flow to venous return. This creates a hypoxic environment within the tumour which actually promotes the proliferation of cancer cells and drives mechanisms for the cancer cells to adapt and metastasise. Low oxygen levels within the tumour also compromises the effectiveness of radiation therapy. I have not seen anything explaining the mechanism of oxygen level influencing chemotherapy but certainly the rate of blood flow through the tumour is a key factor in chemotherapy effectiveness.

So the priority to improve chemotherapy and radiation therapy effectiveness (and ferroptosis) is to increase blood flow through the tumour tissue. Exercise does this in two ways:

1. Acute exercise increases blood pressure and, interestingly, vasoconstriction of the arterioles entering cancerous growths does not occur in response to exercise as it does in most of the

other tissues of the body. This means that any exercise induced increase in blood pressure results in direct increase in blood flow through the tumour tissue delivering more blood and oxygen to enhance the radiation therapy effectiveness as well as delivering more chemotherapy agent to also improve effectiveness. This increased blood flow also delivers more "endogenous" medicine such as anti-cancer cytokines, hormones, natural killer and other T cells.

2. Chronic exercise causes adaptations in the microvasculature within tumour tissues of a more organised and effective fluid conduction system. This also contributes to increased tumour tissue perfusion and oxygenation both at rest and during exercise. Exercise appears to "normalise" the dysfunctional microvasculature that develops within tumours as they grow. In part the mechanism is the sheer stress induced by exercise on the blood vessel walls which produces positive adaptations in terms of structure and reduces leakage and thus also has the action of suppressing metastatic processes.'

In addition to aerobic work, resistance exercise will increase the volume of muscle, which then acts like a sink for excess glucose, preventing it reaching the tumour. Regular resistance work is important for every cancer patient, both aerobic and resistance exercise increase the number of GLUT4 receptors in muscle so that blood glucose uptake is not as dependant on insulin. Glucose uptake into contracting muscle normalises, even in the presence of type 2 diabetes. Resistance work has also been shown to improve response to immunotherapy.

EWOT (exercise with oxygen)

Exercising with an oxygen concentrator (e.g. on a static bike) could be more effective than HBOT but never use 100% oxygen with treatment. Most oxygen concentrators deliver about 90% oxygen which is safe. Stop immediately if you feel dizzy or faint.

Conclusion

Ferroptosis is a new dawn in cancer treatment. Dr Ahmed Elsakka, Dr Mark Rosenberg and Dr Daniel Thomas have already seen some great results in the clinic. In the future I hope that I can set up some formal training and we can see many more clinics dedicated to delivering this new specialism. I will provide updates on developments as research evolves on the best timing and duration of treatment, but there will be much variability between patients depending on the stage and aggressiveness of the tumour. Some may wish to try it for a few days, every now and then, others may want to try it for extended periods.

I welcome people's experiences and I would kindly request you allow me to gather your data on my upcoming Starve Cancer App to discover the best combinations for different cancer subtypes for the benefit of all.

Summary

To summarise my protocol – Starve it. Stop it spreading. Snuff it out.

Starve it with the Metro Map combination of drugs and supplements, stop it spreading by blocking growth factors, lastly snuff it out with a Kill Phase by oxidising the cancer cells. This will encourage the immune system to be switched on without relying on immunotherapies, which can cause hyper-progression. If you have found the science a struggle, please do consider my online course, it is more in-depth about diet, the workings of the immune system and more specific about the drugs and supplements for different cancers.

1. Starve the cancer by using all four modalities; exercise, diet, supplements and the off-label drugs. Lifestyle modifications are just as important as the drugs.

   a) Stick to a low glycaemic diet at all times. No cheating! Avoid all simple sugars. Look up The Montignac Method for a list of the rough glycaemic indexes of foods, but remember that this is a diet designed for weight loss/cardiovascular health and not cancer. Montignac died aged 63 of prostate cancer, which is fuelled by fat and protein. You will need to cut out more foods from your diet than this, but view dietary changes as treatment. With any luck you will be able to add the occasional treat back in the future.

   If your cancer is glutamine-driven, cut out red meat, even poultry (asparagine) and reduce other protein (even beans contain glutamate) and eat a mainly pescatarian diet.

All cancers need fat so cut out saturated fats too. Instead, take sea buckthorn oil and supplement with omega-3 oils for their anti-inflammatory and lipid-modulating effects. Avoid a really 'extreme' diet. Be sensible.

b) Include intermittent fasting (time-restricted feeding) into your regime, but not for extended periods while you have cancer. Fast for one or two days a week or stop eating after six o'clock in the evening until 11 o'clock or midday the next. Cut down on portion sizes, particularly in the evening. Set achievable targets but aim to be tough on your cancer and 'go for it' for three months.

c) Exercise. Fifteen minutes after every meal, go for a brisk walk and clench those buttocks! Do more exercise if you can. Avoid 'extreme' exercising, which will only deplete your immunity. Going for a walk 15 minutes after supper rather than watching TV on the sofa will pay dividends. Otherwise the bad stuff just stays in the system to be used as fuel by the cancer overnight.

d) Investigate off label drugs in my Facebook group. My top recommended drugs to starve cancer are: aspirin, metformin, lipophilic statins, dipyridamole, mebendazole, doxycycline and niclosamide. Be selective. All of these drugs have 'pleiotropic effects' (they have many targets). Use ones with a low risk of side effects. Combine drugs and supplements that target different pathways rather than the same pathway, or there will not be synergy. Do not 'self-hack' and self-prescribe, as dosages need to be carefully and gradually increased. Beware of drug interactions and always check with a health professional before taking any of these.

2. Add supplements. Include berberine, gymnema sylvestre, chromium picolinate, hydroxycitrate, luteolin, vitamins A, B, D, K, magnesium, ursolic acid, curcumin, EGCG, resveratrol, glucosamine sulphate, niacin, omega-3 and omega-7. Remember to monitor blood glucose levels with a glucometer. For most healthy individuals, normal blood sugar levels are currently set between 4.0 to 5.4 mmol/L (72 to 99 mg/dL) when fasting. Up to 7.8mmol/L (140mg/dL) 2 hours after

eating is considered normal but not ideal when you have cancer. This needs to be lower. Post prandial levels should not drop below a reading of four. This type of dieting is dangerous for Type 1 diabetics.

3. 'Pulse' a stronger NSAID (etodolac, celecoxib, diclofenac or the liposomal version of ibuprofen) with a statin to trigger apoptosis. For the best cancer-killing effect I believe this strategy should also be combined with low dose metronomic chemotherapy and intravenous vitamin C. Add other glutathione-lowering drugs and oxygen therapies if this is not enough to reduce (kill) the tumours.

4. Be proactive. Do not wait until your cancer is progressing before taking action. You will only make your task bigger and harder to contain. It is with dismay that I regularly see people waiting for cancer to return before doing anything. Prevention. Prevention. Prevention.

5. Discover the individual metabolic drivers of your cancer by researching PubMed for clues. Type in 'Metabolic Phenotype' then your cancer (e.g., melanoma) into Google. Look for words in the articles that correspond to words on my Metro Map to work out whether it is glucose, glutamine, lactate, ketone (SREBP-1), fat-driven or all of these. Prostate cancer, for example, uses glutaminolysis, arginine and lipogenesis (fatty acid synthesis). But not glycolysis until in its later stages, so intravenous vitamin C and 2-DG or DCA, for example, would not be a priority. It is still worth blocking the glycolysis pathway (with IVC) to prevent it rerouting once the OXPHOS pathway has been blocked. Drugs that target more than one side of the triangle should be included in every programme.

6. Find out the genetic changes in your tumour (the histology). Mutations and over-expressed genes make the cancer cell hungrier than ever for certain nutrients and they each affect the metabolism in different ways.

   Oncogenes turn on cancer cells and suppressor genes turn them off. When oncogenes are switched on in cancer, it is like having the gas pedal in the car permanently stuck down, allowing the cancer to progress.

If suppressor genes are turned off it is like taking the brakes off the car: it allows the cancer to progress unchecked. Both oncogenes and suppressor genes can be changed 'epigenetically', in other words by changing the environmental stimuli around the cell. Little strands of 'microRNA' carry information from outside the cell into the cell to influence the genes and how they behave. Diet, supplements, exercise and the drugs all affect the activity of the genes and can switch them off or turn them on. Having a BRCA gene mutation does not mean you automatically need to undergo surgery.

While all cancers share some common metabolic properties, they also have distinct sensitivities depending on their oncogenic mutation profiles. This knowledge is important for personalising your diet and treatment:

- P13K/Akt increases glucose transport (Glut receptors), glycolysis and lipogenesis.

- The p53 gene, a tumour suppressor, guards normal mitochondrial oxidative phosphorylation. When deleted or mutated, common in a great many cancers, it promotes the switch to glycolysis, the fermentation of glucose in the cytoplasm. It also controls the xCT antiporter.

- MYC stimulates mitochondrial glutaminolysis and glutamine addiction as well as glycolysis and fatty acid oxidation.[327]

- The Src gene regulates glycolysis. Src-3 increases oestrogen metabolism.[328]

- HER2 and EGFR increase glycolysis, glutaminolysis and fat metabolism.

327 Camarda R, Zhou Z, Kohnz RA, *et al.* Inhibition of fatty acid oxidation as a therapy for MYC-overexpressing triple-negative breast cancer. Nature medicine. 2016;22(4): 427-432. doi: 10.1038/nm.4055.

328 Subhamoy Dasgupta et al Metabolic enzyme PFKFB4 activates transcriptional coactivator SRC-3 to drive breast cancer Nature 03 April 2018

- Braf mutations love ketones.[329]
- Ras activates greater glucose consumption, lactate accumulation and reduced mitochondrial activity (less OXPHOS)[330]
- Kras, a more aggressive Ras oncogene, makes the cell more dependent on glucose and glutamine. This mutation is present in the majority of pancreatic cancers and these cancers use a process called 'macropinocytosis' to grab nutrients from its surroundings. This process is likely upregulated in many advanced (stage IV) cancers as they become more aggressive. (See the action of dipyridamole and chloroquine which will both help block this).

7. Demand to have regular metabolic markers of your disease so that you can chart your progress.
   - Antigen markers (CA15-3 is a marker for breast cancer, CA19-9 antigen may be elevated in the blood of some patients with gastrointestinal tumours. CA-125 is a marker for monitoring ovarian cancer, CEA, SCC, etc.)
   - TM2PK test (also known as PKM2).
   - Levels of lactate dehydrogenase (LDH).
   - A PET scan will show glucose uptake. Other tracers can track glutamine (protein), phosphocholine (fat) and ketone uptake on PET scans but unfortunately these are only just being introduced. One day these tests will be standard.
   - Measuring the lactate produced to glucose consumed (mol/mol) ratio will determine the glycolytic efficiency of your tumour.
   - Scans to detect oxygen consumption will reveal the 'Reverse Warburg Effect', an increase in oxidative phosphorylation (super-charged mitochondria) with an increase in lactate uptake. This is visible on special MRIs tracking the oligomycine-sensitive oxygen consumption rate (mitoOCR).

329 Kang H-B, Fan J, Lin R, et al. Metabolic rewiring by oncogenic BRAF V600E links ketogenesis pathway to BRAF-MEK1 signaling. Molecular cell. 2015;59(3): 345-358. doi: 10.1016/j.molcel.2015.05.037.
330 Bos JL (1989) Ras oncogenes in human cancer: a review. Cancer Res49: 4682-4689

- The presence of the following in your tumour suggests it is using ketones (so avoid the ketogenic diet):

  Succinyl CoA: 3 Oxoacid CoA Transferase (OXCT1),

  3-hydroxybutyrate dehydrogenase 1 and 2 (BDH1 and BDH2)

  Acetyl-CoA acetyltransferase 1 (ACAT1).

To date, none of these tests (bar the glucose PET, LDH and antigen markers) are regularly used. It falls to us, the patients, to demand these tests and push for better treatment and services.

8. Visit a practitioner in functional medicine. Undergo micronutrient status tests, thyroid checks, DHEA levels and stool tests (for parasites) as well as genetic tests. Understand your body, your cancer, what your body is lacking or what you need less of. We are all different.

9. Combine therapies.
   - Take targeted genetic drugs if available to weaken and reduce the fast-dividing cells.
   - Take immunotherapy drugs with caution, knowing that they work best only when your microbiome is healthy[331] (especially with sufficient levels of bifidobacteria) and when the abnormal metabolism and growth factors have been normalised. Otherwise, you may end up taking ever greater amounts, becoming increasingly toxic, to try and overcome the cancer, eventually reaching a point where the immune system simply fails. Side effects of immunotherapy drugs are overwhelming inflammation and autoimmunity.[332]

10. Other treatments can be added to your protocol to increase the chances of ridding yourself of cancer (e.g., photodynamic therapy, High Intensity Frequency Ultrasound, stereotactic radiotherapy – cyberknife or Proton Beam, hyperthermia).

---

331 Gut bacteria can dramatically amplify cancer immunotherapy. UChicago News Nov 6th, 2015

332 Kroschinsky F, Stölzel F, von Bonin S, *et al.* New drugs, new toxicities: severe side effects of modern targeted and immunotherapy of cancer and their management. Critical Care. 2017; 21:89. doi: 10.1186/s13054-017-1678-1.

11. Target growth factors and MMPs with supplements and drugs. The role of the extracellular matrix and blocking Matrix Metalloproteinases (MMPs) as well as FGF, VEGF, PDGF are not fully appreciated. Blocking these is critical to halting growth. Remember it is usually metastatic spread that kills the patient.

12. Block oestrogen, which drives certain cancers, especially for cervical, uterine, breast, prostate, lung and brain cancers. Indole-3-carbinol or DIM, melatonin, metformin and of course tamoxifen. The latter two also block IGF-1.[333]

13. Investigate drugs/supplements to target the abnormal signalling pathways your tumour reveals (Sonic Hedgehog, Wnt, Notch). This information should be available from your oncologist or search medical journals online.

14. Boost immunity. Consider taking cimetidine for three months after treatment if you have shifted to a more Th2 immune response as I had (test IL5 and IL12 and TNF beta responses). Various Chinese mushrooms (e.g. maitake, Turkey tail) will help stimulate a better immune response. Melatonin works particularly well with IL2 (interleukin 2) for treatment in some cancers e.g. kidney.

15. Oxygenate using intravenous vitamin C in high dose, two or three times a week, ensuring you are also blocking fat and glutamine pathways too unless you are activating ferroptosis. On its own, or used only with glycolysis inhibitors, this treatment will fail. Look into including HIIT exercise, exercise with oxygen, HBOT (hyperbaric oxygen therapy) or ozone infusions.

16. Avoid stress whenever possible. Meditation, visualisations, yoga, pilates, relaxing baths, do whatever it takes! If you are particularly stressed, propranolol may be a good choice to help block cancer spread (MMP-2 and 9 inhibitor, VEGF inhibitor) as well as calm you down (remember it cannot be taken with dipyridamole). Cortisol levels are highest in the morning. (Sometimes I take propranolol

---

333 Professor Ben Williams cured his brain cancer using tamoxifen as part of his mix (it is also an IGF-1 inhibitor). Tamoxifen can eventually cause endometrial cancer, by upregulating the glycolytic pathways, but Professor Williams doesn't have an endometrium. These glycolytic pathways can be blocked in other ways to prevent this metabolic shift, e.g., using berberine and metformin.

in the morning, dypridamole in the evening – always check with a physician).

17. Understand the stage of your disease and do your own research. Oncologists make decisions on your behalf. Do they expect you to recover, or are they offering palliative care under the banner of curative treatment? Put yourself in the driving seat. Find out what they are really thinking. You need the truth, not reassuring platitudes, to make the best decisions. Remember the stats do not apply to you. Ask questions, be annoying! Understand what the oncologist realistically expects to achieve from treatment. Is he working towards a cure or merely believing he is watching the slow motion 'car crash', merely trying to minimise the impact? If you are brave, ask them for a rough idea of prognosis (this is more to gauge their expectations, not your own) but remember it is 100% out of date and wrong! Do not be disheartened but let this guide your level of action. The worse the prognosis, the more action you need to take.

18. Be organised. See my website *www.howtostarvecancer.com*. Make a list of what you're taking and when you should be taking it. Make a note of supplier's websites and phone numbers for re-ordering. Devote one hour a week to ensuring pills are organised for the upcoming week. I am designing an App that will help you track progress and make suggestions.

19. Listen to your intuition but do not always 'follow your gut.' Your gut may well be telling you to eat sugar! (Those naughty critters in your intestines send pleading messages to your brain), particularly if you suddenly adopt a low sugar diet and add cancer starving drugs and supplements.

20. Keep an open mind! There will be lots of people telling you to avoid chemotherapy at all costs and to avoid all drugs. There are benefits to both. Avoid polarised views on this as you may be missing something important. Remember, metronomic low-dose chemotherapy is completely different to the maximum tolerated dose of chemotherapy that is usually given.

Cancer is complicated. But not as complicated as the pharmaceutical industry would have you believe. It will take a few read-throughs to get the scale of the input required and I realise this is all a huge amount of information to take in if you have just been diagnosed. I urge you to consult with a growing number of functional medicine practitioners, join my facebook group: (www.facebook.com/groups/off.label. drugsforcancer) and visit my website for further help if this is all too overwhelming (*www.howtostarvecancer.com*).

Beating cancer needs dedication and if you are committed, I firmly believe almost all cancers, even stage IV (unless organ damage is too severe) can be reversed and that it is possible to achieve long-term remission (a 'cure') without the huge toxic doses of chemotherapy and radiotherapy as per current standard of care. Immune systems will be less damaged and it will be far easier to regain full health if this approach were adopted, which is surely the ultimate goal for every patient.

Oncologists are obliged to prescribe only 'approved' drugs, but imagine if they were allowed to use their training, experience and expertise to guide and personalise treatments using safe off label drugs as well? Surely the goal is to save lives? Instead, patients continue to die in droves, with oncologists forced to follow out-of-date formulaic regimes and wait for the General Medical Council and NICE to approve the use of off label drug combinations. Will their shackles ever come off?

The world desperately needs more 'revolting' doctors willing to treat the body holistically, and more integrative practitioners who can provide intravenous vitamin C, ozone, ultraviolet blood irradiation, hyperthermia, hyperbaric oxygen and even offer faecal transplants to the very sick. A clinic that provides the correct nutrition for the individual so that he or she can learn what to avoid and what to eat during their period of healing would be revolutionary. I dream of running my own health clinic one day, offering everything a cancer patient needs to nurse them back to health.

Today I continue to take berberine and/or metformin and half an aspirin daily, and I still rattle with about 15 key supplements and many friends still call me Maracas. I look after my gut with a good diet, and I take occasional probiotics and prebiotics to keep my immune system functioning optimally. I regularly use time-restricted feeding, not eating for 16 or 18 hours between meals, then a couple of times a year I fast for a few days to regenerate immune stem cells. If I become concerned that I am running low on immunity, I take a short term (couple of weeks) boost of cimetidine and book in for some intravenous vitamin C. If I panic that cancer might be coming back, which does happen (I am only human), I take my cocktail of dipyridamole, statin, a strong NSAID, metformin and berberine for a few weeks. Despite discovering in 2020 that I have had cystic fibrosis all my life, I have great lung function and remain healthy.

I hope that after reading this book you are not daunted by the task ahead. There are a lot of drugs and supplements in my protocol, but you will get used to taking them. Always, of course, under medical guidance. Do not give up, as tipping the balance from cancer destroying you, to you destroying the cancer, might be the simple addition of one or two more low-toxicity drugs. Give it time to work; it may take several months, but put in the effort and the rewards are immense. My body is rejuvenated; I feel better, fitter and stronger than ever and younger than I did fifteen years ago! Believe in yourself. You can achieve this too. Go on! Do it.

Find strength and solidarity through my Facebook groups and together let's ignite a global revolution – it is long overdue.

Useful References and Further Reading

Organised by the George Yu Foundation for Nutrition and Health and the Reichhart family, experts in cancer metabolism across the globe converged in Baltimore for the *Tripping Over the Truth Retreat* (2017). Their talks are now available online. Speakers included Dr George Yu, Jane McLelland, Travis Christofferson, Professor Thomas Seyfried, Young Hee Ko Ph.D., Dr Gregory Riggins, Dr Akbar Khan, Dr Nasha Winters, Miriam Kalamian, Dr Laurent Schwartz and many others.

Go to *www.howtostarvecancer.com* or *YuFoundation.org* for details.

Discussions and interpretations of research articles relating to the drugs and supplements mentioned in my book can be found in my Facebook group and on my website *www.howtostarvecancer.com*.

The following references are taken from the Care Oncology Clinic website:

1. Hanahan D, Weinberg RA. The hallmarks of cancer. Cell 100(1), 57-70 (2000). Crossref, Medline, CAS

2. Hanahan D, Weinberg RA. Hallmarks of cancer: the next generation. Cell 144(5), 646-674 (2011). Crossref, Medline, CAS

3. Warburg O, Wind F, Negelein E. The metabolism of tumors in the body. J. Gen. Physiol. 8, 519-530 (1927). Crossref, Medline, CAS

4. Warburg O. On the origin of cancer cells. Science 123(3191), 309- 314 (1956). Crossref, Medline, CAS

5. De Berardinis RJ, Chandel NS. Fundamentals of cancer metabolism. Sci. Adv. 2(5), e1600200 (2016). Crossref, Medline

6. Vander Heiden MG, Cantley LC, Thompson CB. Understanding the Warburg effect: the metabolic requirements of cell proliferation. Science324(5930), 1029-1033 (2009). Crossref, Medline, CAS

7.   Koppenol WH, Bounds PL, Dang CV. Otto Warburg's contributions to current concepts of cancer metabolism. Nat. Rev. Cancer 11(5), 325-337 (2011). Crossref, Medline, CAS

8.   Pearce EL. Metabolism in T cell activation and differentiation. Curr. Opin. Immunol. 22(3), 314-320 (2010). Crossref, Medline, CAS

9.   Pearce EL, Poffenberger MC, Chang CH, Jones RG. Fueling immunity: insights into metabolism and lymphocyte function. Science 342(6155), 1242454 (2013). Crossref, Medline

10. Rathmell JC. Metabolism and autophagy in the immune system: immunometabolism comes of age. Immunol. Rev. 249(1), 5-13 (2012). Crossref, Medline, CAS

11. Le A, Lane AN, Hamaker M et al. Glucose-independent glutamine metabolism via TCA cycling for proliferation and survival in B cells. Cell Metab. 15(1), 110-121 (2012). Crossref, Medline, CAS

12. Fan J, Kamphorst JJ, Mathew R et al. Glutamine-driven oxidative phosphorylation is a major ATP source in transformed mammalian cells in both normoxia and hypoxia. Mol. Syst. Biol. 9(1), 712 (2013). Crossref, Medline, CAS

13. Krebs HA. Metabolism of amino-acids. Biochem. J. 29(8), 1951-1969 (1935). Crossref, Medline, CAS

14. Geddes WF, Hunter A. Observations upon the enzyme asparaginase. J. Biol. Chem. 77(1), 197-229 (1928). CAS

15. Greenstein JP, Price VE. α-Keto acid-activated glutaminase and asparaginase. J. Biol. Chem. 178(2), 695-705 (1949). Medline, CAS

16. Greenstein JP, Leuthardt FM. Effect of added phosphate on glutamine desamidation in tumors. J. Natl Cancer Inst. 8(4), 161-162 (1948). Medline, CAS

17. Svenneby G, Torgner IA, Kvamme E. Purification of phosphate-dependent pig brain glutaminase. J. Neurochem. 20(4), 1217-1224 (1973). Crossref, Medline, CAS

18. Curthoys NP, Kuhlenschmidt T, Godfrey SS. Regulation of renal ammoniagenesis. Arch. Biochem. Biophys. 174(1), 82-89 (1976). Crossref, Medline, CAS

19. Haser WG, Shapiro RA, Curthoys NP. Comparison of the phosphate-dependent glutaminase obtained from rat brain and kidney. Biochem. J. 229(2), 399-408 (1985). Crossref, Medline, CAS

20. Chiu JF, Boeker EA. Cow brain glutaminase: partial purification and mechanism of action. Arch. Biochem. Biophys. 196(2), 493-500 (1979). Crossref, Medline, CAS

21. Archibald RM. Preparation and assay of glutaminase for glutamine determinations. J. Biol. Chem. 154(3), 657-667 (1944). CAS

22. Heini HG, Gebhardt R, Brecht A, Mecke D. Purification and characterization of rat liver glutaminase. Eur. J. Biochem. 162(3), 541-546 (1987). Crossref, Medline, CAS

23. Smith EM, Watford M. Rat hepatic glutaminase: purification and immunochemical characterization. Arch. Biochem. Biophys. 260(2), 740-751 (1988). Crossref, Medline, CAS

24. Nagase T, Ishikawa K, Suyama M et al. Prediction of the coding sequences of unidentified human genes. XII. The complete sequences of 100 new cDNA clones from brain which code for large proteins in vitro. DNA Res. 5(6), 355-364 (1998). Crossref, Medline, CAS

25. Elgadi KM, Meguid RA, Qian M, Souba WW, Abcouwer SF. Cloning and analysis of unique human glutaminase isoforms generated by tissue-specific alternative splicing. Physiol. Genomics1(2), 51-62 (1999). Medline, CAS

26. Porter LD, Ibrahim H, Taylor L, Curthoys NP. Complexity and species variation of the kidney-type glutaminase gene. Physiol. Genomics 9(3), 157-166 (2002). Crossref, Medline, CAS

27. Sammeth M, Foissac S, Guigó R. A general definition and nomenclature for alternative splicing events. PLoS Comput. Biol. 4(8), e1000147 (2008). Crossref, Medline

28. Brosnan JT, Ewart HS, Squires SA. Hormonal control of hepatic glutaminase. Adv. Enzyme Regul. 35, 131-146 (1995). Crossref, Medline, CAS

29. Kalra J, Brosnan JT. The subcellular localization of glutaminase isoenzymes in rat kidney cortex. J. Biol. Chem. 249(10), 3255-3260 (1974). Medline, CAS

30. Aledo JC, de Pedro E, Gomez-Fabre PM, Nunez de Castro I, Marquez J. Submitochondrial localization and membrane topography of Ehrlich ascitic tumour cell glutaminase. Biochim. Biophys. Acta 1323(2), 173-184 (1997). Crossref, Medline, CAS

31. Cassago A, Ferreira APS, Ferreira IM *et al.* Mitochondrial localization and structure-based phosphate activation mechanism of Glutaminase C with implications for cancer metabolism. Proc. Natl Acad. Sci. USA 109(4), 1092-1097 (2012). Crossref, Medline, CAS

32. Kvamme E, Torgner IA, Roberg B. Kinetics and localization of brain phosphate activated glutaminase. J. Neurosci. Res. 66(5), 951-958 (2001). Crossref, Medline, CAS

33. Shapiro RA, Haser WG, Curthoys NP. The orientation of phosphate-dependent glutaminase on the inner membrane of rat renal mitochondria. Arch. Biochem. Biophys. 243(1), 1-7 (1985). Crossref, Medline, CAS

34. Olalla L, Gutiérrez A, Campos JA *et al.* Nuclear localization of L-type glutaminase in mammalian brain. J. Biol. Chem. 277(41), 38939-38944 (2002). Crossref, Medline, CAS

35. Shen HB, Chou KC. A top-down approach to enhance the power of predicting human protein subcellular localization: Hum-mPLoc 2. 0. Anal. Biochem. 394(2), 269-274 (2009). Crossref, Medline, CAS

36. Emanuelsson O, Nielsen H, Brunak S, von Heijne G. Predicting subcellular localization of proteins based on their N-terminal amino acid sequence. J. Mol. Biol. 300(4), 1005-1016 (2000). Crossref, Medline, CAS

37. Blum T, Briesemeister S, Kohlbacher O. MultiLoc2: integrating phylogeny and gene ontology terms improves subcellular protein

localization prediction. BMC Bioinformatics 10(1), 1-11 (2009). Crossref, Medline

38. Mooney C, Wang Y, Pollastri G. SCLpred: protein subcellular localization prediction by N-to-1 neural networks. Bioinformatics 27(20), 2812-2819 (2011). Crossref, Medline, CAS

39. Lin WZ, Fang JA, Xiao X, Chou KC. iLoc-Animal: a multi- label learning classifier for predicting subcellular localization of animal proteins. Mol. Biosyst. 9(4), 634-644 (2013). Crossref, Medline, CAS

40. Shapiro RA, Farrell L, Srinivasan M, Curthoys NP. Isolation, characterization, and in vitro expression of a cDNA that encodes the kidney isoenzyme of the mitochondrial glutaminase. J. Biol. Chem. 266(28), 18792-18796 (1991). Medline, CAS

41. Srinivasan M, Kalousek F, Curthoys NP. In vitro characterization of the mitochondrial processing and the potential function of the 68-kDa subunit of renal glutaminase. J. Biol. Chem. 270(3), 1185- 1190 (1995). Crossref, Medline, CAS

42. Vaca Jacome AS, Rabilloud T, Schaeffer-Reiss C *et al.* N-terminome analysis of the human mitochondrial proteome. Proteomics 15(14), 2519-2524 (2015). Crossref, Medline, CAS

43. Chung-Bok MI, Vincent N, Jhala U, Watford M. Rat hepatic glutaminase: identification of the full coding sequence and characterization of a functional promoter. Biochem. J. 324(1), 193-200 (1997). Crossref, Medline, CAS

44. Gómez-Fabre PM, Aledo JC, Del Castillo-Olivares A *et al.* Molecular cloning, sequencing and expression studies of the human breast cancer cell glutaminase. Biochem. J. 345(2), 365-375 (2000). Crossref, Medline, CAS

45. Campos-Sandoval JA, López de la Oliva AR, Lobo C *et al.* Expression of functional human glutaminase in baculovirus system: affinity purification, kinetic and molecular characterization. Int. J. Biochem. Cell Biol. 39(4), 765-773 (2007). Crossref, Medline, CAS

46. de la Rosa V, Campos-Sandoval JA, Martín-Rufián M *et al.* A novel glutaminase isoform in mammalian tissues. Neurochem. Int. 55(1- 3), 76-84 (2009). Crossref, Medline, CAS

47. Martín-Rufián M, Tosina M, Campos-Sandoval JA *et al.* Mammalian glutaminase Gls2 gene encodes two functional alternative transcripts by a surrogate promoter usage mechanism. PLoS ONE 7(6), e38380 (2012). Crossref, Medline, CAS

48. Ota T, Suzuki Y, Nishikawa T *et al.* Complete sequencing and characterization of 21, 243 full-length human cDNAs. Nat. Genet. 36(1), 40-45 (2004). Crossref, Medline

49. Häussinger D, Gerok W, Sies H. Regulation of flux through glutaminase and glutamine synthetase in isolated perfused rat liver. Biochim. Biophys. Acta 755(2), 272-278 (1983). Crossref, Medline, CAS

50. Meijer AJ. Channeling of ammonia from glutaminase to carbamoyl- phosphate synthetase in liver mitochondria. FEBS Lett. 191(2), 249-251 (1985). Crossref, Medline, CAS

51. McGivan JD, Lacey JH, Joseph SK. Localization and some properties of phosphate-dependent glutaminase in disrupted liver mitochondria. Biochem. J. 192(2), 537-542 (1980). Crossref, Medline, CAS

52. Although the compounds may have substantial off-targets, the natural products investigated in this manuscript by Lee and coworkers remain the only small molecules so far reported to have potent selectivity for liver-type glutaminase over kidney-type glutaminase.

    Lee YZ, Yang CW, Chang HY *et al.* Discovery of selective inhibitors of glutaminase-2, which inhibit mTORC1, activate autophagy and inhibit proliferation in cancer cells. Oncotarget 5(15), 6087-6101 (2014). Crossref, Medline

53. Curthoys NP, Watford M. Regulation of glutaminase activity and glutamine metabolism. Annu. Rev. Nutr. 15, 133-159 (1995). Crossref, Medline, CAS

54. A number of key structural features of GLS are described which significantly impact its catalytic activities. Li Y, Erickson JW,

Stalnecker CA *et al.* Mechanistic basis of glutaminase activation: a key enzyme that promotes glutamine metabolism in cancer cells. J. Biol. Chem. 291(40), 20900-20910 (2016). Crossref, Medline, CAS

55. The initial discovery of 968 by Wang *et al.* introduced one of two important inhibitors to the field. Wang JB, Erickson JW, Fuji R *et al.* Targeting mitochondrial glutaminase activity inhibits oncogenic transformation. Cancer Cell 18(3), 207-219 (2010). Crossref, Medline, CAS

56. Hu W, Zhang C, Wu R, Sun Y, Levine A, Feng Z. Glutaminase 2, a novel p53 target gene regulating energy metabolism and antioxidant function. Proc. Natl Acad. Sci. USA 107(16), 7455-7460 (2010). Crossref, Medline, CAS

57. Ramachandran S, Pan CQ, Zimmermann SC *et al.* Structural basis for exploring the allosteric inhibition of human kidney type glutaminase. Oncotarget 7(36), 57943-57954 (2016). Medline

58. McDermott *et al.* designed heterocyclic derivatives of bis-2-(5-phenylacetamido-1, 2, 4-thiadiazol-2-yl)ethyl sulfide (BPTES) with superior pharmacological properties relative to CB-839. This is the only current nonpatent publication describing a large number of such compounds.

    McDermott LA, Iyer P, Vernetti L *et al.* Design and evaluation of novel glutaminase inhibitors. Bioorganic Med. Chem. 24(8), 1819-1839 (2016). Crossref, Medline, CAS

59. Thangavelu K, Chong QY, Low BC, Sivaraman J. Structural basis for the active site inhibition mechanism of human kidney- type glutaminase (KGA). Sci. Rep. 4, 3827 (2014). Crossref, Medline, CAS

60. Ferreira AP, Cassago A, Goncalves K de A *et al.* Active glutaminase C self-assembles into a supratetrameric oligomer that can be disrupted by an allosteric inhibitor. J. Biol. Chem. 288(39), 28009- 28020 (2013). Crossref, Medline, CAS

61. Thangavelu K, Pan CQ, Karlberg T *et al.* Structural basis for the allosteric inhibitory mechanism of human kidney-type glutaminase (KGA) and its regulation by Raf-Mek-Erk signaling

in cancer cell metabolism. Proc. Natl Acad. Sci. USA 109(20), 7705-7710 (2012). Crossref, Medline, CAS

62. DeLaBarre B, Gross S, Fang C *et al.* Full-length human glutaminase in complex with an allosteric inhibitor. Biochemistry 50(50), 10764-10770 (2011). Crossref, Medline, CAS

63. Patel M, McGivan JD. Partial purification and properties of rat liver glutaminase. Biochem. J. 220(2), 583-590 (1984). Crossref, Medline, CAS

64. Møller M, Nielsen SS, Ramachandran S *et al.* Small angle x-ray scattering studies of mitochondrial glutaminase C reveal extended flexible regions, and link oligomeric state with enzyme activity. PLoS ONE 8(9), e74783 (2013). Crossref, Medline

65. Katt WP, Cerione RA. Glutaminase regulation in cancer cells: a druggable chain of events. Drug Discov. Today. 19(4), 450-457 (2014). Crossref, Medline, CAS

66. Lukey MJ, Wilson KF, Cerione RA. Therapeutic strategies impacting cancer cell glutamine metabolism. Future Med. Chem. 5(14), 1685-1700 (2013). Link, CAS

67. DeBerardinis RJ, Cheng T. Q's next: the diverse functions of glutamine in metabolism, cell biology and cancer. Oncogene 29(3), 313-324 (2010). Crossref, Medline, CAS

68. Tennant DA, Duran RV, Gottlieb E. Targeting metabolic transformation for cancer therapy. Nat. Rev. Cancer 10(4), 267-277 (2010). Crossref, Medline, CAS

69. Cairns RA, Harris IS, Mak TW. Regulation of cancer cell metabolism. Nat. Rev. Cancer 11(2), 85-95 (2011). Crossref, Medline, CAS

70. Hensley CT, Wasti AT, DeBerardinis RJ. Glutamine and cancer: cell biology, physiology, and clinical opportunities. J. Clin. Invest. 123(9), 3678-3684 (2013). Crossref, Medline, CAS

71. Erickson JW, Cerione RA. Glutaminase: a hot spot for regulation of cancer cell metabolism? Oncotarget 1(8), 734-740 (2010). Crossref, Medline

72. Cline MS, Craft B, Swatloski T *et al.* Exploring TCGA pan-cancer data at the UCSC Cancer Genomics Browser. Sci. Rep. 3, 2652 (2013). Crossref, Medline

73. Cancer Genome Atlas Research Network, Weinstein JN, Collisson EA *et al.* The cancer genome atlas pan-cancer analysis project. Nat. Genet. 45(10), 1113-1120 (2013). Crossref, Medline

74. Seltzer MJ, Bennett BD, Joshi AD *et al.* Inhibition of glutaminase preferentially slows growth of glioma cells with mutant IDH1. Cancer Res. 70(22), 8981-8987 (2010). Crossref, Medline, CAS

75. Emadi A, Jun SA, Tsukamoto T, Fathi AT, Minden MD, Dang CV. Inhibition of glutaminase selectively suppresses the growth of primary acute myeloid leukemia cells with IDH mutations. Exp. Hematol. 42(4), 247-251 (2014). Crossref, Medline, CAS

76. Willems L, Jacque N, Jacquel A *et al.* Inhibiting glutamine uptake represents an attractive new strategy for treating acute myeloid leukemia. Blood 122(20), 3521-3532 (2013). Crossref, Medline, CAS

77. Katt WP, Ramachandran S, Erickson JW, Cerione RA. Dibenzophenanthridines as inhibitors of glutaminase C and cancer cell proliferation. Mol. Cancer Ther. 11(6), 1269-1278 (2012). Crossref, Medline, CAS

78. Introduces CB-839, a potent BPTES derivative currently considered to be the best-in-class molecule for inhibiting GLS. Gross MI, Demo SD, Dennison JB *et al.* Antitumor activity of the glutaminase inhibitor CB-839 in triple-negative breast cancer. Mol. Cancer Ther. 13(4), 890-901 (2014). Crossref, Medline, CAS

79. Huang F, Zhang Q, Ma H, Lv Q, Zhang T. Expression of glutaminase is upregulated in colorectal cancer and of clinical significance. Int. J. Clin. Exp. Pathol. 7(3), 1093-1100 (2014). Medline

80. Gameiro PA, Yang J, Metelo AM *et al.* In vivo HIF-mediated reductive carboxylation is regulated by citrate levels and sensitizes VHL-deficient cells to glutamine deprivation. Cell Metab. 17(3), 372-385 (2013). Crossref, Medline, CAS

81. Shroff EH, Eberlin LS, Dang VM *et al.* MYC oncogene overexpression drives renal cell carcinoma in a mouse model through glutamine metabolism. Proc. Natl Acad. Sci. USA 112(21), 6539-6544 (2015). Crossref, Medline, CAS

82. van den Heuvel AP, Jing J, Wooster RF, Bachman KE. Analysis of glutamine dependency in non-small cell lung cancer. Cancer Biol. Ther. 13(12), 1185-1194 (2012). Crossref, Medline, CAS

83. Hernandez-Davies JE, Tran TQ, Reid MA *et al.* Vemurafenib resistance reprograms melanoma cells towards glutamine dependence. J. Transl. Med. 13(1), 1-11 (2015). Crossref, Medline, CAS

84. Roy S, Maity P. Modulation of metastatic potential of B16F10 melanoma cells by acivicin: synergistic action of glutaminase and potentiation of cisplatin cytotoxicity. Asian Pacific J. Cancer Prev. 8(2), 301-306 (2007). Medline

85. Son J, Lyssiotis CA, Ying H *et al.* Glutamine supports pancreatic cancer growth through a KRAS-regulated metabolic pathway. Nature496(7443), 101-105 (2013). Crossref, Medline, CAS

86. Cheng T, Sudderth J, Yang C *et al.* Pyruvate carboxylase is required for glutamine-independent growth of tumor cells. Proc. Natl Acad. Sci. USA108(21), 8674-8679 (2011). Crossref, Medline, CAS

87. Lu W, Pelicano H, Huang P. Cancer metabolism: is glutamine sweeter than glucose?Cancer Cell 18(3), 199-200 (2010). Crossref, Medline, CAS

88. Yudkoff M, Pleasure D, Cregar L *et al.* Glutathione turnover in cultured astrocytes: studies with [15N]glutamate. J. Neurochem. 55(1), 137-145 (1990). Crossref, Medline, CAS

89. Shanware NP, Mullen AR, DeBerardinis RJ, Abraham RT. Glutamine: pleiotropic roles in tumor growth and stress resistance. J. Mol. Med. 89(3), 229-236 (2011). Crossref, Medline, CAS

90. Gao P, Tchernyshyov I, Chang TC *et al.* c-Myc suppression of miR-23a/b enhances mitochondrial glutaminase expression and glutamine metabolism. Nature 458(7239), 762-765 (2009). Crossref, Medline, CAS

91. Martín-Rufián M, Nascimento-Gomes R, Higuero A *et al.* Both GLS silencing and GLS2 overexpression synergize with oxidative stress against proliferation of glioma cells. J. Mol. Med. 92(3), 277- 290 (2014). Crossref, Medline, CAS

92. Antonyak MA, Wilson KF, Cerione RA. R(h)oads to microvesicles. Small GTPases 3(4), 219-224 (2013). Crossref

93. Santana SM, Antonyak MA, Cerione RA, Kirby BJ. Cancerous epithelial cell lines shed extracellular vesicles with a bimodal size distribution that is sensitive to glutamine inhibition. Phys. Biol. 11(6), 65001 (2014). Crossref

94. Gaglio D, Metallo CM, Gameiro PA *et al.* Oncogenic K-Ras decouples glucose and glutamine metabolism to support cancer cell growth. Mol. Sys. Biol. 7(1), 1-15 (2011).

95. Weinberg F, Hamanaka R, Wheaton WW *et al.* Mitochondrial metabolism and ROS generation are essential for Kras-mediated tumorigenicity. Proc. Natl Acad. Sci. USA 107(19), 87889-8793 (2010). Crossref

96. Davidson SM, Papagiannakopoulos T, Olenchock BA *et al.* Environment impacts the metabolic dependencies of Ras-driven non-small cell lung cancer. Cell Metab. 23(3), 517-528 (2016). Crossref, Medline, CAS

97. Hensley CT, Faubert B, Yuan Q *et al.* Metabolic heterogeneity in human lung tumors. Cell 164(4), 681-694 (2016). Crossref, Medline, CAS

98. Laterza OF, Curthoys NP. Effect of acidosis on the properties of the glutaminase mRNA pH-response element binding protein. J. Am. Soc. Nephrol. 11(9), 1583-1588 (2000). Medline, CAS

99. Katt WP, Antonyak MA, Cerione RA. Simultaneously targeting tissue transglutaminase and kidney type glutaminase sensitizes cancer cells to acid toxicity and offers new opportunities for therapeutic intervention. Mol. Pharm. 12(1), 46-55 (2015). Crossref, Medline, CAS

100. Huang W, Choi W, Chen Y *et al.* A proposed role for glutamine in cancer cell growth through acid resistance. Cell Res. 23(5), 724-727 (2013). Crossref, Medline, CAS

101. Wise DR, DeBerardinis RJ, Mancuso A *et al.* Myc regulates a transcriptional program that stimulates mitochondrial glutaminolysis and leads to glutamine addiction. Proc. Natl Acad. Sci. USA105(48), 18782-18787 (2008). Crossref, Medline, CAS

102. Rathore MG, Saumet A, Rossi JF *et al.* The NF-kappa B member p65 controls glutamine metabolism through miR-23a. Int. J. Biochem. Cell Biol. 44(9), 1448-1456 (2012). Crossref, Medline, CAS

103. Reynolds MR, Lane AN, Robertson B *et al.* Control of glutamine metabolism by the tumor suppressor Rb. Oncogene 33(5), 556-566 (2014). Crossref, Medline, CAS

104. McGuirk S, Gravel SP, Deblois G *et al.* PGC-1α supports glutamine metabolism in breast cancer. Cancer Metab. 1(1), 1-11 (2013). Crossref, Medline

105. Lukey MJ, Greene KS, Erickson JW, Wilson KF, Cerione RA. The oncogenic transcription factor c-Jun regulates glutaminase expression and sensitizes cells to glutaminase-targeted therapy. Nat. Commun. 7, 11321 (2016). Crossref, Medline, CAS

106. Sebastián C, Zwaans BM, Silberman DM *et al.* The histone deacetylase SIRT6 is a tumor suppressor that controls cancer metabolism. Cell151(6), 1185-1199 (2012). Crossref, Medline, CAS

107. Polletta L, Vernucci E, Carnevale I *et al.* SIRT5 regulation of ammonia-induced autophagy and mitophagy. Autophagy 11(2), 253-270 (2015). Crossref, Medline

108. Redis RS, Vela LE, Lu W *et al.* Allele-specific reprogramming of cancer metabolism by the long non-coding RNA CCAT2. Mol. Cell. 61(4), 520-534 (2016). Crossref, Medline, CAS

109. Szeliga M, Obara-Michlewska M, Matyja E *et al.* Transfection with liver-type glutaminase cDNA alters gene expression and reduces survival, migration and proliferation of T98G glioma cells. Glia 57(9), 1014-1023 (2009). Crossref, Medline

110. Szeliga M, Zgrzywa A, Obara-Michlewska M, Albrecht J. Transfection of a human glioblastoma cell line with liver- type

glutaminase (LGA) down-regulates the expression of DNA-repair gene MGMT and sensitizes the cells to alkylating agents. J. Neurochem. 123(3), 428-436 (2012). Crossref, Medline, CAS

111. Xiang L, Xie G, Liu C *et al*. Knock-down of glutaminase 2 expression decreases glutathione, NADH, and sensitizes cervical cancer to ionizing radiation. Biochim. Biophys. Acta 1833(12), 2996-3005 (2013). Crossref, Medline, CAS

112. Suzuki S, Tanaka T, Poyurovsky MV *et al*. Phosphate-activated glutaminase (GLS2), a p53-inducible regulator of glutamine metabolism and reactive oxygen species. Proc. Natl Acad. Sci. USA 107(16), 7461-7466 (2010). Crossref, Medline, CAS

113. Lamonte G, Tang X, Chen JL *et al*. Acidosis induces reprogramming of cellular metabolism to mitigate oxidative stress. Cancer Metab. 1(1), 23 (2013). Crossref, Medline

114. Xiao D, Ren P, Su H *et al*. Myc promotes glutaminolysis in human neuroblastoma through direct activation of glutaminase 2. Oncotarget 6(38), 40655-40666 (2015). Medline

115. Wang R, Dillon CP, Shi LZ *et al*. The transcription factor Myc controls metabolic reprogramming upon T lymphocyte activation. Immunity 35(6), 871-882 (2011). Crossref, Medline, CAS

116. Thomas AG, O'Driscoll CM, Bressler J, Kaufmann W, Rojas CJ, Slusher BS. Small molecule glutaminase inhibitors block glutamate release from stimulated microglia. Biochem. Biophys. Res. Commun. 443(1), 32-36 (2014). Crossref, Medline, CAS

117. Pinkus LM. Glutamine binding sites. Methods Enzymol. 46, 414-427 (1977). Crossref, Medline, CAS

118. The discovery by Robinson and coworkers of the GLS inhibitor BPTES, which has subsequently been used in numerous preclinical studies. Robinson MM, McBryant SJ, Tsukamoto T *et al*. Novel mechanism of inhibition of rat kidney-type glutaminase by bis-2-(5-phenylacetamido-1, 2, 4-thiadiazol-2-yl)ethyl s u l f i d e (BPTES). Biochem. J. 406(3), 407-414 (2007). Crossref, Medline, CAS

119. Shukla K, Ferraris DV, Thomas AG *et al*. Design, synthesis, and pharmacological evaluation of Bis-2-(5-phenylacetamido-1, 2, 4-thiadiazol-2-yl)ethyl sulfide 3 (BPTES) analogs as glutaminase inhibitors. J. Med. Chem. 55(23), 10551-10563 (2012). Crossref, Medline, CAS

120. BenncttMK,GrossMI,BromleySDetal.WO/2014/089048(2014).

121. Zimmermann SC, Wolf EF, Luu A *et al*. Allosteric glutaminase inhibitors based on a 1, 4-di(5-amino-1, 3, 4-thiadiazol-2-yl) butane scaffold. ACS Med. Chem. Lett. 7(5), 520-524 (2016). Crossref, Medline, CAS

122. 122. Newcomb R, Newcomb M. US20020115698A1 (2002).

123. Di Francesco ME, Jones P, Heffernan T *et al*. WO2016004404A2 (2016).

124. Di Francesco ME, Heffernan T, Soth MJ *et al*. US20160002248A1 (2016).

125. Di Francesco ME, Jones P, Heffernan T *et al*. WO2016004417A1 (2016).

126. Lemieux RM, Popovici-Muller J, Salituro FG, Saunders JO, Travins J, Yan S. US20140142146A1 54 (2014).

127. Lemieux RM, Popovici-Muller J, Salituro FG, Saunders JO, Travins J, Chen Y. US20140142081A1 (2014).

128. Bhavar PK, Vakkalanka SKVS, Viswanadha S, Swaroop MG, Babu G. WO2015101958A2 (2015).

129. Finlay MRV, Ekwuru CT, Charles MD, Raubo PA, Winter JJG, Nissink JWM. WO2015181539A1 (2015).

130. Cianchetta G, Lemieux RM, Cao S, Ding Y, Ye Z. WO2015143340A1 (2015).

131. Mackinnon AL, Rodriguez ML. WO2016014890A1 (2016).

132. Stalnecker CA, Ulrich SM, Li Y *et al*. Mechanism by which a recently discovered allosteric inhibitor blocks glutamine metabolism in transformed cells. Proc. Natl Acad. Sci. USA112(2), 394-399 (2014). Crossref, Medline

133. Gao M, Monian P, Quadri N, Ramasamy R, Jiang X. Glutaminolysis and transferrin regulate ferroptosis. Mol. Cell 59(2), 298-308 (2016). Crossref

- Cancer as a metabolic disease, Seyfried Nutrition and Metabolism, 2010. Visit Website
- Mitochondria and the evolutionary roots of cancer, Davila Phys Biol, 2013. Visit Website
- Cancer metabolism: current perspectives and future direction, Munoz-Pinedo, Cell Death and Disease 2012. Visit Website

Lipid metabolism

- The Role of Statins in Cancer Therapy, Hindler, The Oncologist, 2006. Visit Website
- Statin a day keeps the cancer at bay, Sinh World Journal of Oncology, 2013. Visit Website

Glucose metabolism

- Metformin is Associated with Survival Benefit in Cancer Patients With Concurrent Type 2 Diabetes: A Systemic Review and Meta-Analysis, Ming Yin et al, The Oncologist November 2013. Visit Website
- Diabetes, cancer, and metformin: connections of metabolism and cell proliferation, Gallagher, Annals of the New York Academy of Sciences 2011. Visit Website
- Cancer Risk in Diabetic Patients Treated with Metformin: A systematic Review and Meta-analysis, Noto, PlosOne 2012. Visit Website

Glycolysis Inhibition

- Mebendazole mono-therapy and long term disease control in metastatic adrenocortical carcinoma, Dobrosotskaya, Endocrine Practice 2011. Visit Website

- Mebendazole Elicits a potent anti-tumour Effect on Human Cancer Cell Lines Both in vitro and in Vivo, Roth, Clinical Cancer Research 2002. Visit Website

- Wang C, Schwab LP, Fan M, Seagroves TN, Buolamwini JK. Chemoprevention Activity of Dipyridamole in the MMTV-PyMT Transgenic Mouse Model of Breast Cancer. Cancer prevention research (Philadelphia, Pa). 2013;6(5): 10. 1158/1940-6207. CAPR-12-0345. doi: 10. 1158/1940-6207. CAPR-12-0345.

Index

Note: 'fn' indicates a footnote.